Nutritional Management of Gastrointestinal Diseases

Editors

GERARD E. MULLIN
BERKELEY N. LIMKETKAI

GASTROENTEROLOGY
CLINICS OF NORTH AMERICA

www.gastro.theclinics.com

Consulting Editor
ALAN L. BUCHMAN

March 2021 • Volume 50 • Number 1

ELSEVIER

1600 John F. Kennedy Boulevard • Suite 1800 • Philadelphia, Pennsylvania, 19103-2899
http://www.theclinics.com

GASTROENTEROLOGY CLINICS OF NORTH AMERICA Volume 50, Number 1
March 2021 ISSN 0889-8553, ISBN-13: 978-0-323-76163-5

Editor: Kerry Holland
Developmental Editor: Karen Solomon

Gastroenterology Clinics of North America (ISSN 0889-8553) is published quarterly by Elsevier Inc., 360 Park Avenue South, New York, NY 10010-1710. Months of issue are March, June, September, and December. Business and Editorial Offices: 1600 John F. Kennedy Blvd., Suite 1800, Philadelphia, PA 19103-2899. Customer Service Office: 6277 Sea Harbor Drive, Orlando, FL 32887-4800. Periodicals postage paid at New York, NY and additional mailing offices. Subscription prices are $365.00 per year (US individuals), $100.00 per year (US students), $945.00 per year (US institutions), $391.00 per year (Canadian individuals), $100.00 per year (Canadian students), $997.00 per year (Canadian institutions), $463.00 per year (international individuals), $220.00 per year (international students), and $997.00 per year (international institutions). Foreign air speed delivery is included in all *Clinics* subscription prices. All prices are subject to change without notice. **POSTMASTER:** Send address changes to *Gastroenterology Clinics of North America*, Elsevier Health Sciences Division, Subscription Customer Service, 3251 Riverport Lane, Maryland Heights, MO 63043. **Telephone: 1-800-654-2452 (U.S. and Canada); 314-447-8871 (outside U.S. and Canada). Fax: 314-447-8029. E-mail: journalscustomerservice-usa@elsevier.com (for print support); journalsonlinesupport-usa@elsevier.com (for online support).**

Reprints. For copies of 100 or more, of articles in this publication, please contact the Commercial Reprints Department, Elsevier Inc., 360 Part Avenue South, New York, New York 10010-1710. Tel. 212-633-3874, Fax: 212-633-3820, E-mail: reprints@elsevier.com.

Gastroenterology Clinics of North America is also published in Italian by Il Pensiero Scientifico Editore, Rome, Italy; and in Portuguese by Interlivros Edicoes Ltda., Rua Commandante Coelho 1085, 21250 Cordovil, Rio de Janeiro, Brazil.

Gastroenterology Clinics of North America is covered in *MEDLINE/PubMed (Index Medicus), Excerpta Medica, Current Contents/Clinical Medicine, Science Citation Index, ISI/BIOMED*, and *BIOSIS*.

Contributors

CONSULTING EDITOR

ALAN L. BUCHMAN, MD, MSPH, FACP, FACN, FACG, AGAF
Professor of Clinical Surgery, Medical Director, Intestinal Rehabilitation and Transplant Center, The University of Illinois at Chicago/UI Health, Chicago, Illinois, USA

EDITORS

GERARD E. MULLIN, MD
Associate Professor of Medicine, Division of Gastroenterology and Hepatology, Johns Hopkins School of Medicine, Baltimore, Maryland, USA

BERKELEY N. LIMKETKAI, MD, PhD
Associate Clinical Professor, Division of Digestive Diseases, David Geffen School of Medicine at UCLA, Los Angeles, California, USA

AUTHORS

MAAZA ABDI, MD
Director of Telemedicine Gastroenterology, Johns Hopkins Hospital, Baltimore, Maryland, USA

ANDRES ACOSTA, MD, PhD
Consultant, Division of Gastroenterology and Hepatology, Department of Medicine, Mayo Clinic, Rochester, Minnesota, USA

VENKATA S. AKSHINTALA, MD
Baltimore, Maryland, USA

ASHWIN N. ANANTHAKRISHNAN, MD, MPH
Division of Gastroenterology, Massachusetts General Hospital and Harvard Medical School, Boston, Massachusetts, USA

KATHY BULL-HENRY, MBA, MD
Director of Endoscopy, Johns Hopkins Bayview Medical Center, Assistant Professor of Medicine, Johns Hopkins Hospital, Baltimore, Maryland, USA

JOY W. CHANG, MD, MS
Clinical Lecturer, Division of Gastroenterology and Hepatology, Department of Internal Medicine, University of Michigan, Ann Arbor, Michigan, USA

NAUEEN A. CHAUDHRY, MD
Gastroenterology Fellow, Division of Gastroenterology and Hepatology, Department of Medicine, University of Florida, Gainesville, Florida, USA

LAWRENCE J. CHESKIN, MD, FACP, FTOS
Professor and Chair, Nutrition and Food Studies, George Mason University, Fairfax, Virginia, USA; Adjunct Professor, Johns Hopkins School of Medicine, Baltimore, Maryland, USA

EVAN S. DELLON, MD, MPH
Professor, Division of Gastroenterology and Hepatology, Department of Internal Medicine, University of North Carolina School of Medicine, Chapel Hill, North Carolina, USA

SHANTI L. ESWARAN, MD
Associate Professor, Division of Gastroenterology, Department of Internal Medicine, University of Michigan, Ann Arbor, Michigan, USA

CHRISTOPHER FAIN, DO
Director of Inpatient Gastroenterology, Assistant Professor of Medicine, Johns Hopkins Hospital, Baltimore, Maryland, USA

SINA GALLO, PhD, MSc, RD
Associate Professor, Foods and Nutrition, University of Georgia, Athens, Georgia, USA

PETER H.R. GREEN, DO
Phyllis & Ivan Seidenberg Professor of Medicine, Director, Celiac Disease Center at Columbia University, New York, New York, USA

SANDEEP K. GUPTA, MD
Attending Faculty, Section of Pediatric Gastroenterology, Hepatology, Nutrition, Riley Hospital for Children at IU Health, Indiana University School of Medicine, Indianapolis, Indiana, USA

EMILY HALLER, MS, RDN
Registered Dietitian Nutritionist, Division of Gastroenterology and Hepatology, Department of Internal Medicine, University of Michigan, Ann Arbor, Michigan, USA

JAMES P. HAMILTON, MD
Division of Gastroenterology and Hepatology, Johns Hopkins School of Medicine, Baltimore, Maryland, USA

KIMBERLY N. HARER, MD, ScM
Clinical Lecturer, Division of Gastroenterology, Department of Internal Medicine, University of Michigan, Ann Arbor, Michigan, USA

GLENN HARVIN, MD
Associate Professor of Medicine, Chief, Division of Gastroenterology, Hepatology and Nutrition, Department of Internal Medicine, Brody School of Medicine, East Carolina University, Greenville, North Carolina, USA

EMILY HON, MD
Assistant Professor of Clinical Pediatrics, Division of Pediatric Gastroenterology, Hepatology, and Nutrition, Riley Hospital for Children at IU Health, Indianapolis, Indiana, USA

MARIA DANIELA HURTADO A, MD, PhD
Senior Associate Consultant, Division of Endocrinology, Diabetes, Metabolism, and Nutrition, Department of Medicine, Mayo Clinic Health System La Crosse, Wisconsin, USA; Mayo Clinic, Rochester, Minnesota, USA

RICHARD J.M. INGRAM, BMBS(Hons), MRCP, PhD
Division of Gastroenterology, University of Calgary, Calgary, Alberta, Canada

CHELSEA JACOBS, DO
Internal Medicine Resident, Department of Medicine, University of Florida, Gainesville, Florida, USA

KAVIN A. KANTHASAMY, MD
Division of Gastroenterology, Johns Hopkins Medical Institutions, Baltimore, Maryland, USA

AHYOUNG KIM, MD
Division of Gastroenterology and Hepatology, Johns Hopkins School of Medicine, Baltimore, Maryland, USA

ARUNKUMAR KRISHNAN, MBBS
Division of Gastroenterology and Hepatology, Johns Hopkins School of Medicine, Baltimore, Maryland, USA

BERKELEY N. LIMKETKAI, MD, PhD
Associate Clinical Professor, Division of Digestive Diseases, David Geffen School of Medicine at UCLA, Los Angeles, California, USA

LAURA E. MATARESE, PhD, RDN, LDN, CNSC, FADA, FASPEN, FAND
Professor of Medicine, Division of Gastroenterology, Hepatology and Nutrition, Department of Internal Medicine, Brody School of Medicine, East Carolina University, Greenville, North Carolina, USA

GERARD E. MULLIN, MD
Associate Professor of Medicine, Division of Gastroenterology and Hepatology, Johns Hopkins School of Medicine, Baltimore, Maryland, USA

ALYSSA M. PARIAN, MD
Assistant Professor of Medicine, Division of Gastroenterology and Hepatology, Johns Hopkins School of Medicine, Baltimore, Maryland, USA

MAITREYI RAMAN, MD, MSc, FRCPC
Division of Gastroenterology, University of Calgary, Calgary, Alberta, Canada

S. DEVI RAMPERTAB, MD
Division of Gastroenterology and Hepatology, Associate Professor, Department of Medicine, University of Florida, Gainesville, Florida, USA

SAMARA RIFKIN, MD, ScM
Clinical Lecturer, Department of Medicine, Division of Gastroenterology and Hepatology, University of Michigan School of Medicine, Ann Arbor, Michigan, USA

JOANN ROMANO-KEELER, MD, MS
Assistant Professor, Division of Neonatology, Department of Pediatrics, University of Illinois at Chicago, Chicago, Illinois, USA

ALEXA N. SASSON, MD, FRCPC
Division of Gastroenterology, University of Toronto, Toronto, Ontario, Canada

KATE SCARLATA, MPH, RDN
Registered Dietitian Nutritionist, Founder, For a Digestive Peace of Mind, LLC, Medway, Massachusetts, USA

VIKESH K. SINGH, MD, MSc
Baltimore, Maryland, USA

JUN SUN, PhD
Professor, Division of Gastroenterology and Hepatology, Department of Medicine, University of Illinois Cancer Center, Chicago, Illinois, USA

TINSAY A. WORETA, MD, MPH
Division of Gastroenterology and Hepatology, Johns Hopkins School of Medicine, Baltimore, Maryland, USA

JILEI ZHANG, PhD
Research Associate, Division of Gastroenterology and Hepatology, Department of Medicine, University of Illinois at Chicago, Chicago, Illinois, USA

ELINOR ZHOU, MD
Gastroenterology Fellow, Division of Gastroenterology and Hepatology, Johns Hopkins School of Medicine, Baltimore, Maryland, USA

Contents

Nutrition Tools for the Practicing Gastroenterologist   1

Kate Scarlata and Emily Haller

> There are several online tools, books, and applications available to enhance the application of nutrition interventions for gastroenterologists and patients with gastrointestinal (GI) disorders. Nutritional health may be compromised in GI patients because of the nature of the disease impacting use of nutritional substrates or reducing oral intake. Protein-calorie malnutrition can result from insufficient intake, malabsorption of nutrients, and increased energy expenditure, all of which can occur in certain GI conditions. Eating disorders and disordered eating, and food insecurity, also impact nutritional status. Therapeutic nutrition interventions should be implemented with guidance of a registered dietitian with expertise in their application.

Nutritional Considerations in the Hospital Setting   15

Christopher Fain, Kathy Bull-Henry, and Maaza Abdi

> Malnutrition and issues of nutrition are common in hospitalized patients. Identifying patients at nutritional risk can help to improve hospital-related outcomes. Specialized nutritional support in the form of oral nutritional supplementation, enteral nutrition, and parenteral nutrition is essential to meeting the nutritional needs of many patients. Disease-specific nutritional considerations are fundamental to the quality care of hospitalized patients. Many vitamin, macronutrient, and micronutrient deficiencies are relevant in hospital setting.

All Things Gluten: A Review   29

Naueen A. Chaudhry, Chelsea Jacobs, Peter H.R. Green, and S. Devi Rampertab

> Gluten is a common dietary component with a complex protein structure. It forms incomplete products of digestion, which have the potential to mount an immune response in genetically predisposed individuals, resulting in celiac disease. It also has been linked with nonceliac gluten sensitivity and irritable bowel syndrome due to wheat allergy. A gluten-free diet is an effective treatment of these conditions; however, it can lead to micro-nutrient and mineral deficiencies and a macronutrient imbalance with higher sugar and lipid intake. Recent popularity has led to greater availability, but increasing cost, of commercially available gluten-free products.

Obesity affects 2 of 5 Americans, and nearly 1 of 10 is considered severely obese, with the greatest risk of morbidity and mortality. A reduction in body weight of 2% to 5% can lead to improvements in cardiovascular health, with weight loss maintenance associated with the best health outcomes. Lifestyle interventions that focus on changes in diet and physical activity behaviors are best to maintain weight loss. This article provides a review of the treatment of adult obesity with a focus on dietary interventions.

The highly variable response to obesity therapies justifies the search for treatment strategies that are best suited to individual patients to enhance their effectiveness and tolerability via precision medicine. Precision medicine development in recent years has been driven by the emergence of powerful methods to characterize patients ("omic" assays). Current available information has revealed that there are numerous intermediary processes that contribute to obesity and have provided a framework for partially comprehending the mechanisms behind the heterogeneity of obesity and its clinical consequences. Some of these processes have or are currently being targeted to individualize obesity therapy with some success.

Acute pancreatitis (AP) remains among the most common gastrointestinal disorders leading to hospital admission. Optimizing nutritional support and maintaining gut function is instrumental in recovery of patients with AP. Enteral nutrition remains one of the only interventions with demonstrated mortality benefit in AP largely through preservation of gut function, serving to preserve the gut barrier as means to mitigate immune dysregulation and systemic inflammation inherent to AP. Practice variation remains in timing, route, and composition of nutritional support. This review highlights contemporary evidence regarding optimal nutritional support in AP and provides recommendations for management in line with current consensus opinions.

With the increasing global prevalence of inflammatory bowel diseases, research in this field is expanding to better understand the multifactorial etiologies of this complex disease. Nutrition and diet, as modifiable risk factors, have been shown to play an important role in disease activity and prognosis. This article reviews the role of nutrition in inflammatory bowel disease, including appropriate nutrition screening in this at-risk population, and associated micronutrient deficiencies. We provide recommendations on dosing supplementation. We briefly review diet as a risk factor for inflammatory bowel disease and the currently proposed published dietary intervention studies.

Dietary supplements have increasingly gained popularity over the years not only to replete micronutrient deficiencies but for their use in treatment of disease. The popularity of dietary supplements for inflammatory bowel diseases (IBD) arises from their perceived ease of use, potential disease-modifying benefits, and perceived safety. Overall, randomized controlled trials have not consistently shown a benefit of fish oil for the maintenance of remission with Crohn's disease. The inconsistency of these findings highlights the need for more studies that are powered to clarify the context in which omega-3 fatty acids might have a role in the treatment algorithm of IBD.

Irritable bowel syndrome (IBS) affects 10% to 15% of the population and often is difficult to treat with available pharmacologic agents. Dietary therapies for IBS are of particular interest because up to 90% of IBS patients exclude certain foods to improve their gastrointestinal symptoms. Among the available dietary interventions for IBS, the low FODMAP diet has the greatest evidence for efficacy. Although dietary therapies rapidly are becoming first-line treatment of IBS, gastroenterologists need to be aware of the negative effects of prescribing restrictive diets and red flag symptoms of maladaptive eating patterns.

Intestinal failure is a debilitating, complex disorder associated with loss of portions of intestine or loss of intestinal function. Short bowel syndrome is the most common form of intestinal failure and results in inability to maintain nutritional, fluid, and electrolyte status while consuming a regular diet. Nutrition interventions to treat short bowel syndrome include enteral and parenteral nutrition, intestinal rehabilitation techniques to enhance absorptive capacity of remnant bowel, and surgical reconstruction designed to provide more surface area for absorption. These therapies are interrelated services to restore nutritional status through the safest most effective therapy consistent with patient lifestyle and wishes.

Nonalcoholic fatty liver disease (NAFLD) has become one of the most common causes of chronic liver disease worldwide. The prevalence of NAFLD has grown proportionally with the rise in obesity, sedentary lifestyle, unhealthy dietary patterns, and metabolic syndrome. Currently, in the absence of approved pharmacologic treatment, the keystone of treatment is lifestyle modification focused on achieving a weight loss of 7%–10%, cardiovascular exercise, and improving insulin sensitivity. The primary aim of this review is to outline the effect of different dietetic approaches against NAFLD and highlight the important micronutrient components in the management of NAFLD.

GASTROENTEROLOGY
CLINICS OF NORTH AMERICA

SERIES OF RELATED INTEREST

Gastrointestinal Endoscopy Clinics of North America
(Available at: https://www.giendo.theclinics.com)
Clinics in Liver Disease
(Available at: https://www.liver.theclinics.com)

THE CLINICS ARE AVAILABLE ONLINE!
Access your subscription at:
www.theclinics.com

Foreword

Nutrition and the Gastrointestinal Tract: Where It all Begins and Ends

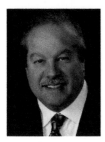

Alan L. Buchman, MD, MSPH
Consulting Editor

Nutrition starts with and ends with the gastrointestinal tract; under normal circumstances, food enters the body via the digestive system and exits via the digestive system, albeit often in a different form. Nutritional intake can affect gastrointestinal functioning, and gastrointestinal function or dysfunction can affect nutrient intake. The gastrointestinal system also plays host to the intestinal microbiome, which may alter nutrient intake and absorption or be altered by nutrient intake and absorption.

In this issue of *Gastroenterology Clinics of North America*, Drs Mullin and Limketkai have assembled a group of investigator authors who explore nutritional management of various digestive diseases, including celiac disease and food allergies, eosinophilic esophagitis, inflammatory bowel disease, irritable bowel syndrome, pancreatitis, and intestinal failure, where obviously nutrition plays an important role. Less obvious, but no less important, is the role of the gastrointestinal tract on the development and management of obesity and its complications and how nutritional interactions with the intestinal microbiome play a role in disease development and potential management.

Understanding the appropriate role of nutrition in gastrointestinal disease management is critically important so that the importance of nutrition is neither exaggerated nor underappreciated. We can approach patient nutritional queries with appropriate answers, which may even be counter to what the patient has read on the Internet or heard from their friends; as such, "fake" (nutritional) news stops with the

Gastroenterol Clin N Am 50 (2021) xiii–xiv
https://doi.org/10.1016/j.gtc.2020.12.002
0889-8553/21/© 2020 Published by Elsevier Inc.

gastroenterologist, and we can better educate our patients about what we know that just isn't so and what we don't know that we still need to learn.

Alan L. Buchman, MD, MSPH
Intestinal Rehabilitation and Transplant Center
Department of Surgery/UI Health
University of Illinois at Chicago
840 South Wood Street
Suite 402 (MC958)
Chicago, IL 60612, USA

E-mail address:
buchman@uic.edu

Preface

The Inextricable Relationship Between Nutrition and Gastrointestinal Health

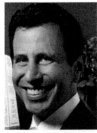
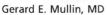

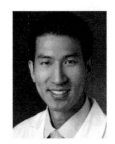

Gerard E. Mullin, MD   Berkeley N. Limketkai, MD, PhD
Editors

The primary raison d'être of the digestive system is the processing, metabolism, and absorption of nutrients. As such, gastrointestinal health and disease strongly drive the body's nutritional status. The presence of intestinal inflammation in inflammatory bowel disease (IBD) or celiac disease, or a deficit in intestinal surface area in short bowel syndrome, often leads to nutrient malabsorption. Pancreatitis and compromise in the synthesis or release of pancreatic enzymes cause maldigestion of macronutrients. On a more macroscopic scale, functional gastrointestinal disorders can deter individuals from eating normally and thus reduce calorie consumption. All these processes place the individual at risk for protein-calorie malnutrition and nutrient deficiencies that have the potential to disrupt function in all organ systems.

Inversely, nutrition also plays a defining role in gastrointestinal health. The building blocks, cofactors, and energy that derive from nutrients help maintain the integrity and function of enterocytes and other cells of the digestive system. Nutrients themselves can serve as antigens or pathophysiologic triggers in conditions such as food allergies and sensitivities and celiac disease. Particular nutrients serve as substrates for proinflammatory and anti-inflammatory metabolic pathways. Nutrients can also indirectly act on gastrointestinal health through its impact on the gut microbiota and metabolome. There is emerging evidence that the gut microbiome has a major controlling influence on many systemic processes, such as the liver, lung, cardiovascular, kidney, immune, central nervous system, and likely others. Collectively, the digestive tract and its constituent microbiota not only assimilate nutrients into energy but also transform our food into signals for cellular health and vibrance.

Given the intricate and inextricable relationship between nutrition and gastrointestinal health, an in-depth treatise on this topic would require volumes. Nonetheless,

Gastroenterol Clin N Am 50 (2021) xv–xvi
https://doi.org/10.1016/j.gtc.2020.12.001
0889-8553/21/© 2020 Published by Elsevier Inc.

this issue strives to balance between providing meaningful updates on the more common gastrointestinal conditions and discussing cutting-edge topics. Some articles are devoted to nutrition in the management of IBD, irritable bowel syndrome, acute pancreatitis, esophageal disorders, nonalcoholic fatty liver disease, and other conditions. Other articles focus on emerging concepts, such as the potential role for precision medicine in obesity, the life-long impact of nutrition on the gut microbiome, and dietary risk modification of colorectal cancer. The article authors are recognized experts in their respective fields, and we are reassured that they provide informative and thought-provoking discussions on nutrition in gastroenterology. We hope you enjoy reading this issue as much as we have.

Gerard E. Mullin, MD
Division of Gastroenterology and Hepatology
Johns Hopkins University School of Medicine
600 North Wolfe Street
Baltimore, MD 21287, USA

Berkeley N. Limketkai, MD, PhD
Division of Digestive Diseases
David Geffen School of Medicine at UCLA
100 UCLA Medical Plaza, Suite 345
Los Angeles, CA 90095, USA

E-mail addresses:
gmullin1@jhmi.edu (G.E. Mullin)
berkeley.limketkai@gmail.com (B.N. Limketkai)

Nutrition Tools for the Practicing Gastroenterologist

Kate Scarlata, MPH, RDN[a],*, Emily Haller, MS, RDN[b]

KEYWORDS

- Nutrition • Malnutrition • Nutrition assessment • Dietitian
- Gastrointestinal disorders

KEY POINTS

- Evidenced-based nutrition is emerging for gastrointestinal conditions.
- Disordered eating and overt eating disorders, such as anorexia nervosa and bulimia, are more common in individuals with gastrointestinal (GI) disorders than healthy control subjects.
- A comprehensive assessment is essential to provide an individualized nutrition treatment plan and is best guided by a registered dietitian with GI expertise.

INTRODUCTION

Challenging gastrointestinal (GI) conditions often require a multifaceted approach for treatment. Research and the application of nutrition interventions for GI conditions are growing exponentially, with evidenced-based guidelines for irritable bowel syndrome (IBS), celiac disease (CD), eosinophilic esophagitis (EoE), and inflammatory bowel disease (IBD), to name a few. Another area of mounting interest is the intersection of diet, modulation of the gut microbiome, and health outcomes. As this area of science progresses, individualized diet therapies may be guided by personal metabolomic and fecal microbial sequencing. Patients and GI practitioners can benefit from a variety of tools and resources to navigate therapeutic diets to aid symptom management

Scarlata disclosures: Published low FODMAP diet books and educational materials, FODY Food Company paid advisor and equity, Epicured-Employee and equity, A2 milk company paid educational content, Green Valley Organics paid educational content, Enjoy life Foods paid educational content, Salix pharmaceuticals paid educational content.
[a] For a Digestive Peace of Mind, LLC, 11 Pine Street, Medway, MA 02053, USA; [b] Division of Gastroenterology, Michigan Medicine, University of Michigan, 3912 Taubman Center, 1500 East Medical Center Drive, Ann Arbor, MI 48109, USA
* Corresponding author.
E-mail address: kate@katescarlata.com
Twitter: @KateScarlata_RD (K.S.)

and meet their patient's nutritional needs. Referring patients to a registered dietitian (RD) with GI expertise is your best nutrition resource. If you do not have access to an RD in your clinical setting, consider hiring one for your practice or finding one with digestive health expertise to refer to in your local community. To help you or your patients locate a dietitian near you, refer to **Table 1** for resources.

Nutritional assessment in GI patients should include screening for malnutrition risk, disordered eating, and eating disorders (ED). A full review of the medical history, medication, and supplement use, along with an assessment of nutrient intake, socioeconomic status, and lifestyle factors, aids in the creation of a comprehensive assessment and tailored nutrition intervention. Dietitians have the necessary time allotment (initial assessments are 1 hour) and expertise to individualize a nutrition care plan. Personalized nutrition care is essential in GI disorders because some conditions result from or contribute to other comorbid diseases. For example, nutrition recommendations can be individualized to meet comorbid conditions, such as diabetes with carbohydrate modifications, and gastroparesis with fat, fiber, and food particle size adaptions.

NUTRITION RISK SCREEN AND ASSESSMENT

Disordered eating is common in GI disorders; a systematic review of GI patients revealed that 23.43% displayed eating patterns that were suggestive of disordered eating.[1] Disordered eating can present with food restriction, skipping meals, or fasting. Avoidant/restrictive food intake eating disorder (ARFID) is a diagnosis of eating or feeding disturbance because of lack of interest in eating, avoidance of sensory characteristics of food, and/or fear of adverse eating consequences (eg, digestive distress) and does not involve concerns about body shape or size, or fear of gaining weight.[2] Research by Zia and colleagues[3] found that approximately 21% of a functional GI disorder patient sample met the criteria for ARFID. In a retrospective study of GI patients referred to GI behavioral health providers from Michigan Medicine, 12.6% of the cohort met criteria for ARFID.[4] Moreover, patients with a past or current history of an ED frequently report GI symptoms and meet the criteria for functional gut disorders.[5] Given many individuals with ED avoid health care settings, a gastroenterologist appointment may be the first setting that the ED is assessed and/or observed.

Table 1 Where to find a dietitian	
Web Site	**Dietitian Expertise**
Academy of Nutrition and Dietetics; find an expert https://www.eatright.org/find-an-expert	Registered dietitian listing for a variety of disease states, including gastrointestinal
For a Digestive Peace of Mind FODMAP Dietitian Registry https://www.katescarlata.com/fodmapdietitians	Low FODMAP diet knowledgeable dietitians
International Foundation for Gastrointestinal Disorders Dietitian listing https://www.iffgd.org/dietitian-listing.html	Dietitians with GI expertise
International Federation of Eating Disorder Dietitians http://www.eddietitians.com	Dietitians with eating disorder expertise

It is imperative this opportunity for appropriate assessment and care is not missed. One study of individuals with ED found 98% fit the criteria for a functional gut disorder; therefore, it is likely that gastroenterologists will benefit from tools to assess for ED and disordered eating or refer to a dietitian for assessment.[6] When disordered eating or an ED is of concern, a specialist with ED expertise should be involved in the patient's care (see **Table 1** to find a suitable dietitian expert). Self-guided elimination diets can result in severe food restriction and in some cases, malnutrition, as observed in patients in clinical practice. This reiterates the importance of proper nutritional education and assessment. Nutrition screening tools can quickly identify those at risk for malnutrition (**Table 2**) and in need of escalation of care and nutrition intervention. Food insecurity (FI) is a prevalent public health problem affecting one in eight US households. Screening for FI should be considered to best help patients receive supportive services (see **Table 2** for an FI screening tool).[7] Patients who struggle with FI, which includes limited access to nutritionally adequate foods, require additional resources if specialty foods are required. A referral to a social worker or patient navigator can provide a patient with support, information, and resources to assist with overcoming this barrier to care.

Various screening tools are available for the practicing gastroenterologist to use and screen for risk of malnutrition, disordered eating and ED, and FI (see **Table 2** for a summary of key resources). Once nutrition risk is identified, a comprehensive nutrition

Table 2 Nutrition screening tools	
Assessment	**Tool**
Nutrition screening for malnutrition and nutrition risk	Malnutrition Screening Tool (MST)[8] A validated tool to screen adult patients for the risk of malnutrition in the inpatient and outpatient setting Includes 2 questions: Have you recently lost weight without trying? Have you been eating poorly because of a decreased appetite? Malnutrition Universal Screening Tool[9] A validated screening tool for malnutrition suitable for adults in acute and community settings
Assessment for eating disorder or disordered eating	Eating Attitudes Test 26[10] Eating disorder screening tool Nine Question ARFID nutritional status tool[11]
Food insecurity	Hunger Vital Sign TM Two-Question Screening for Food Insecurity[12] Two questions: "Within the past 12 mo we worried whether our food would run out before we got money to buy more." Was that often true, sometimes true, or never true for you/your household? "Within the past 12 mo the food we bought just didn't last and we didn't have money to get more." Was that often, sometimes, or never true for you/your household?

assessment should be performed by a dietitian to provide interventions tailored to the patient.

IRRITABLE BOWEL SYNDROME

IBS accounts for up to half the visits with gastroenterologists and often requires several therapeutic interventions.[13] The low FODMAP diet has been shown to manage symptoms in up to 50% to 70% of patients with IBS and has in part validated the patient experience that food triggers symptoms.[14,15] One study revealed that up to 84% of individuals with IBS perceive food-related symptoms.[16] Patients with IBS are interested in holistic approaches to treatment. A pilot study from the Netherlands explored a shared decision model of IBS management, where patients were presented with 10 different treatment modalities. Most patients favored holistic approaches, and the top three selected interventions were peppermint oil, probiotics, and the low FODMAP diet.[17] Research reveals that a dietitian-guided low FODMAP diet is not challenging for the patient. One study showed that 60% of patients found the low FODMAP diet easy to follow, 65% could easily find suitable products to eat, and 43% were able to incorporate the diet easily into their life.[18] The low FODMAP diet education is much more than providing a high and low FODMAP food list. Dietitians provide menu and grocery store planning to enhance application and understanding of this complex diet intervention. In the absence of a dietitian, an individual should be provided with more than a one-page handout of foods to avoid. A longer list of foods allowed, sample menu, and resources, such as appropriate downloadable telephone applications, books, and Web sites, sets a patient up for better success. **Table 3** provides various IBS resources for the practicing gastroenterologist and their patients.

CELIAC DISEASE

CD is an immune-mediated enteropathic condition that occurs in about 1.4% of people globally.[19] The current treatment is a gluten-free diet. Nutritional deficiencies affect up to 20% to 38% of patients with CD and may arise because of malabsorption in untreated CD or the gluten-free diet.[20] Many food products using gluten-free flours are devoid of enrichment and are often made with refined flours, such as white rice flour, providing less fiber and minerals than their whole wheat alternatives. Micronutrients often lacking in a gluten-free diet include iron; folic acid; vitamins A, B_6, B_{12}, D, E, and K; copper; and zinc.[20] Patients with CD should be encouraged to consume naturally occurring, nutrient-dense gluten-free foods to best meet their needs. A dietitian assessment can identify any nutritional shortcomings and provide diet modifications to meet needs better.

Maladaptive eating is common in CD; one cohort of adolescent subjects with CD identified more than 53.3% with maladaptive eating behaviors.[21] As with many GI disorders, assessing for overt ED, reduced food-related quality of life, FI (gluten-free food products are more expensive than their gluten-containing counterparts), and maladaptive eating is important. If your practice setting does not allow enough time for these important assessments, refer to a dietitian with GI expertise or alternatively an ED specialist, as indicated. **Table 4** provides several resources for living gluten-free and with CD for provider and patients.

EOSINOPHILIC ESOPHAGITIS

EoE is a chronic immune-mediated disorder that is increasing in prevalence in adult and pediatric populations worldwide.[22] Common symptoms of EoE in adults include

Table 3 Educational resources and tools for IBS	
Educational Tool	**Description**
Books The Low FODMAP Diet Step by Step, by Kate Scarlata, MPH, RDN and Dede Wilson (recipe developer) The IBS Elimination Diet and Cookbook, by Patsy Catsos, MS, RDN	Both books provide easy to read, 3 phases of the low FODMAP diet; tips to meet nutrient needs; and covers meal planning, grocery shopping, and recipes. Designed for American audience. Step by step programs that can be used adjunctively with dietitian or independently, if necessary.
Community Support IBSPatient.org	Community forum and podcast. Provides numerous downloadable resources including letters to the employer about working from home, restroom access card, current IBS clinical trial links, and more.
General information Web sites The International Foundation for Gastrointestinal Disorders https://www.iffgd.org/, http://www.aboutibs.org	Informs, assists, and supports people with GI disorders. Provides information about GI disorders (symptoms, causes, how to prepare for tests, and more) and ways to find a doctor and dietitian.
Nutritional information Web sites Monash University www.monashfodmap.com Kate Scarlata, MPH, RDN www.katescarlata.com Patsy Catsos, MS, RDN https://www.ibsfree.net Myginutrition.com FODMAP Friendly https://fodmapfriendly.com/	Detailed information on low FODMAP science, IBS topics, recipes, and more.
Best Low FODMAP Diet App Monash University low FODMAP Diet app	Ability to filter for the country you reside in. Tailor to fit individual tolerances because it can filter for specific FODMAP sensitivities. Updated regularly with latest FODMAP food analysis.

dysphagia, food impaction, heartburn, and chest pain and occur because of esophageal dysfunction.[22] There are several treatment options for individuals diagnosed with EoE: proton pump inhibitors; two-, four-, or six-food elimination diets (SFED); swallowed topical steroids; and most recently immune-modifying biologic agents.[23] Long-term therapy to prevent disease recurrence and esophageal complications is required.[22]

A little more than two decades ago, the use of an elemental diet in children highlighted the ability of nutrition therapy to treat EoE.[24] Peterson and colleagues demonstrated the efficacy of an elemental formula in adults, with 72% achieving complete or near-complete disease remission. However, there was a high dropout rate of 41%.[25] The unpalatable taste and high cost with lack of insurance coverage of hypoallergenic, amino acid–based formulas are major limitations to implementing this therapy routinely in clinical practice.[22]

A more popular, and still effective, diet strategy for the treatment of EoE is the use of an empiric elimination diet. The empiric SFED consists of whole foods but excludes the top six food allergen groups including dairy, wheat, soy, eggs, fish/shellfish, and

Table 4
Educational resources and tools for celiac disease

Educational Tool	Description
Booklets for practice 　Celiac Disease Nutrition Guide, 3rd edition, 　　by Tricia Thompson, MS, RD	These booklets can be purchased in bulk for patient use. https://www.eatrightstore.org/product-type/booklets-workbooks/celiac-disease-nutrition-guide-3rd-ed-packs-of-10
Books 　Gluten Free: The Definitive Resource 　　Guide, 5th edition, by Shelley Case, RD	Comprehensive guide on the gluten-free diet.
Real Life with Celiac Disease, by Melinda Dennis, MS, RD and Daniel Leffler, MD	Case study style approach to living with celiac disease, sharing aspects of the disease that patients may experience.
Cookbook 　America's Test Kitchen, editor. The How 　　Can It Be Gluten Free Cookbook Volume 　　2: New Whole-Grain Flour Blend, 75+ 　　Dairy-Free Recipes	Delicious gluten-free recipes from America's Test Kitchen.
National Celiac Association https://nationalceliac.org	Resources, such as "ask the dietitian," gluten-free restaurant listing, gluten-free recipes, and FAQ section. Provides inks to local support groups.
Celiac Disease Foundation https://celiac.org	Resource for celiac disease for researchers, health care providers, and patients. Provides information on clinical trials, how to find a health care practitioner, and testing for celiac disease. Gluten-free diet reviewed in detail from label reading, dining out, menu plans, and more.
Beyond Celiac https://www.beyondceliac.org/	Comprehensive celiac disease and gluten-free diet information including recipes, baking and cooking tips, food safety, gluten-free training for food service professionals, symptom checklist, and more.
Gluten Free Watchdog https://www.glutenfreewatchdog.org	Founded by dietitian Tricia Thompson, MS, RD this Web site provides unbiased reporting of gluten-free food testing for consumers.
The Celiac Society Web site for clinicians https://www.theceliacsociety.org/	The Society for the Study of Celiac Disease is the professional organization of physicians, nurses, dietitians, and allied health professionals in the United States, Canada, and Mexico who specialize in the treatment of celiac disease and other gluten-related disorders.
Apps Find gluten-free restaurants https://www.findmeglutenfree.com https://glutenfreepassport.com https://nationalceliac.org/gluten-free-restaurants/	Apps for gluten-free diet followers to find suitable restaurants in their local area or when traveling.

(continued on next page)

Table 4 *(continued)*	
Educational Tool	Description
What companies use "purity protocol oats?" https://www.glutenfreewatchdog.org/news/ oats-produced-under-a-gluten-free-purity- protocol-listing-of-suppliers-and- manufacturers/	Oat consumption is a concern for those living with celiac disease caused by cross- contamination. This listing provides companies that offer oats grown and processed in a way that minimizes gluten exposure.

peanuts/tree nuts. SFED has shown efficacy in the treatment of EoE, with histologic remission in 73% of adults.[26] Food-reintroduction protocols require repeated endoscopies with biopsies after reintroducing one or two foods. An esophagogastroduodenoscopy is required to assess response to the diet and after the reintroduction of food groups to identify triggers; symptoms alone are not valid predictors of a histologic response.[27] The goal of the reintroductions is to identify causative food triggers and expand the patient's diet.

Milk, wheat, egg, and soy have been identified as the most common food triggers for EoE, and most of the patients (65%–85%) who respond to the SFED have just one or two causative foods identified.[28] To shorten the overall time to complete the food reintroduction process and reduce the number of endoscopies, the four-food elimination diet was investigated and proved to be successful, with 54% of adult patients achieving histologic remission.[28] Recently a "step-up" approach has been tested with the goal of reducing the number of esophagogastroduodenoscopies and dietary restrictions. Histologic remission rates of 44%, 60%, and 80% were observed for adults who did the step-up approach from the two-, four-, or six-food elimination diets, respectively.[29]

Comprehensive nutrition education on nutrition label reading, cross-contamination, and acceptable allergen-friendly food products should be provided to any patient who is going to undertake an elimination diet. With the restriction of multiple food groups comes the risk of nutrient deficiencies, unintentional weight loss, and reduced quality of life.[30,31] Patients should be educated on acceptable foods and provided with sound resources they can use while undergoing an elimination diet; many of these resources are found in **Table 5**. A hypoallergenic multivitamin with minerals is also recommended.[30] Success on an empiric elimination diet requires a multidisciplinary approach and includes gastroenterologists, allergists, dietitians, and nurses.

INFLAMMATORY BOWEL DISEASE

An estimated 1.3% of Americans reported being diagnosed with IBD (Crohn disease or ulcerative colitis) in 2015, a rise from 0.9% in 1999.[33] IBD is a global disease that is experiencing a growth in prevalence worldwide, particularly in westernized countries. Individuals with IBD are concerned about the role of diet in their digestive condition. "What should I eat?" is one of the most common questions asked to gastroenterologists.[34] Given the high prevalence of conflicting and misinformation on the Internet, it is essential that clinicians take the time to answer this question and ideally refer their patients with IBD to a dietitian. Patients require a more thorough answer than "Eat what you can tolerate."

Decreased oral intake, reduced absorption caused by resections or inflammation, increased output of stool or effluent, and drug-nutrient interactions can contribute

Table 5
Educational resources and tools for EoE and food allergy

Educational Tool	Description
Books: Allergy-Free and Easy Cooking: 30-Minute Meals without Gluten, Wheat, Dairy, Eggs, Soy, Peanuts, Tree Nuts, Fish, Shellfish, and Sesame, by Cybele Pascal The Allergy-Free Pantry: Make Your Own Staples, Snacks, and More Without Wheat, Gluten, Dairy, Eggs, Soy or Nuts, by Colette Martin	Cookbooks that provide recipes that are free from the top allergens.
Web sites: https://www.foodallergy.org/	Trusted source of food allergy information, programs, research, and resources.
University of Michigan GI Dietitians Pinterest Boards for the 2-, 4-, and 6-food elimination diets https://www.pinterest.com/UMGIdietitians/6-food-elimination-diet-for-eoe/	Pinterest boards with product suggestions that are suitable for the 2-, 4-, and 6-food elimination diets. Great for visual learners.
Yummly.com	Recipe index where users can select and filter out food allergies and preferences.
Clinician Resource: Dietary Therapy and Nutrition Management of Eosinophilic Esophagitis: Work Group Report of the American Academy of Allergy, Asthma, and Immunology[32]	A work group report that addresses the potential challenges of implementing a chosen dietary therapy for the management of EoE. Provides tools and guidance for effective implementation to health care professionals caring for patients with EoE.
Apps Ipiitt	Food allergy app with barcode reader.
Allergy Food Translator	The app translates allergies into French, German, or Spanish.
Yummly	Recipe index that has the option to select and filter out food allergies and preferences.
Biteappy	Great for finding allergy-friendly restaurants worldwide.

to micronutrient deficiencies. Micronutrient levels should be checked when there is a concern for a deficiency and supplemented when low. Vitamin D status should be checked regularly and supplemented to within normal limits.[35] One of the most common manifestations of IBD is anemia, with iron deficiency anemia and anemia of chronic disease being the two most common causes.[36] It is recommended that individuals with iron deficiency anemia receive appropriate iron supplementation, either oral or parenteral.[37]

Nutrition research for inducing and maintaining remission, outside of exclusive enteral nutrition therapy for IBD, has been nonconclusive. A 2019 Cochrane review assessed dietary interventions for Crohn disease and ulcerative colitis and concluded the effects of diet interventions are uncertain at this time, and firm conclusions could not be drawn because of limitations of the available studies.[38] A 2018 Cochrane review suggests that exclusive enteral nutrition is superior to corticosteroids in pediatric Crohn disease and is slightly inferior for the induction of remission in adults.[39] The

Crohn's Disease Exclusion Diet is a whole-food diet combined with partial enteral nutrition that has shown the ability to induce remission in mild-to-moderate Crohn disease in a randomized controlled trial.[40] Therapeutic diets for IBD are of interest to patients and providers. Several diets have been reported to be efficacious in small case series, including the specific carbohydrate diet, IBD anti-inflammatory diet, Crohn's Disease Exclusion Diet, and semivegetarian diet.[41] We await larger randomized clinical trials to help expand the clinical application of nutrition interventions for IBD.

The Enhanced Recovery After Surgery Society guidelines should be used to optimize recovery for patients undergoing elective surgery for best postsurgical outcomes.[42] A low FODMAP diet for symptomatic patients with quiescent disease has shown to be effective for IBS-like symptomology.[43] Maintaining a long-term low FODMAP elimination diet is not the goal and patients should be instructed to engage in all three phases to help liberalize the diet as much as possible while managing IBS symptoms. Dietary recommendations should be tailored individually in IBD and consider many factors including but not limited to disease activity, age, food tolerance/intolerance, laboratory findings, clinical symptoms, and the patient's goals. Educational tools and resources for IBD are found in **Table 6**.

Table 6 Educational resources and tools for IBD	
Educational Tool	**Description**
Books: Breaking the Vicious Cycle: Intestinal Health Through Diet, by Elaine Gloria Gottschall (1994) Nutrition in Immune Balance (NIMBAL) Therapy, by David L Suskind (2015)	Books on the specific carbohydrate diet.
Web sites Crohn's and Colitis Foundation https://www.crohnscolitisfoundation.org/	The Crohn's & Colitis Foundation of America is a nonprofit, volunteer-driven organization whose mission is to cure Crohn disease and ulcerative colitis, and to improve the quality of life of children and adults affected by these diseases.
I'llBeDetermined https://www.ibdetermined.org/ibd-information/ibd-diet.aspx Nutrition in Immune Balance (NiMBAL) https://www.nimbal.org/education/the-specific-carbohydrate-diet-	IBD resources and information, discussion boards, and patient personal stories. Specific carbohydrate diet information.
Clinician Resources: Nutrition Resources for Healthcare Providers by the Crohn's and Colitis Foundation https://site.crohnscolitisfoundation.org/science-and-professionals/programs-materials/nutritional-resources-for.html	Online CME education modules, nutrition fact sheets, such as the Crohn's & Colitis Foundation's IBD Anemia Care Pathway and Common Micronutrient Deficiencies in IBD, Foundation-led Research Studies.
Apps: My IBD Manager by the American Gastroenterological Association	The app offers tools and features for patients, including a treatment tracker to help monitor dosing, schedules, and supplements; a symptom tracker to monitor pain and progress; and a food log to monitor diet and nutritional intake.

SUMMARY

Individuals with GI conditions are interested in nutritional approaches for treatment management. As clinicians, it is imperative that we provide evidence-based resources and tools to help them navigate this approach to care as seamlessly as possible. Having an RD with GI expertise is your best resource, but when access is limited, there are several apps, books, Web sites, and online communities to support you and your patients.

CLINICS CARE POINTS

- The success of nutrition therapy relies on a patient's engagement in the process, motivation to adhere to specific nutrition interventions, understanding of how to avoid specific food groups when applicable (for example a gluten free diet for celiac disease, an elimination diet for EoE), and the financial means to remain on a specialized diet.
- Regardless of the digestive condition and the practicing gastroenterologist's good intentions, providing a patient with a simple list of "avoid these foods" or "eat this not that" has the potential to cause more harm than good as there are many nuances when it comes to nutrition therapy that require an in-depth discussion and patients benefit from personalization as well as educational resources.
- A guided, systematic reintroduction of foods is required for patients who are doing an elimination diet such as the low FODMAP diet or the 2-, 4-, or 6-food elimination diet. The low FODMAP diet reintroduction requires patients to monitor GI symptoms to assess their specific tolerance while those with EoE will require EGDs to assess response to diet therapy and identify their specific food trigger(s) as foods are reintroduced.
- Selecting a particular nutrition intervention is best guided by a registered dietitian who can provide a complex nutrition assessment to best inform the most appropriate nutritional approach.
- Growing data links eating disorder risk in people with GI conditions, screening for disordered eating and eating disorders in this population should be part of any GI assessment.

DISCLOSURE

None.

REFERENCES

1. Satherley R, Howard R, Higgs S. Disordered eating practices in gastrointestinal disorders. Appetite 2015;84:240–50.
2. American Psychiatric Association. Diagnostic and statistical manual of mental disorders. 5th edition. Washington, DC: American Psychiatric Publishing; 2013.
3. Zia JK, Riddle M, DeCou CR, et al. Prevalence of eating disorders, especially DSM-5's avoidant restrictive food intake disorder, in patients with functional gastrointestinal disorders: a cross-sectional online survey. Gastroenterology 2017;152(5 Suppl 1):S715–6.
4. Harer KN, Jagielski CH, Riehl ME, et al. 272 – Avoidant/restrictive food intake disorder among adult gastroenterology behavioral health patients: demographic and clinical characteristics. Gastroenterology 2019;156(6):S-53.

5. Wang X, Luscombe GM, Boyd C, et al. Functional gastrointestinal disorders in eating disorder patients: altered distribution and predictors using ROME III compared to ROME II criteria. World J Gastroenterol 2014;20(43):16293–9.
6. Boyd C, Abraham S. Kellow J. Psychological features are important predictors of functional gastrointestinal disorders in patients with eating disorders. Scand J Gastroenterol 2005;40(8):929–35.
7. Coleman-Jensen A, Rabbitt M, Gregory C, et al. Household food security in the United States in 2015. Report No.: ERR-215. Washington, DC: US Department of Agriculture; 2016.
8. Ferguson M, Capra S, Bauer J, et al. Development of a valid and reliable malnutrition screening tool for adult acute hospital patients. Nutrition 1999;15(6): 458–64.
9. Malnutrition Advisory Group (MAG). A standing Committee of the British Association for Parenteral and Enteral Nutrition (BAPEN). The 'MUST' Explanatory booklet. A Guide to the 'malnutrition universal screening tool' ('MUST') for adults. BAPEN; 2003. Available at: https://www.bapen.org.uk/pdfs/must/must_explan.pdf.
10. Eating attitudes test (EAT-26). 2009-2017. Available at: www.EAT-26.com. Accessed February 9, 2020.
11. Zickgraf HF, Ellis JM. Initial validation of the Nine Item Avoidant/Restrictive Food Intake disorder screen (NIAS): a measure of the three restrictive eating patterns. Appetite 2018;123:32–42.
12. Available at: https://hungerandhealth.feedingamerica.org/wp-content/uploads/2017/11/Food-Insecurity-Toolkit.pdf. Accessed February 16, 2020.
13. Gunn MC, Cavin AA, Mansfield JC. Management of irritable bowel syndrome. Postgrad Med J 2003;79:154–8.
14. Halmos EP, Power VA, Shepherd SJ, et al. A diet low in FODMAPs reduces symptoms in irritable bowel syndrome. Gastroenterology 2014;146(1):67–75.
15. Eswaran SL, Chey WD, Han-Markey T, et al. A randomized controlled trial comparing the low FODMAP diet vs. modified NICE guidelines in US adults with IBS-D. Am J Gastroenterol 2016;111(12):1824–32.
16. Böhn L, Störsrud S, Törnblom H. Self-reported food-related gastrointestinal symptoms in IBS are common and associated with more severe symptoms and reduced quality of life. Am J Gastroenterol 2013;108(5):634–41.
17. Otten MH, Holierhoek Y, Stellingwerf F, et al. Reduce IBS project: multiple therapy choices and shared decision-making give IBS patients self management and better quality of life. Gastroenterology 2017;5(152):S45.
18. de, Roest RH, Dobbs BR, Chapman BA, et al. The low FODMAP diet improves gastrointestinal symptoms in patients with irritable bowel syndrome: a prospective study. Int J Clin Pract 2013;67:895–903.
19. Singh P, Arora A, Strand A, et al. Global prevalence of celiac disease: systematic review and meta-analysis. Clin Gastroenterol Hepatol 2018;16(6):823–36.
20. Di Nardo G, Villa MP, Conti L, et al. Nutritional deficiencies in children with celiac disease resulting from a gluten-free diet: a systematic review. Nutrients 2019; 11(7):1588.
21. Cadenhead JW, Wolf RL, Lebwohl B, et al. Diminished quality of life among adolescents with coeliac disease using maladaptive eating behaviors to manage a gluten free diet; a cross-sectional, mixed-methods study. J Hum Nutr Diet 2019;32(3):311–20.
22. Gonsalves NP, Aceves SS. Diagnosis and treatment of eosinophilic esophagitis. J Allergy Clin Immunol 2020;145(1):1–7.

23. Spergel JM, Dellon ES, Liacouras CA, et al. Summary of the updated international consensus diagnostic criteria for eosinophilic esophagitis: AGREE conference. Ann Allergy Asthma Immunol 2018;121(3):281–4.

24. Kelly KJ, Lazenby AJ, Rowe PC, et al. Eosinophilic esophagitis attributed to gastroesophageal reflux: improvement with an amino acid-based formula. Gastroenterology 1995;109(5):1503–12.

25. Peterson KA, Byrne KR, Vinson LA, et al. Elemental diet induces histologic response in adult eosinophilic esophagitis. Am J Gastroenterol 2013;108(5): 759–66.

26. Lucendo AJ, Arias Á, González-cervera J, et al. Empiric 6-food elimination diet induced and maintained prolonged remission in patients with adult eosinophilic esophagitis: a prospective study on the food cause of the disease. J Allergy Clin Immunol 2013;131(3):797–804.

27. Dellon ES, Gonsalves N, Hirano I, et al. ACG clinical guideline: evidenced based approach to the diagnosis and management of esophageal eosinophilia and eosinophilic esophagitis (EoE). Am J Gastroenterol 2013;108(5):679–92.

28. Molina-infante J, Arias A, Barrio J, et al. Four-food group elimination diet for adult eosinophilic esophagitis: a prospective multicenter study. J Allergy Clin Immunol 2014;134(5):1093–9.e1.

29. Molina-infante J, Arias Á, Alcedo J, et al. Step-up empiric elimination diet for pediatric and adult eosinophilic esophagitis: the 2-4-6 study. J Allergy Clin Immunol 2018;141(4):1365–72.

30. Doerfler B, Bryce P, Hirano I, et al. Practical approach to implementing dietary therapy in adults with eosinophilic esophagitis: the Chicago experience. Dis Esophagus 2015;28(1):42–58.

31. Taft TH, Kern E, Keefer L, et al. Qualitative assessment of patient reported outcomes in adults with eosinophilic esophagitis. J Clin Gastroenterol 2011;45(9): 769–74.

32. Groetch M, Venter C, Skypala I, et al. Dietary therapy and nutrition management of eosinophilic esophagitis: a work group report of the American Academy of Allergy, Asthma, and Immunology. J Allergy Clin Immunol Pract 2017;5(2): 312–24.e29.

33. Dahlhamer JM, Zammitti EP, Ward BW, et al. Prevalence of inflammatory bowel disease among adults aged ≥18 years—United States, 2015. MMWR Morb Mortal Wkly Rep 2016;65(42):1166–9. Available at: https://www.cdc.gov/mmwr/volumes/65/wr/mm6542a3.htm.

34. Lewis JD, Abreu MT. Diet as a trigger or therapy for inflammatory bowel diseases. Gastroenterology 2017;152(2):398–414.e6.

35. Parizadeh SM, Jafarzadeh-esfehani R, Hassanian SM, et al. Vitamin D in inflammatory bowel disease: from biology to clinical implications. Complement Ther Med 2019;47:102189.

36. Kaitha S, Bashir M, Ali T. Iron deficiency anemia in inflammatory bowel disease. World J Gastrointest Pathophysiol 2015;6(3):62–72.

37. Forbes A, Escher J, Hébuterne X, et al. ESPEN guideline: clinical nutrition in inflammatory bowel disease. Clin Nutr 2017;36(2):321–47.

38. Limketkai BN, Iheozor-ejiofor Z, Gjuladin-hellon T, et al. Dietary interventions for induction and maintenance of remission in inflammatory bowel disease. Cochrane Database Syst Rev 2019;2:CD012839.

39. Narula N, Dhillon A, Zhang D, et al. Enteral nutritional therapy for induction of remission in Crohn's disease. Cochrane Database Syst Rev 2018;4:CD000542.

40. Levine A, Wine E, Assa A, et al. Crohn's disease exclusion diet plus partial enteral nutrition induces sustained remission in a randomized controlled trial. Gastroenterology 2019;157(2):440–50.e8.

41. Hou JK, Lee D, Lewis J. Diet and inflammatory bowel disease: review of patient-targeted recommendations. Clin Gastroenterol Hepatol 2014;12:1592–600.

42. Gustafsson UO, Scott MJ, Hubner M, et al. Guidelines for perioperative care in elective colorectal surgery: Enhanced Recovery After Surgery (ERAS) Society recommendations: 2018. World J Surg 2019;43(3):659–95.

43. Colombel JF, Shin A, Gibson PR. AGA clinical practice update on functional gastrointestinal symptoms in patients with inflammatory bowel disease: expert review. Clin Gastroenterol Hepatol 2019;17(3):380–90.e1.

Nutritional Considerations in the Hospital Setting

Christopher Fain, DO[a],*, Kathy Bull-Henry, MBA, MD[b], Maaza Abdi, MD[c]

KEYWORDS

- Nutrition • Hospital • Malnutrition • Nutritional risk • Specialized nutrition support
- Disease-specific considerations • Micronutrient and vitamin deficiencies

KEY POINTS

- Malnutrition is common in the hospital setting and is associated with morbidity, mortality, increased length of stay, infections, and postoperative complications.
- Nutritional risk calculations can be used to target hospitalized patients that need nutritional support to improve outcomes.
- Pragmatic protocols and measures for enteral and parenteral nutrition are essential.
- Practical, evidenced-based management of hospitalized patients with specific gastrointestinal and liver disease can improve outcomes.
- Many nutrient deficiencies are important in hospitalized patients.

INTRODUCTION

The growing need for physician training in diet and nutrition is increasingly being recognized by major societies and being encouraged as part of standard gastroenterology fellowship training.[1,2] Probably nowhere is that need for training more important than in the hospital, where patient stays are often complicated by nutritional issues. The purpose of this review is to focus on the practical issues and management of nutrition related hospital issues: malnutrition, specialized nutritional support, disease-specific nutritional considerations, and relevant micronutrient and vitamin deficiencies seen in the hospital.

MALNUTRITION IN THE HOSPITAL

Malnutrition in the hospital is associated with increased morbidity, mortality, length of stay, infections, and postoperative complications.[3] Malnutrition, however, remains

[a] Johns Hopkins Hospital, 600 North Wolfe Street, 461 Blalock, Baltimore, MD 21287, USA;
[b] Johns Hopkins Bayview Medical Center, Johns Hopkins Hospital, 4940 Eastern Avenue, Baltimore, MD 21224, USA; [c] Gastroenterology, Johns Hopkins Hospital, 600 North Wolfe Street, Halsted 415, Baltimore, MD 21287, USA
* Corresponding author.
E-mail address: cfain1@jhmi.edu

Gastroenterol Clin N Am 50 (2021) 15–28
https://doi.org/10.1016/j.gtc.2020.10.015
0889-8553/21/Published by Elsevier Inc.
gastro.theclinics.com

difficult to define. The Academy of Nutrition and Dietetics and the American Society for Parenteral and Enteral Nutrition in 2012 defined malnutrition as having 2 more of the following 6 characteristics[4]:

- Insufficient energy intake
- Weight loss
- Loss of muscle mass
- Loss of subcutaneous fat
- Localized or generalized fluid accumulation that may mask weight loss
- Diminished functional status as measured by handgrip strength

A more recent multidisciplinary international committee divided malnutrition into 3 categories[5]:

- Starvation-related malnutrition
- Chronic disease–related malnutrition with low-grade inflammation
- Acute disease-related malnutrition characterized by a high degree of inflammation

Nutritional risk assessment, in contrast, is a practical concept because it is characterized by disease severity and nutritional status, both of which are important to outcomes and the need for nutritional therapy.[6,7] Nutritional risk is also more easily defined than malnutrition as it uses objective parameters. Nutritional risk scores can be used to identify patients with high risk scores to direct nutritional support to improve outcomes and to avoid unnecessary nutritional support in those with low scores.[6,8,9] The 2 assessment tools that are available to determine nutritional risk are the Nutritional Risk Score 2002 and the NUTRIC Score (**Table 1**).

SPECIALIZED NUTRITIONAL SUPPORT: ORAL NUTRITION SOLUTIONS, ENTERAL NUTRITION AND PATERNAL NUTRITION

Oral Nutritional Solutions

Oral nutrition solutions (ONS) can be particularly helpful in hospitalized patients with poor oral intake, appetite, and/or malnourishment. ONS comes in a variety of forms (liquids, powders, puddings, thickened, etc), types (low lactose, fiber containing, high protein, etc), and varying calories densities. ONS interventions have been shown to decrease hospital costs, length of stay, complications, and mortality, as well as 30-day readmissions.[10,11]

Enteral Nutrition

Enteral nutrition (EN) formulas differ primarily on osmolarity, calorie density, protein content, and electrolytes and can be categorized into standard, concentrated, and predigested, previously called semielemental or elemental, formulas. Concentrated formulas differ primarily from standard formulas on calorie content. The calorie density of standard formulas is 1 cal/mL, whereas that of concentrated formulas is 1.5 to 2.0 cal/mL. Predigested formulas, in contrast, contain short chain peptides and less complex carbohydrates when compared with standard formulations.

The preponderance of the evidence suggests that standard formulations are appropriate for most patients with some patient-specific exceptions. Concentrated formulations are helpful in patients needing fluid restriction, and predigested formulations can be helpful in patients with thoracic duct leaks, in those with significant issues of maldigestion or malabsorption, or in patients with severe diarrhea despite efforts to correct the underlying medical condition. Even renal formulations are unlikely to benefit most renal patients, except in those with significant electrolyte abnormalities.

Table 1
Nutritional risk factors scoring systems: NRS 2002 and NUTRIC scores

NRS 2002 (Reference[6])	
Impaired Nutritional Status	**Severity of Disease**
Absent score 0: Normal nutritional status	Absent score 0: Normal nutritional requirements
Mild score 1: Weight loss >5% in 3 mo OR Food intake <50%–75% of normal requirement in preceding week	Mild score 1: Hip fracture Chronic patients in particular with acute complications: cirrhosis, COPD Chronic hemodialysis, diabetes, oncology
Moderate score 2: Weight loss >5% in 2 mo OR BMI 18.5–20.5 + impaired general condition OR Food intake 25%–50% of normal requirement in preceding week	Moderate score 2: Major abdominal surgery, stroke Severe pneumonia, hematologic malignancy
Severe score 3: Weight loss >5% in 1 mo (15% in 3 mo) OR BMI 18.5+ impaired general condition OR Food intake <25% of normal requirement in preceding week	Severe score 3: Head injury Bone marrow transplantation Intensive care patients (APACHE II >10)

NUTRIC Score: Factors Used to Determine Score

Factors (Reference[7])	NUTRIC Points			
	0	1	2	3
Age (years)	<50	50–74	≥75	-
APACHE II score	<15	15–19	20–27	≥28
Baseline SOFA score	<6	6–9	≥10	-
No. of comorbidities	0–1	≥2	-	-
Days in hospitals to ICU admits	0	≥1	-	-
IL-6 (μ/mL)	0–399	≥400	-	-

APACHE, Acute Physiologic and Chronic Health Evaluation; BMI, body mass index; COPD, chronic obstructive pulmonary disease; ICU, intensive care unit; NRS-2002, Nutritional Risk Score 2002; SOFA, Simplified Organ Failure Assessment.
If age ≥70 years, add 1 point (for NRS-2002).
Total score = (Points for nutritional status) + (Points for disease severity) + (Points for age) (for NRS-2002).
Total score is from 6 separate factors (for NUTRIC Score).

From McClave SA, DiBaise JK, Mullin GE, Martindale RG. ACG clinical guideline: nutrition therapy in the adult hospitalized patient. American Journal of Gastroenterology. 2016;111(3):315-334.

In 1 trial, renal patients were be able to tolerate a much higher concentration of protein, 2.5 g protein/kg body weight, than previously thought.[12]

In terms of application, delivery and monitoring of EN, standard EN clinical protocols should be developed in hospitals, and several points are worth noting. As a part of the monitoring protocols, auscultation for bowel sounds and monitoring of gastric residual volumes should be discouraged because neither practice correlates well with tolerance of tube feeds. Instead, nutritional experts recommend checking for EN tolerance every 12 hours and monitoring for abdominal signs indicative of intolerance, such as significant distention, discomfort, nausea, and vomiting.[13]

While EN is running, the patient's bedrest should be elevated at 30° to 45° to minimize aspiration. Continuous feedings should be considered in those patients that are especially at high risk of vomiting, reflux or aspiration. The evidence to support placing tubes past the pylorus to prevent aspiration is weak.[14] Common indications for jejunal tube feeds are shown in **Table 2**.

Diarrhea in the hospital is quite common and is often multifactorial and not related to tube feedings.[15] Other more common causes of diarrhea in the hospital, including infections, digestive diseases, and medications, including liquid medications that contain sorbitol, should be sought first before discontinuing a tube feed and changing formulations.

Total Parenteral Nutrition

An exhaustive review of total parenteral nutrition (TPN) is beyond the scope of this article. Instead, common indications, contradictions, and complications and practical inpatient issues related to the application are discussed. Common indications, contraindications and complications for TPN are shown in **Table 3**. Peripheral parenteral nutrition can be considered in patients with good, stable venous access, who have no significant fluid restrictions, cannot meet their nutritional needs orally or via EN, and generally require nutritional support for less than 1 to 2 weeks. Peripheral parenteral nutrition is particularly helpful in patients needing to remain off oral feeding for procedures for an extended period of time and who have some underlying malnourishment but can resume oral intake within 1 week.

As a matter of practical concern, these authors recommend the development of inpatient protocols for the initiation of TPN. These protocols should include the training of specialized TPN case managers, dieticians, nurses and physicians, processes to cycle TPN and patient education. Also, before committing a patient to central venous access for planned outpatient TPN, insurance coverage and an outpatient provider with expertise in TPN care must be determined. The inpatient TPN protocols should also include clinical scenarios that Medicare will and likely will not cover.[16]

DISEASE-SPECIFIC CONSIDERATIONS
Small Bowel Syndrome

The nutritional needs, including the need for total paternal nutrition, of a patient with short gut are largely dependent on the length of the remaining small bowel and

| Table 2 | |
Indications for jejunal feeding	
Indicated	Gastroparesis or delayed gastric empty
	Proximal obstructions
	Proximal enterocutaneous fistulas
Possibly indicated	Severe pancreatitis (to avoid pancreatic stimulation)
	To prevent aspiration (evidence weak)
	Severe reflux disease (such as in scleroderma)

Table 3	
Common indications, contraindications and complications of TPN	
Indications	Enteral feeding not an option
	Gut failure
	High output fistulas (>500 mL/d) or uncontrolled high output ostomies
	Bowel obstructions
	Prolonged bowel rest necessary
Contrain-dications	Poor short-term prognosis
	Functioning gastrointestinal gut
	Risks outweigh benefits
	Severe cardiac and metabolic derangements
Compli-cations	Metabolic complications (hyperglycemia, electrolyte disturbances, metabolic acidosis, hyperlipidemia)
	Line associated thrombosis
	Line infections
	Line insertion complications (pneumothorax, hemorrhage, skin infection, etc)
	Metabolic bone disease
	PN-associated liver disease

whether there is loss of ileum versus jejunum, the ileocecal valve, and part or all of the colon and whether there is intestinal continuity.[17,18] The ileum is much more adept at regaining function than the jejunum and having at least a partial colon can be equivalent to about 50 cm of small bowel. The prognosis thus is generally best for those with a jejunal–ileocolonic anastomoses and least for end jejunostomies.

The general principle guiding the nutritional management of patients with small bowel syndrome is a hyperphagia diet, one that involves caloric intake 1.5 to 2.0 times a standard diet.[19] General diet recommendations include 5 to 6 smaller meals, consisting of complex carbohydrates (60%), fats (20%–30%), proteins (20%–30%), and minimal simple sugars.[20] Oral rehydration solutions might especially be necessary in those without a colon or without small bowel to large bowel continuity. Chewing feed well is mandatory.

Fiber can also help to slow the transit of food for greater absorption of nutrients, can aid in adaption, and can provide an additional source of calories via short chain fatty acids in those with an intact colon. Medium chain triglycerides, which are devoid of essential fatty acids, and are absorbed in both the small and large intestines, can be used as an additional source of calories in patient struggling to maintain weight goals. TPN is generally indicated in all patients in the initial phase of small bowel syndrome and in those with uncontrollable high output ostomies or that have failed oral or EN nutritional attempts.

Vitamin B_{12} deficiency is common in short bowel syndrome when more than 50 to 60 cm is resected.[21] Vitamin B_{12} injections in these patients often become requisite. Resection of ileum of more than 100 cm leads to bile acid deficiencies, which then leads to both fat and fat vitamin malabsorption and deficiencies. Zinc deficiency, and less so copper and selenium deficiency, is common in those with excessive diarrhea.[20]

Inflammatory Bowel Disease

Malnutrition in inflammatory bowel disease (IBD) is often related to poor oral intake and appetite from symptomology, especially nausea and abdominal pain. Thus, disease control is essential in improving the nutrition of patients with IBD. For hospitalized patients with IBD with significantly active disease, protein intake generally should be increased to 1.2 to 1.5 g/kg/d because catabolism, steroid use, and protein losses in stools can all contribute to significant loss of protein mass in these patients.[22]

TPN is generally reserved for obstructions, short gut syndrome, proximal high output fistulas, or high output ostomies and those that have failed oral diet or EN. TPN should not be considered an effective monotherapy for Crohn's disease.[23] For any significantly malnourished IBD patient needing surgery, as in any presurgical patient that is significantly malnourished, consideration should be made to improve nutrition, including with TPN, by delaying the surgery for 7 to 14 days to improve surgical outcomes.[24] See the section on Nutrition in Critically Ill and Surgical Patients elsewhere in this article.

Vitamin and mineral deficiencies should be checked regularly in patients with IBD, especially in those who are hospitalized frequently. Deficiencies should be considered in specific clinic scenarios. Patients with significant diarrhea, including high output ostomies or with high output fistulas, are at risk for zinc deficiency. Those with extensive ileal resection or ileal disease are risk for vitamin B_{12} deficiency and fat-soluble vitamin deficiency. Iron deficiencies should be considered in those with anemia, with chronic blood loss, and with extensive proximal small disease. Folate deficiencies should be considered in those with anemia or who are on drugs, such as methotrexate and sulfasalazine, that cause folate deficiency.

Physicians often confuse low residue versus low fiber diets. A low residue diet is any diet that decreases stool output by limiting fibrous meats, dairy products, and most fruits and vegetables.[25] A small prospective trial showed no differences in outcomes, including rates of flares, in patients on a low residue diet versus a standard Italian diet.[26] However, what is not known is whether a low residue diet could affect inpatient outcomes, especially symptoms and length of stay. Low fiber diets should be considered in any patients with intestinal strictures because fiber could potentially cause an obstruction at the site of narrowing.

Acute Pancreatitis

There is substantial evidence that early oral feeding with a low fat, soft diet in patients without significant ileus or nausea and with mild acute pancreatitis is safe and shortens hospital stays.[27] Patients with moderate to severe acute pancreatitis often have difficulty tolerating diet from anorexia, ileus, pain, gastroduodenal inflammation, and/or partial gastric outlet obstructions from fluid collections. Aggressive inpatient management, when possible of those associated conditions, can help improve appetite and oral intake.

Generally, EN feeding should be initiated early in admission in patients with severe pancreatitis when there is poor oral intake. EN feeding protects the gut barrier from bacterial translocation; decreases overall complications, including mortality, infections, and organ failure; and avoids the significant complications of TPN.[28,29] A recent Expert Statements and Practical Guidance for Nutrition guideline recommends starting EN as early as 24 to 72 hours when oral intake is poor.[27] This practice is supported by a Cochrane review.[30]

The preponderance of evidence suggests the noninferiority in outcomes of nasogastric to nasojejunal (NJ) feeding, although this recommendation may not be based on adequately powered studies and appropriate NJ tube location was not always confirmed.[31] In patients with severe pancreatitis and necrosis, consideration should be made for NJ feeding, which may cause less pancreatic stimulation.[32] Standard formulas are as effective and as tolerated as predigested ones.[27] Predigested formulas, which are generally more expensive, should be reserved only for those with intolerance to standard formulas.

NJ tubes should also be used in those with delayed gastric emptying or in those with partial gastric outlet obstructions from gastroduodenal inflammation. Efforts should be made to minimize narcotics, which can cause gastrointestinal dysfunction, limiting oral intake and EN. Judicious use of gastrointestinal neuromodulators should be considered to control abdominal pain. These medications may have the additional effect of controlling nausea and vomiting. TPN should generally be reserved for those that did not tolerate EN or have contraindications to EN such as bowel obstruction.

Gastroparesis

Patients hospitalized with gastroparesis can experience long and complicated hospital stays.[33] Nutritional management of these patients generally begins with supportive care, especially control of nausea and vomiting, which is usually best accomplished with around the clock antiemetics, temporary use of prokinetics such as metoclopramide (Reglan) or erythromycin, frequent small meals, and minimizing medications that will exacerbate symptoms, especially narcotics.[34] Endocrinology consults can be particularly helpful in hospitalized gastroparetics with difficult to control blood sugars.

Diet diaries should be kept by both patients and nursing and nutritional support staff, and physicians should review these diaries daily, as well as a patient's verbal account of oral intake. Endoscopic methods, including pyloric directed botulinum toxin (Botox), postpyloric feeding tubes, and gastric peroral endoscopic myotomies should be considered in severe cases. TPN should generally only be considered in those that have failed or have contraindications to EN. Gastrointestinal neuromodulators, such as buspirone (dyspeptic symptoms/increased gastric accommodation) and mirtazapine (pain, nausea, and vomiting) can be initiated in the hospital to help in the management of chronic symptoms.[35]

Scleroderma

Malnutrition is very common in scleroderma and is responsible for as many as 20% of the associated deaths from this disease.[36] Nutrition in scleroderma is complicated by the fact that it can involve any part of the gastrointestinal tract. Poor nutrition in a patient with scleroderma can be related to difficulty opening the mouth and chewing food, sicca syndrome, dysphagia or esophageal dysmotility, severe gastroesophageal reflux disease, gastroparesis, small intestinal bacterial overgrowth, and chronic intestinal pseudo-obstruction. Appropriate management of patients hospitalized for gastrointestinal scleroderma should be directed at all these areas including aggressive oral care, proton pump inhibitor and lifestyle management of gastroesophageal reflux disease, prokinetic therapy (metoclopramide and pyridostigmine [Mestinon]) for issues of dysmotility and antibiotic therapy for small intestinal bacterial overgrowth.

Diets restrictive in simple sugars, fruit juices, sugar alcohols, and fibers may help to improve small intestinal bacterial overgrowth symptoms.[37] Lactose should generally be avoided because secondary intolerance is common in these patients. EN should be considered in those with poor oral intake, but may be limited by underlying gastroparesis, small bowel dysmotility, small intestinal bacterial overgrowth, or complete intestinal failure, for which then PN is recommended.

Severely Malnourished and Refeeding Syndrome

Patients with severe malnutrition, especially those with rapid weight loss or whose ideal body weight is less than 70%, are at particular risk for refeeding syndrome.[38,39] Refeeding syndrome is characterized by hypophosphatemia, which is initially caused by depleted stores of phosphate from starvation. When feeding is initiated in these patients, the hypophosphatemia is then exacerbated by carbohydrate intake, which leads to increased insulin secretion, which increases the metabolism of phosphate and drives phosphate into cells. The resultant severe hypophosphatemia can then cause both cardiac and respiratory failure. The refeeding syndrome is generally managed by first repleting deficient electrolytes, vitamins and minerals—a process that often can be done in the first 24 to 48 hours. The caloric intake is then slowly increased over the course of days while monitoring closely for electrolyte disturbances and signs of cardiorespiratory distress.[39,40]

Alcoholic Hepatitis

Malnutrition in very common in patients with alcoholic hepatitis.[41,42] Numerous factors can contribute to this malnutrition, including higher resting energy expenditure and poor oral intake from anorexia, nausea, encephalopathy, and early satiety from delayed gastric emptying from ascites.[43,44] Although alcohol abstinence is the key to improvement in patients with moderate to severe alcoholic hepatitis, malnutrition probably affects important outcomes in these patients including infection, encephalopathy, histology, and mortality.[45]

Malnutrition was shown to be an independent predictor of mortality in those with moderate alcoholic hepatitis and is associated with mortality in severe alcoholic hepatitis.[42,45] A multicenter study showed that a lower calorie intake of 21.5 kcal/kg/d was significantly associated with death in these patients.[46] A systemic review that was limited by a high risk of bias suggested that nutritional therapy could decrease hepatic encephalopathy, infection rates, and mortality, but called for higher quality studies.[47] Based on the available evidence, the Expert Statements and Practical Guidance for Nutrition guidelines suggest that nutritional therapy should be offered to those with severe alcoholic hepatitis who cannot meet nutrition needs by spontaneous food intake to improve outcomes.[45]

The American Gastroenterological Association recommends 1.5 g protein/kg body weight and 30 to 40 kcal/kg per body weight as nutritional goals for those with significant alcoholic hepatitis.[48] For those unable to meet these goals spontaneously, EN is favored over PN because it helps to maintain gut integrity, which has possible implications in pathogenesis of alcoholic hepatitis.[49] PN should generally be avoided in these patients given its inherent risks as well as its pathogenesis in liver disease.[50] Other key practical nutritional measures for hospitalized patients with alcoholic hepatitis are to address common vitamin and micronutrient deficiencies (especially B vitamins, thiamine, and zinc), avoid prolonged periods of fasting and foods that make early satiety worse (high fiber), provide frequent snacks, especially at night time and in morning (to decrease gluconeogenesis/breakdown of protein), and consider feeding tubes in those unable to eat on their own violation.[44]

Post Gastric and Pancreatic Surgery

Dumping syndrome is caused by the loss of the pyloric sphincter and occurs in 15% to 20% of patients after partial gastrectomy and up to 70% of early postgastric bypass patients.[51,52] Most patients only experience the early dumping syndrome, which occurs 10 to 30 minutes after food intake, and is caused by the rapid emptying of hyperosmolar chyme into the small bowel, leading to rapid shifts of fluid into the lumen of the small bowel. This process leads to the characteristic signs and symptoms of the syndrome: abdominal pain, nausea, weight loss, bloating, and explosive diarrhea. First-line management is dietary and includes small, more frequent meals that are high in

Table 4
Important macro and micronutrient and vitamin deficiencies in hospitalized patients

Nutrient	Cause of Deficiency	Clinical Implications
Thiamine B$_1$	Alcoholism, severe malnutrition	Wet beriberi—heart failure and low vascular resistance Wernicke's encephalopathy—nystagmus, ophthalmoplegia and ataxia Korsakoff's psychosis—hallucinations, impaired memory, confabulation
Niacin B$_3$	Carcinoid syndrome	Pellagra—dementia, pigmented dermatitis on sun exposed area, and diarrhea
Vitamin B$_{12}$	Reduced intestinal absorption; pernicious anemia, pancreatic insufficiency, atrophic gastric, small intestinal bacterial overgrowth and ileal disease	Megaloblastic anemia Demyelination of nerves—ataxia, depression and psychosis
Vitamin B$_6$ and folate	Medication associated Vitamin B$_6$: isoniazid, cycloserine, penicillamine, theophylline Folate: sulfasalazine, phenytoin, methotrexate	Vitamin B$_6$—stomatitis, angular cheilosis, glossitis, irritability, confusion, anemia Folate—megaloblastic anemia
Zinc	Excessive gastrointestinal losses Severe diarrhea, high output fistulas and ostomies	Poor wound healing, dermatitis around orifices and extremities, glottis, alopecia, and corneal clouding
Iron	Chronic blood loss and proximal gastrointestinal diseases	Microcytic anemia, glossitis, koilonychias
Ceruloplasmin	Advanced liver disease Nephrotic syndrome Wilson's disease Copper deficiency from malnutrition	Altered copper metabolism
Essential fatty acids	Severe malabsorption, enterocutaneous fistulas, cystic fibrosis, long-term TPN with no fat emulsion, carnitine deficiency, extreme fat free oral or EN diet	Hyperlipidemia, abnormal liver function tests, thrombocytopenia, bleeding, scaly rash, hair depigmentation, poor wound healing
Chromium	Long term TPN with no replacement	Hyperglycemia and impaired glucose tolerance

fiber and protein and low in carbohydrates, especially simple sugars.[53] Liquid intake should only occur 30 minutes after solid food intake.

Delayed gastric emptying occurs in 14% to 40% of patients after pancreaticoduo-denectomy and is associated with poor intake that leads to lengthy hospitalizations and readmissions.[54] There are limited data on how to best treat this condition in these patients, but an initial trial with prokinetics and small, frequent meals with oral nutritional supplements should be attempted. Jejunal feeding tubes are reserved for those who fail conservative measures.

Achalasia

Achalasia is a motility disorder characterized by solid and liquid dysphagia, regurgitation, and variable amounts of weight loss with an average loss of 20 $\pm$ 16 pounds.[55] The precise mechanism of weight loss in achalasia is unclear but does seem to be influenced by its phenotype with those with type II achalasia experiencing the most weight loss.[56] For those patients who are not immediate candidates for more definitive therapies such as endoscopic peroral endoscopic myotomies, pneumatic dilations or Heller myotomy, endoscopic botulinum toxin to the lower esophageal sphincter, and a diet that consists of eating small, frequent, low fiber meals with a higher liquid content has been suggested.[57]

Nutrition in Critically Ill and Surgical Patients

Early oral intake after surgery has been shown to reduce lengths of stays, infection rates, mortality, anastomotic dehiscence, and resumption of bowel function.[58–60] Whereas studies show early EN (<48 hours) in postsurgical patients decrease overall complications, early PN increases them and thus should generally be avoided except in severely malnourished patients.[61–63]

Well-nourished people can tolerate periods of fasting up to 14 days, whereas those who are significantly malnourished have more complications when critically ill or after surgery.[24,61,62,64,65] A couple of general principles can be made based on these facts. First, TPN is generally only initiated for well-nourished postsurgical and critically ill patients when they cannot meet caloric needs from either oral intake or EN after 10 to 14 days. Earlier initiation of TPN can be considered in more severely malnourished people who are not tolerating EN. Second, elective surgery should generally be withheld for 7 to 14 days to provide specialized nutritional support in severely malnourished patients. EN is favored over TPN unless caloric needs cannot be met in that fashion.

MACRONUTRIENT, MICRONUTRIENT, AND VITAMIN DEFICIENCIES

Clinicians should be familiar with the many clinical manifestations and associated clinical scenarios of macronutrient, micronutrient and vitamin deficiencies. Some deficiencies are more common, more pronounced or clinically relevant in hospitalized patients. These are described in **Table 4**.

SUMMARY

Issues of malnutrition and nutrition are common and essential to the quality care and outcomes of hospitalized patients. Educational programs should develop training programs for practical application of nutritional management in health and disease. Although malnutrition is more difficult to define, a more practical concept—nutritional risk—can be especially useful to identify patients who would benefit from nutritional support. Hospitals should develop specialized, multidisciplinary teams and protocols for specialized nutritional support. Understanding when specialized nutritional support can help or harm a patient is also critical. Finally, physicians should familiarize themselves with the disease-specific nutritional issues that hospitalized patients face, including relevant macronutrient, micronutrient, and vitamin deficiencies, for optimal management.

ACKNOWLEDGMENTS

Murewa Oguntimein, PhD, MHS, CHES, for editorial support.

CLINICS CARE POINTS

- Nutritional risk scores can be used to identify patients with high risk scores to direct nutritional support to improve outcomes and to avoid unnecessary nutritional support in those with low scores.
- The initiation of inpatient TPN should include protocols that verify insurance coverage and make sure there is a committed outpatient provider to direct the care of TPN before central venous access is obtained.
- TPN is generally only initiated for well-nourished postsurgical and critically ill patients when they cannot meet caloric needs from either oral intake or EN after 10 to 14 days. Earlier initiation of TPN can be considered in more severely malnourished people who are not tolerating EN or oral intake.
- It is imperative that the physician taking care of a hospitalized patient's nutritional needs knows the disease specific considerations related to nutrition and also knows the clinical manifestations and clinical scenarios for common macronutrient, micronutrient and vitamin deficiencies.

DISCLOSURE

No individual disclosures.

REFERENCES

1. Micic D, McDonald EK, Stein AC, et al. How to obtain training in nutrition during the gastroenterology fellowship. Gastroenterology 2018;154(3):467–70.
2. Daley BJ, Cherry-bukowiec J, Van Way CW, et al. Current status of nutrition training in graduate medical education from a survey of residency program directors. JPEN J Parenter Enteral Nutr 2016;40(1):95–9.
3. McClave SA, DiBaise JK, Mullin GE, et al. ACG clinical guideline: nutrition therapy in the adult hospitalized patient. Am J Gastroenterol 2016;111(3):315–34.
4. White JV, Guenter P, Jensen G, et al. Consensus statement: Academy of Nutrition and Dietetics and American Society for Parenteral and Enteral Nutrition: characteristics recommended for the identification and documentation of adult malnutrition (undernutrition). JPEN J Parenter Enteral Nutr 2012;36(3):275–83.
5. Jensen GL, Compher C, Sullivan DH, et al. Recognizing malnutrition in adults: definitions and characteristics, screening, assessment, and team approach. JPEN J Parenter Enteral Nutr 2013;37(6):802–7.
6. Heyland DK, Dhaliwal R, Jiang X, et al. Identifying critically ill patients who benefit the most from nutrition therapy: the development and initial validation of a novel risk assessment tool. Crit Care 2011;15(6):R268.
7. Kondrup J, Johansen N, Plum L, et al. Incidence of nutritional risk and causes of inadequate nutritional care in hospitals. Clin Nutr 2002;21(6):461–8.

8. Jie B, Jiang Z-M, Nolan MT, et al. Impact of preoperative nutritional support on clinical outcome in abdominal surgical patients at nutritional risk. Nutrition 2012;28(10):1022–7.
9. Starke J, Schneider H, Alteheld B, et al. Short-term individual nutritional care as part of routine clinical setting improves outcome and quality of life in malnourished medical patients. Clin Nutr 2011;30(2):194–201.
10. Elia M, Normand C, Laviano A, et al. A systematic review of the cost and cost effectiveness of using standard oral nutritional supplements in community and care home settings. Clin Nutr 2016;35(1):125–37.
11. Mullin GE, Fan L, Sulo S, et al. The association between oral nutritional supplements and 30-day hospital readmissions of malnourished patients at a US academic medical center. J Acad Nutr Diet 2019;119(7):1168–75.
12. Scheinkestel C, Kar L, Marshall K, et al. Prospective randomized trial to assess caloric and protein needs of critically Ill, anuric, ventilated patients requiring continuous renal replacement therapy. Nutrition 2003;19(11–12):909–16.
13. Parrish CR, McCray S. Part I enteral feeding barriers: pesky bowel sounds & gastric residual volumes. Nutrition issues in gastroenterology, Series 2019;183:35–50.
14. Bridges M, Parrish CR. Part III jejunal feeding: the tail is wagging the Dog(ma) dispelling myths with physiology, evidence, and clinical experience. Pract Gastroenterol 2019;185:32–54.
15. Parrish CR, McCray S. Part II enteral feeding: eradicate barriers with root cause analysis and focused intervention. Pract Gastroenterol 2019;184:15.
16. Allen P. Medicare coverage for home parenteral nutrition–an oxymoron? Part I. Pract Gastroenterol 2016;158:34–50.
17. Jeong S-H, Lee H-J, Bae H-J, et al. Factors affecting postoperative dietary adaptation in short bowel syndrome. Hepatogastroenterology 2009;56(93):1049–52.
18. Carbonnel F, Cosnes J, Chevret S, et al. The role of anatomic factors in nutritional autonomy after extensive small bowel resection. JPEN J Parenter Enteral Nutr 1996;20(4):275–80.
19. Carroll RE, Benedetti E, Schowalter JP, et al. Management and complications of short bowel syndrome: an updated review. Curr Gastroenterol Rep 2016;18(7):40.
20. Parrish CR, DiBaise J. Short bowel syndrome in adults–part 2. Nutrition therapy for short bowel syndrome in the adult patient. Pract Gastroenterol 2014;134:40–51.
21. Booth C. The metabolic effects of intestinal resection in man. Postgrad Med J 1961;37(434):725.
22. Forbes A, Escher J, Hébuterne X, et al. ESPEN guideline: clinical nutrition in inflammatory bowel disease. Clin Nutr 2017;36(2):321–47.
23. Triantafillidis JK, Papalois AE. The role of total parenteral nutrition in inflammatory bowel disease: current aspects. Scand J Gastroenterol 2013;49(1):3–14.
24. Weimann A, Braga M, Carli F, et al. ESPEN guideline: clinical nutrition in surgery. Clin Nutr 2017;36(3):623–50.
25. Shah ND. Low residue vs. low fiber diets in inflammatory bowel disease: evidence to support vs. habit? Pract Gastroenterol 2015;39(7):48–57.
26. Levenstein S, Prantera C, Luzi C, et al. Low residue or normal diet in Crohn's disease: a prospective controlled study in Italian patients. Gut 1985;26(10):989–93.
27. Arvanitakis M, Ockenga J, Bezmarevic M, et al. ESPEN guideline on clinical nutrition in acute and chronic pancreatitis. Clin Nutr 2020;39(3):612–31.

28. Yi F, Ge L, Zhao J, et al. Meta-analysis: total parenteral nutrition versus total enteral nutrition in predicted severe acute pancreatitis. Intern Med 2012;51(6): 523–30.
29. Al-Omran M, AlBalawi ZH, Tashkandi MF, et al. Enteral versus parenteral nutrition for acute pancreatitis. Cochrane Database Syst Rev 2010;(1):CD002837.
30. Petrov MS, Pylypchuk RD, Uchugina AF. A systematic review on the timing of artificial nutrition in acute pancreatitis. Br J Nutr 2008;101(6):787–93.
31. Chang Y-s, Fu H-q, Xiao Y-m, et al. Nasogastric or nasojejunal feeding in predicted severe acute pancreatitis: a meta-analysis. Crit Care 2013;17(3):R118.
32. Uppal D. Pragmatic management of nutrition in severe acute pancreatitis. Pract Gastroenterol 2018;179:21.
33. Wang X, Han X, Guo X, et al. The effect of periodontal treatment on hemoglobin A1c levels of diabetic patients: a systematic review and meta-analysis. PloS one 2014;9:e108412.
34. Parrish CR, McCray S. Gastroparesis and nutrition: the art. Pract Gastroenterol 2011;99(4):26–41.
35. Drossman DA, Tack J, Ford AC, et al. Neuromodulators for functional gastrointestinal disorders (disorders of gut– brain interaction): a Rome foundation working team report. Gastroenterology 2018;154(4):1140–71. e1141.
36. Chatterjee S. Nutritional implications of GI-related scleroderma. Pract Gastroenterol 2016;40(1):35–46.
37. Krause L, Becker MO, Brueckner CS, et al. Nutritional status as marker for disease activity and severity predicting mortality in patients with systemic sclerosis. Ann Rheum Dis 2010;69(11):1951–7.
38. Mehanna HM, Moledina J, Travis J. Refeeding syndrome: what it is, and how to prevent and treat it. BMJ 2008;336(7659):1495–8.
39. Mehler PS, Winkelman AB, Andersen DM, et al. Nutritional rehabilitation: practical guidelines for refeeding the anorectic patient. J Nutr Metab 2010;2010:625782.
40. Boateng AA, Sriram K, Meguid MM, et al. Refeeding syndrome: treatment considerations based on collective analysis of literature case reports. Nutrition 2010; 26(2):156–67.
41. Mendenhall CL, Anderson S, Weesner RE, et al. Protein-calorie malnutrition associated with alcoholic hepatitis: veterans administration cooperative study group on alcoholic hepatitis. Am J Med 1984;76(2):211–22.
42. Mendenhall C, Roselle GA, Gartside P, et al. 119 VACSG, 275. Relationship of protein calorie malnutrition to alcoholic liver disease: a reexamination of data from two Veterans administration cooperative studies. Alcohol Clin Exp Res 1995;19(3):635–41.
43. John WJ, Phillips R, Ott L, et al. Resting energy expenditure in patients with alcoholic hepatitis. JPEN J Parenter Enteral Nutr 1989;13(2):124–7.
44. Aday AW, Mitchell MC. Food for thought: importance of nutrition in alcoholic hepatitis. Pract Gastroenterol 2018;42(3):30–6.
45. Plauth M, Bernal W, Dasarathy S, et al. ESPEN guideline on clinical nutrition in liver disease. Clin Nutr 2019;38(2):485–521.
46. Moreno C, Deltenre P, Senterre C, et al. Intensive enteral nutrition is ineffective for patients with severe alcoholic hepatitis treated with corticosteroids. Gastroenterology 2016;150(4):903–10. e908.
47. Fialla AD, Israelsen M, Hamberg O, et al. Nutritional therapy in cirrhosis or alcoholic hepatitis: a systematic review and meta-analysis. Liver Int 2015;35(9): 2072–8.

48. Mitchell MC, Friedman LS, McClain CJ. Medical management of severe alcoholic hepatitis: expert review from the clinical practice updates committee of the AGA institute. Clin Gastroenterol Hepatol 2017;15(1):5–12.
49. Puri P, Thursz M. Intensive enteral nutrition in alcoholic hepatitis: more food for thought. Gastroenterology 2016;150(4):803.
50. Xu Z-W, Li Y-S. Pathogenesis and treatment of parenteral nutrition-associated liver disease. Hepatobiliary Pancreat Dis Int 2012;11(6):586–93.
51. Eagon JC, Kelly KA, Miedema BW. Postgastrectomy syndromes. Surg Clin North Am 1992;72(2):445–65.
52. Mallory GN, Macgregor AM, Rand CS. The influence of dumping on weight loss after gastric restrictive surgery for morbid obesity. Obes Surg 1996;6(6):474–8.
53. Ukleja A. Dumping syndrome. Pract Gastroenterol 2006;30(2):32.
54. Kamarajah SK, Bundred JR, Marc OS, et al. A systematic review and network meta-analysis of different surgical approaches for pancreaticoduodenectomy. HPB (Oxford) 2020;22(3):329–39.
55. Fisichella PM, Raz D, Palazzo F, et al. Clinical, radiological, and manometric profile in 145 patients with untreated achalasia. World J Surg 2008;32(9):1974–9.
56. Patel D, Naik R, Slaughter J, et al. Weight loss in achalasia is determined by its phenotype. Dis Esophagus 2018;31(9):doy046.
57. Patel DA, Vaezi MF. Achalasia and nutrition: is it simple physics or biology. Pract Gastroenterol 2016;40(11):42–8.
58. Andersen HK, Lewis SJ, Thomas S. Early enteral nutrition within 24h of colorectal surgery versus later commencement of feeding for postoperative complications. Cochrane Database Syst Rev 2006;(4):CD004080.
59. Lewis SJ, Andersen HK, Thomas S. Early enteral nutrition within 24 h of intestinal surgery versus later commencement of feeding: a systematic review and meta-analysis. J Gastrointest Surg 2009;13(3):569.
60. Osland E, Yunus RM, Khan S, et al. Early versus traditional postoperative feeding in patients undergoing resectional gastrointestinal surgery: a meta-analysis. JPEN J Parenter Enteral Nutr 2011;35(4):473–87.
61. Koretz RL, Avenell A, Lipman TO, et al. Does enteral nutrition affect clinical outcome? A systematic review of the randomized trials: CME. Am J Gastroenterol 2007;102(2):412–29.
62. Casaer MP, Mesotten D, Hermans G, et al. Early versus late parenteral nutrition in critically ill adults. N Engl J Med 2011;365(6):506–17.
63. Doig GS, Simpson F, Sweetman EA, et al. Early parenteral nutrition in critically ill patients with short-term relative contraindications to early enteral nutrition: a randomized controlled trial. JAMA 2013;309(20):2130–8.
64. Rosenthal MD, Vanzant EL, Martindale RG, et al. Evolving paradigms in the nutritional support of critically ill surgical patients. Curr Probl Surg 2015;52(4):147.
65. Singer P, Blaser AR, Berger MM, et al. ESPEN guideline on clinical nutrition in the intensive care unit. Clin Nutr 2019;38(1):48–79.

All Things Gluten: A Review

Naueen A. Chaudhry, MD[a], Chelsea Jacobs, DO[b],
Peter H.R. Green, DO[c], S. Devi Rampertab, MD[a],*

KEYWORDS

- Gluten • Gluten-free diet • Celiac disease • Gluten sensitivity
- Irritable bowel syndrome • Nutrition

KEY POINTS

- Gluten protein present in wheat-based products, produces incomplete products of digestion which can mount intestinal and extra-intestinal host responses.
- Immune-mediated responses include celiac disease and gluten ataxia, but there can be allergic responses such as "Bakers' asthma", non-celiac gluten sensitivity and wheat sensitive IBS.
- A gluten free diet is the only definitive treatment for immune-mediated responses to gluten. It has become more accessible, although more expensive, over the past two decades.
- Recognition of celiac disease is important to prevent chronic complications of malabsorption and malnutrition, as well as future risk of small bowel lymphoma or adenocarcinoma.
- Measurement of urinary gluten immunogenic peptides (GIP's) can be helpful to determine gluten exposure and compliance with gluten free diet.

INTRODUCTION

Gluten has become a household name over the past 2 decades, given the rising global popularity of the gluten-free diet (GFD). Patients often are curious about the impact of a GFD on their gastrointestinal symptoms; hence, it is a common topic of discussion during clinic visits. The benefits of a wheat-free diet in patients with celiac sprue initially were described by the Dutch pediatrician Dr. Willem-Karel Dicke in 1941.[1] The timing was impacted by food shortages, including wheat, during World War II, which resulted in malnutrition in most children. Dicke observed, however, an improvement in diarrhea, skin rashes, and a return to normal growth curve in children with celiac sprue. This was the first steppingstone toward understanding of the pathology of

[a] Division of Gastroenterology and Hepatology, Department of Medicine, University of Florida, 1329 Southwest 16th Street, Suite 5251, Gainesville, FL 32608, USA; [b] Department of Medicine, University of Florida, 1329 Southwest 16th Street, Suite 5251, Gainesville, FL 32608, USA; [c] Celiac Disease Center at Columbia University, 180 Fort Washington Avenue, New York, NY 10032, USA
* Corresponding author.
E-mail address: Devi.Rampertab@medicine.ufl.edu

Gastroenterol Clin N Am 50 (2021) 29–40
https://doi.org/10.1016/j.gtc.2020.10.007
0889-8553/21/© 2020 Elsevier Inc. All rights reserved.

celiac disease (CeD), and the GFD remains the mainstay of treatment to this day. This review discusses gluten and its role in immunogenicity and its impact on gastrointestinal diseases as well as everyday practical aspects of the GFD.

WHAT IS GLUTEN?

Gluten, a protein found naturally within wheat seeds, has amassed significant hype in modern dietary trends. Once water-soluble components and starch are washed off from wheat, what remains is gluten protein. It is a vital component in the baking process, contributing texture and elasticity, and is composed of several complex protein structures using disulfide bonds, gliadins, and glutenins.[2] Given the intricacy of this protein structure, gluten is incompletely broken down by digestive enzymes, resulting in fragmented gluten. These incomplete components have the capacity to evoke a significant host response. The glutamine and proline-rich component gliadin has been identified as the commonly responsible immunomodulating component leading to amplified gut permeability.[3,4] The binding of gliadin to the chemokine receptor CXCR3 triggers zonulin release and subsequent disassembly of the intercellular tight junctions. At this point, gliadin is able to enter the lamina propria, and in certain individuals the recognition of this foreign antigen leads to varying degrees of immune response.[3] This mechanism is not understood fully, given the variance in gluten fragmentation during digestion. It has been proposed that ω-5 gliadin is the offending agent in IgE-mediated wheat allergy, or bakers' asthma.[5] Other gluten components can lead to a more robust immune response after dietary exposure, resulting in antibodies against tissue transglutaminase (tTGs), endomysium (antiendomysial antibodies), or directly to gliadin (antigliadin antibodies), leading to what is known as CeD.

WHAT IS THE GLUTEN-FREE DIET?

The GFD is the only effective treatment of CeD and can induce complete remission.[6–8] The content of gluten in foods is described in parts per million (ppm), corresponding to milligrams per kilogram. In 2013, the Food and Drug Administration (FDA) released a gluten-free labeling rule (**Box 1**), intending to help consumers identify gluten-free foods easily. To earn this voluntary label, the food must contain inherently 20 ppm or less of gluten, or, if gluten exposure is unavoidable, it must be below 20 ppm gluten.[9] Within this ruling, foods that contain whole or refined gluten-containing grains (barley, rye, triticale, wheat, kamut, or spelt) may not use the claim. The limit of 20 ppm may not be all that significant, because it is the level of gluten that can be detected reliably and consistently by analytical methods, thus ensuring the ability of the FDA to regulate its 2013 rule.[9]

As brought to attention in the FDA recommendations, the avoidance of foods that naturally contain gluten and the significant amount of cross-contamination in the

---

Box 1
Food and Drug Administration 2013 requirement for gluten-free labeling on foods

- It inherently does not contain gluten (eg, water or fresh carrots).
- It does not contain a whole gluten-containing grain (eg, barley or spelt).
- It does not contain a refined gluten-containing grain (eg, wheat flower).
- It may inc.lude gluten-containing grains if processed appropriately to remove gluten with the final product not exceeding 20 ppm of gluten

manufacturing of processed foods[10] are both concerns. In some cases, individuals with CeD may be more sensitive to gluten, causing them to have persistent symptoms despite adhering to gluten-free labeled foods. These patients are labeled as nonresponsive CeD, as opposed to refractory CeD, where patients are truly refractory to dietary treatment. In cases of nonresponsive CeD, where a GFD has been followed for 12 months and the patient remains symptomatic, it may be necessary to eliminate the offending agent more aggressively. A gluten contamination elimination diet is a stricter diet that eliminates gluten contamination fully by advocating for naturally gluten-free foods and eliminating processed food.[11–13]

CELIAC DISEASE

CeD is an autoimmune disorder characterized by a systemic response to dietary gluten in genetically predisposed individuals,[8,14,15] which has clinical manifestations of small bowel enteropathy associated with gastrointestinal as well as nongastrointestinal symptoms.[16] In a majority of patients, it is associated with the expression of HLA haplotypes DQ2 and DQ8[14,16] (**Fig. 1**). The presence of these alleles, however, does not represent CeD in the absence of an immune response,[5] which can be triggered by the binding of deamidated gliadin peptides (DAPs) to antigen-presenting cells.

Incidence and Prevalence

King and colleagues[17] recently demonstrated an increasing reported incidence of CeD in the Western Hemisphere. Population-based studies from Asia, Africa, and Latin America, however, were lacking to provide a global overview. This increase in reported

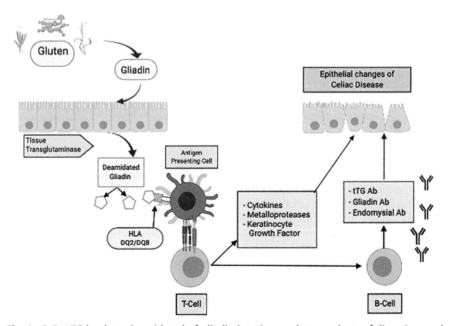

Fig. 1. CeD: tTG leads to deamidated of gliadin into incomplete products of digestion, such as DAPs. In genetically predisposed individuals with HLA DQ2 or DQ8, these then are presented to gliadin-reactive T cells and subsequently lead to a cell-mediated and antibody-mediated immune response, resulting in small bowel epithelial cell injury. Ab, antibody. (created by Biorender.)

incidence also can be attributed to availability and acceptability of reliable noninvasive diagnostic testing (eg, antiendomysial antibody), which have emerged as more efficient and economic tools in the diagnosis of CeD.[18,19]

According to Kim and colleagues,[20] the prevalence of CeD in North America has remained stable over time. The global seroprevalence of CeD is 1.4%, and biopsy-based prevalence is 0.7%, based on a metanalysis by Singh and colleagues.[21] They further discuss that the pooled global prevalence of CeD is on the rise, based on rates reported in studies from 1991 to 2000 (0.6%) compared with 2011 to 2016 (0.8%). The highest seroprevalence is reported in Asia (1.8%) and the lowest in Africa (1.1%), which can be related to dietary patterns of gluten intake in the regions. Biopsy-confirmed studies have reported higher prevalence (1.5 times) in women compared with men and prevalence twice as high in children compared with adults. This metanalysis again highlights the lack of population-based prevalence data on CeD from several countries, which is needed for a more comprehensive overview.[21]

Disease Presentation and Complications

Because a majority of patients present with nonspecific GI complaints, CeD should be suspected in patients presenting with erratic bowel habits representative of irritable bowel syndrome (IBS), bloating, and postprandial abdominal pain.[15] The American College of Gastroenterology provides comprehensive guidelines on clinical scenarios that warrant testing for CeD.[22] They recommend patients with diarrhea, weight loss, and malabsorption, especially those with history of diabetes or with a first-degree relative with CeD (even if asymptomatic), should undergo testing. Children can present with growth retardation, delayed bone mineral density, and enamel defects[4] in the setting of malabsorption, which can be irreversible if not identified early and managed.[4] CeD should be excluded in patients with other autoimmune conditions apart from diabetes, such as Sjögren syndrome, Hashimoto thyroiditis and selective IgA deficiency, and genetic syndromes, for example, Down, Turner, and Williams syndromes.[14,15]

A GFD is the only effective treatment of CeD[22] and works by decreasing small bowel inflammation, hence reducing the risk of long-term complications.[16] Mucosal healing can take up to 2 years and sometimes longer than 5 years, especially in patients with Marsh III lesions on histology.[23] Furthermore, healing often is delayed and incomplete in adults compared with the pediatric population.[24,25] Although complications of malnutrition, such as anemia,[4,26,27] muscle wasting, bone loss, and delayed wound healing, remain the main concern in CeD patients noncompliant with a GFD, they also are at high risk for refractory CeD and malignancy.[16] It is suggested that women with CeD have a higher miscarriage risk.[28,29] Lymphoma, small bowel adenocarcinoma, and oropharyngeal malignancy have been associated with CeD.[30,31] This poses a long-term health concern for CeD patients who are noncompliant with GFD due to unrecognized disease, personal choice, or financial contraints.[32]

GLUTEN-FREE DIET AS TREATMENT IN PATIENTS WITHOUT CELIAC DISEASE
Autoimmune Diseases

Apart from CeD, another autoimmune disease associated with gluten exposure is gluten ataxia.[33,34] The pathogenesis is the development of antibodies against the Purkinje cells, and it is responsive to GFD treatment.[35] Dermatitis herpetiformis is an erythematous, intensely pruritic papular symmetric rash on the face, the extensor surfaces of the elbows and knees, and the buttocks, which is caused by IgA deposition in skin.[36] It often is considered pathognomonic for CeD, and a GFD is recommended treatment.[5]

Allergic Conditions and Hypersensitivity

The prevalence of nonceliac gluten sensitivity (NCGS) is difficult to determine due to a lack of validated biomarkers[4] and has been estimated to be both higher and lower than CeD, based on different studies.[37] NCGS originally was described by the Salerno Experts' Criteria[38] as intestinal and extraintestinal manifestations related to the ingestion of gluten-containing foods in subjects who are not affected by either CeD or wheat allergy. In an update of their recommendations in 2017,[39] however, they recognize another group of patients who present with IBS-like symptoms associated with a wheat allergy and, hence, who also benefit from GFD. This group is less likely to self-report gluten sensitivity than NCGS. Because wheat also contains fructans, patients with wheat-sensitive IBS also report improvement of symptoms with a low FOD-MAP (fermentable oligosaccharides, disaccharides, and monosaccharides, and polyols) diet, whereas those with NCGS do not.[34] The ease of implementation of GFD compared with the low FODMAPs diet is unclear due to a lack of comparative studies.[40] Although wheat avoidance is part of the 6-food elimination diet commonly used for eosinophilic esophagitis, there is no clear role of gluten in the pathogenesis.[34]

Other

There is no strong evidence to recommend GFD in other endocrinological, rheumatological, or psychiatric conditions or for enhancement in athletic performance.[41]

THE CURRENT SOCIAL IMPLICATIONS OF A GLUTEN-FREE DIET

The GFD has emerged as one of the most popular diets in human history.[41] Its use has increased steadily in those without CeD over the past of decades due to multiple reasons, for example, its public perception as a healthier diet, increasing ease of availability of gluten-free products, and even as a preventive measure against the development of CeD.[20] Patients with NCGS, wheat-sensitive IBS, and wheat allergy benefit from the improvement of their symptoms with a GFD as well. The major reason for the increasing popularity of this diet, however, has been through popular media, including celebrity endorsements, including athletes; magazines; social media; and television.[42] This diet has not shown any improvement in gastrointestinal health or performance in people without gluten allergy or sensitivity.[41] A survey of dietary habits, however, reported 23% of people globally practicing gluten avoidance, with a noticeable geographic variation, the most common in Latin America (31%) and least common in Europe (15%).[42] In the United States, market research by the Mintel Group reports a 136% increase from 2013 to 2015 in the gluten-free market, with most products purchased by consumers without CeD. Although an increasing percentage of Americans believe that the GFD is a fad (47% in 2015), approximately 21% of them seek gluten-free products while grocery shopping.[6]

Commercially available gluten-free products can be 240% more expensive than wheat-based food items and are even more costly at health food stores (123%) and online compared with regular grocery stores and upscale markets.[32] There was no noticeable geographic cost variation in this pattern, although the included UK and Northeastern US cities offered greater availability of gluten-free products. This study noted a variation in cost depending on the type of food items compared, with gluten-free pasta noticeably the most expensive at twice the price of regular pasta.[32] This is an interesting finding because another review reveals that gluten-free plain pasta fares on average 0.5 stars less than regular pasta on the Health Star Rating for nutritional content. In contrast, breads and breakfast cereals did not show a significant difference.[43] Lee and colleagues[32] further suggest the use of naturally available gluten-free foods rather than commercially available products to ease the economic cost burden of the GFD on patients.

NUTRITIONAL OVERVIEW OF THE GLUTEN-FREE DIET

A GFD offers no additional nutritional benefits in the absence of documented gluten allergy or intolerance.[41] A study by Kim and colleagues,[44] using data from National Health and Nutrition Examination Survey from 2009 to 2014, concluded that although being on a GFD may be beneficial in weight management, there was no significant difference in terms of the prevalence of metabolic syndrome and cardiovascular disease risk score in gluten-free followers without CeD. Additionally, many gluten-free foods not only are deficient in several nutrients[41] but also, due to their composition, are higher in lipids,[45] salt, and sugar content[46–48] **(Table 1)**. It is recommended that gluten-free flours, such as amaranth, quinoa, and buckwheat, should be present in gluten-free product formulation due to their high nutritional value; however, this suggestion has not been widely adapted by the industry.[49]

Macronutrients

The GFD often is low in dietary fiber due to the composition of most gluten-free products and also self-avoidance of grains and fiber in diet.[41,50] Given the role of dietary fiber in the prevention of colorectal cancer, cardiovascular disease, and diabetes,[50] this can be a concerning risk factor for nonceliac patients on a GFD. Similarly, the increased lipid content of most gluten-free foods, especially breads and flour,[49] can further add to cardiovascular disease risk. With regard to carbohydrates, CeD patients are at a higher obesity risk due to the high glycemic index[51] and glycemic load of a GFD. The most common source of proteins in GFD is animal food and pseudocereals,[50] which are good-quality options.

Table 1		
Nutritional concerns for celiac disease and gluten-free diet		
	Celiac	**Gluten-Free Diet**
Underlying etiology	Malabsorption due to enteropathy	Dietary modification of nutritional intake
Macronutrients abnormalities	• ↓ Lipid loss due to steatorrhea	• ↓ Dietary fiber • ↑ Lipids • ↑ Glycemic load
Vitamin and mineral deficiencies	• Iron • Calcium • Magnesium • Zinc • Folic acid, riboflavin, niacin, thiamine, vitamin B_{12} • Vitamin D • Fat-soluble vitamins (A, D, E, and K)	• Iron • Calcium • Magnesium • Zinc • Folate • Thiamine • Riboflavin • Niacin

↑ Increased
↓ Decreased

Micronutrients

Fruit and vegetable servings need to be increased to at least 5 servings per day[46] in CeD patients to prevent micronutrient deficiencies (see **Table 1**), in addition to recommendations for fish and meat intake.[52] Untreated CeD patients can have vitamin deficiencies, but these can persist subsequently because some studies have shown GFD to be deficient in folate, niacin, riboflavin, and thiamine.[50,53,54] The ones of particular importance are folate, vitamin B_{12}, and vitamin D. Dietary supplementation, with intermittent follow-up of levels, is recommended while on treatment with GFD.[55]

Minerals

Several studies have demonstrated the GFD to be deficient in minerals, especially iron, calcium, magnesium, and zinc.[46,52,55,56] Initial deficiency in CeD can be due to enteropathy (often manifesting as iron deficiency anemia and decreased bone marrow density) and self-corrects after 1 year of GFD. These deficiencies can persist, however, with poor dietary intake. Animal and vegetable foods, including pseudocereals, such as amaranth and quinoa, are good sources of trace elements and minerals.[46]

MEASURING COMPLIANCE WITH A GLUTEN-FREE DIET

Adherence to a GFD, especially in patients with an autoimmune condition, such as CeD, is a lifelong choice and can present its own challenges,[57] because it requires significant adjustments in lifestyle and food choices. White and colleagues[58] have shown that food-related situations at work, food purchases, traveling, and meals with other people were major areas in which patients experienced difficulty, and this could negatively affect their adherence to a GFD. Compliance with a GFD hence can be emotionally exhausting and sometimes a psychological burden, on occasion leading to self-avoidance of social events and travel.[59,60] The compliance rates for GFD in CeD have been reported as widely as 17% to 80%,[61] but, on average, at least one-third of CeD patients do not fully adhere to a GFD.[62] Additionally, approximately 36% to 55% of CeD patients who report adherence to a GFD do not achieve histologic remission, likely due to lapses in gluten intake.[62] Although serologic biomarkers, such as antigliadin antibodies, antiendomysial antibodies, tTGs, and DAPs, are useful in the diagnostic process of CeD, they do not have reliable correlation with histologic findings or patient symptoms[61,63–65] on a GFD. Gluten immunogenic peptides (GIPs), which can trigger the immune response leading to CeD, are resistant to gastrointestinal digestion and can be detected in feces as well as urine.[61] Urinary GIPs can be detected via enzyme-linked immunosorbent assay, but a lateral flow test using a urinary dipstick allows for more convenient testing.[66] Moreno and colleagues[62] successfully demonstrated that point-of-care testing using lateral flow test for urinary GIPs was able to reliably detect greater than 25 mg (ppm) gluten in dietary content. Moreover, they were able to establish a correlation of histologic remission with negative urinary GIPs. CeD patients with detectable GIPs in urine were noted to have more significant intestinal epithelial injury on histology (Marsh II/III on classification). This also allows identifying true cases of refractory CeD[67] versus involuntary dietary gluten exposure leading to persistent symptoms. Handheld devices using the same principle now are available for home use[68,69] for CeD patients to monitor their gluten intake. Lerner and colleagues[70] used crowd-sourced data from one of these devices, Nima®,[68] to study unintentional gluten intake in restaurants by those on a GFD. Their results showed that approximately one-third of restaurant foods labeled as gluten-free tested positive for gluten. Pizza and pasta were the most likely to contain gluten, with more than 50% of samples testing positive. Rates of gluten detection were highest during dinner hours and lowest during breakfast hours. The lowest rates of gluten detection regionally within the United States was in the West and in casual and fast-food restaurants based on the type of restaurant.

SUMMARY

Gluten is a common dietary component that can induce an autoimmune response resulting in intestinal and extraintestinal manifestations due to incomplete products of digestion in genetically predisposed individuals, for example, CeD and gluten ataxia. In other circumstances, it still can cause symptoms in patients with NCGS and wheat-sensitive IBS, and dietary elimination remains an effective management strategy in these circumstances. Given the recent surge in popularity of the GFD, and subsequent easier availability of gluten-free products, it now is followed by many as a trend rather than medical necessity. For individuals who do not suffer from gluten-associated autoimmune diseases, NCGS, or wheat-sensitive IBS, the GFD does not offer additional benefit but can carry the macronutrient and micronutrient imbalance. In addition, market trends confirm that commercially available gluten-free products are more expensive, hence a higher financial burden, than naturally occurring gluten-free foods or gluten-containing products. The recent commercial availability of point-of-care testing has enabled patients to self-monitor their gluten exposure while on a GFD because contamination and poor quality control of gluten-free products can be a confounder. Physicians also can monitor patients and determine if the problem at hand is noncompliance with the GFD or refractory CeD.

CLINICAL CARE POINTS

- A GFD is the only effective treatment of CeD, which can induce histologic remission and subsequently lead to resolution of malabsorption as well as prevention of future complications.
- A GFD is useful in resolving gastrointestinal symptoms in patients with NCGS and wheat-sensitive IBS.
- In patients without autoimmune diseases associated with gluten, NSGS, or wheat-sensitive IBS, a GFD does not offer additional benefit.
- Animal and vegetable sourced foods, including pseudocereals, should be incorporated in a GFD to reduce the risk of potential macronutrient and micronutrient imbalances.
- Point-of-care testing is emerging as a useful tool for both physicians and patients for monitoring of dietary gluten content as well as compliance with GFD.

DISCLOSURE

None of the authors has any financial disclosures for the purpose of this publication.

REFERENCES

1. van Berge-Henegouwen GP, Mulder CJJ. Pioneer in the gluten free diet: Willem-Karel Dicke 1905-1962, over 50 years of gluten free diet. Gut 1993. https://doi.org/10.1136/gut.34.11.1473.
2. Wieser H. Chemistry of gluten proteins. Food Microbiol 2007. https://doi.org/10.1016/j.fm.2006.07.004.

3. Lammers KM, Khandelwal S, Chaudhry F, et al. Identification of a novel immuno-modulatory gliadin peptide that causes interleukin-8 release in a chemokine receptor CXCR3-dependent manner only in patients with coeliac disease. Immunology 2011;132(3):432–40.

4. Leonard MM, Sapone A, Catassi C, et al. Celiac disease and nonceliac gluten sensitivity: A review. JAMA 2017;318(7):647–56.

5. Pietzak M. Celiac disease, wheat allergy, and gluten sensitivity: When gluten free is not a fad. J Parenter Enteral Nutr 2012;36. https://doi.org/10.1177/0148607111426276.

6. Reilly NR. The Gluten-Free Diet: Recognizing Fact, Fiction, and Fad. J Pediatr 2016. https://doi.org/10.1016/j.jpeds.2016.04.014.

7. di Sabatino A, Corazza GR. Coeliac disease. Lancet 2009. https://doi.org/10.1016/S0140-6736(09)60254-3.

8. Lebwohl B, Sanders DS, Green PHR. Coeliac disease. Lancet 2018. https://doi.org/10.1016/S0140-6736(17)31796-8.

9. Federal Register: Food Labeling; Gluten-Free Labeling of Foods. Available at: https://www.federalregister.gov/documents/2013/08/05/2013-18813/food-labeling-gluten-free-labeling-of-foods. Accessed March 9, 2020.

10. Gibert A, Espadaler M, Angel Canela M, et al. Consumption of gluten-free products: Should the threshold value for trace amounts of gluten be at 20, 100 or 200 p.p.m.? Eur J Gastroenterol Hepatol 2006. https://doi.org/10.1097/01.meg.0000236884.21343.e4.

11. Leonard M, Cureton P, Fasano A. Indications and Use of the Gluten Contamination Elimination Diet for Patients with Non-Responsive Celiac Disease. Nutrients 2017;9(10):1129.

12. Hollon JR, Cureton PA, Martin ML, et al. Trace gluten contamination may play a role in mucosal and clinical recovery in a subgroup of diet-adherent non-responsive celiac disease patients. BMC Gastroenterol 2013. https://doi.org/10.1186/1471-230X-13-40.

13. Zanini B, Marullo M, Villanacci V, et al. Persistent Intraepithelial Lymphocytosis in Celiac Patients Adhering to Gluten-Free Diet Is Not Abolished Despite a Gluten Contamination Elimination Diet. Nutrients 2016;8(9):525.

14. Fasano A, Catassi C. Celiac disease. N Engl J Med 2012;367(25). https://doi.org/10.1056/NEJMcp1113994.

15. Kelly CP, Bai JC, Liu E, et al. Advances in diagnosis and management of celiac disease. Gastroenterology 2015;148(6):1175–86.

16. Walker MM, Ludvigsson JF, Sanders DS. Coeliac disease: review of diagnosis and management. Med J Aust 2017;207(4):173–8.

17. King JA, Jeong J, Underwood FE, et al. Incidence of Celiac Disease Is Increasing Over Time. Am J Gastroenterol 2020;1. https://doi.org/10.14309/ajg.0000000000000523.

18. Chorzelski TP, Beutner EH, Sulej J, et al. IgA anti-endomysium antibody. A new immunological marker of dermatitis herpetiformis and coeliac disease. Br J Dermatol 1984;111(4). https://doi.org/10.1111/j.1365-2133.1984.tb06601.x.

19. Dieterich W, Ehnis T, Bauer M, et al. Identification of tissue transglutaminase as the autoantigen of celiac disease. Nat Med 1997;3(7). https://doi.org/10.1038/nm0797-797.

20. Kim HS, Patel KG, Orosz E, et al. Time trends in the prevalence of celiac disease and gluten-free diet in the US population: Results from the national health and nutrition examination surveys 2009-2014. JAMA Intern Med 2016;176(11):1716–7.

21. Singh P, Arora A, Strand TA, et al. Global Prevalence of Celiac Disease: Systematic Review and Meta-analysis. Clin Gastroenterol Hepatol 2018;16(6). https://doi.org/10.1016/j.cgh.2017.06.037.
22. Rubio-Tapia A, Hill ID, Kelly CP, et al. ACG clinical guidelines: Diagnosis and management of celiac disease. Am J Gastroenterol 2013;108(5):656–76.
23. Wahab PJ, Meijer JWR, Mulder CJJ. Histologic follow-up of people with celiac disease on a gluten-free diet: Slow and incomplete recovery. Am J Clin Pathol 2002;118(3). https://doi.org/10.1309/EVXT-851X-WHLC-RLX9.
24. Ciccocioppo R, Kruzliak P, Cangemi GC, et al. The spectrum of differences between childhood and adulthood celiac disease. Nutrients 2015. https://doi.org/10.3390/nu7105426.
25. Husby S, Koletzko S, Korponay-Szabó IR, et al. European society for pediatric gastroenterology, hepatology, and nutrition guidelines for the diagnosis of coeliac disease. J Pediatr Gastroenterol Nutr 2012. https://doi.org/10.1097/MPG.0b013e31821a23d0.
26. Harper JW, Holleran SF, Ramakrishnan R, et al. Anemia in celiac disease is multifactorial in etiology. Am J Hematol 2007. https://doi.org/10.1002/ajh.20996.
27. Abu Daya H, Lebwohl B, Lewis SK, et al. Celiac disease patients presenting with anemia have more severe disease than those presenting with diarrhea. Clin Gastroenterol Hepatol 2013. https://doi.org/10.1016/j.cgh.2013.05.030.
28. Anjum N, Baker PN, Robinson NJ, et al. Maternal celiac disease autoantibodies bind directly to syncytiotrophoblast and inhibit placental tissue transglutaminase activity. Reprod Biol Endocrinol 2009. https://doi.org/10.1186/1477-7827-7-16.
29. Tersigni C, Castellani R, de waure C, et al. Celiac disease and reproductive disorders: Meta-analysis of epidemiologic associations and potential pathogenic mechanisms. Hum Reprod Update 2014. https://doi.org/10.1093/humupd/dmu007.
30. Han Y, Chen W, Li P, et al. Association between coeliac disease and risk of any malignancy and gastrointestinal malignancy: A meta-analysis. Medicine 2015. https://doi.org/10.1097/MD.0000000000001612.
31. Freeman HJ. Adult celiac disease and its malignant complications. Gut Liver 2009;3(4). https://doi.org/10.5009/gnl.2009.3.4.237.
32. Lee AR, Ng DL, Zivin J, et al. Economic burden of a gluten-free diet. J Hum Nutr Diet 2007;20(5):423–30.
33. Hadjivassiliou M, Boscolo S, Davies-Jones GAB, et al. The humoral response in the pathogenesis of gluten ataxia. Neurology 2002. https://doi.org/10.1212/WNL.58.8.1221.
34. Newberry C. The Gluten-Free Diet: Use in Digestive Disease Management. Curr Treat Options Gastroenterol 2019;17(4):554–63.
35. Hadjivassiliou M, Davies-Jones GAB, Sanders DS, et al. Dietary treatment of gluten ataxia. J Neurol Neurosurg Psychiatry 2003. https://doi.org/10.1136/jnnp.74.9.1221.
36. Bolotin D, Petronic-Rosic V. Dermatitis herpetiformis: Part II. Diagnosis, management, and prognosis. J Am Acad Dermatol 2011. https://doi.org/10.1016/j.jaad.2010.09.776.
37. Digiacomo Dv, Tennyson CA, Green PH, et al. Prevalence of gluten-free diet adherence among individuals without celiac disease in the USA: Results from the continuous national health and nutrition examination survey 2009-2010. Scand J Gastroenterol 2013. https://doi.org/10.3109/00365521.2013.809598.
38. Catassi C, Elli L, Bonaz B, et al. Diagnosis of non-celiac gluten sensitivity (NCGS): The salerno experts' criteria. Nutrients 2015;7(6):4966–77.

39. Catassi C, Alaedini A, Bojarski C, et al. The overlapping area of non-celiac gluten sensitivity (NCGS) and wheat-sensitive irritable bowel syndrome (IBS): An update. Nutrients 2017;9(11). https://doi.org/10.3390/nu9111268.

40. Rej A, Sanders DS. Gluten-free diet and its 'cousins' in irritable bowel syndrome. Nutrients 2018;10(11). https://doi.org/10.3390/nu10111727.

41. Palmieri B, Vadalà M, Laurino C. Gluten-free diet in non-celiac patients: Beliefs, truths, advantages and disadvantages. Minerva Gastroenterol Dietol 2019; 65(2):153–62.

42. Newberry C, McKnight L, Sarav M, et al. Going Gluten Free: the History and Nutritional Implications of Today's Most Popular Diet. Curr Gastroenterol Rep 2017; 19(11):54.

43. Wu JHY, Neal B, Trevena H, et al. Are gluten-free foods healthier than non-gluten-free foods? An evaluation of supermarket products in Australia. Br J Nutr 2015. https://doi.org/10.1017/S0007114515002056.

44. Kim HS, Demyen MF, Mathew J, et al. Obesity, Metabolic Syndrome, and Cardiovascular Risk in Gluten-Free Followers Without Celiac Disease in the United States: Results from the National Health and Nutrition Examination Survey 2009–2014. Dig Dis Sci 2017. https://doi.org/10.1007/s10620-017-4583-1.

45. Miranda J, Lasa A, Bustamante MA, et al. Nutritional Differences Between a Gluten-free Diet and a Diet Containing Equivalent Products with Gluten. Plant Foods Hum Nutr 2014. https://doi.org/10.1007/s11130-014-0410-4.

46. Saturni L, Ferretti G, Bacchetti T. The gluten-free diet: Safety and nutritional quality. Nutrients 2010;2(1):16–34.

47. Pellegrini N, Agostoni C. Nutritional aspects of gluten-free products. J Sci Food Agric 2015. https://doi.org/10.1002/jsfa.7101.

48. Fry L, Madden AM, Fallaize R. An investigation into the nutritional composition and cost of gluten-free versus regular food products in the UK. J Hum Nutr Diet 2018;31(1):108–20.

49. Foschia M, Horstmann S, Arendt EK, et al. Nutritional therapy – Facing the gap between coeliac disease and gluten-free food. Int J Food Microbiol 2016;239: 113–24.

50. Vici G, Belli L, Biondi M, et al. Gluten free diet and nutrient deficiencies: A review. Clin Nutr 2016;35(6):1236–41.

51. Lamacchia C, Camarca A, Picascia S, et al. Cereal-based gluten-free food: How to reconcile nutritional and technological properties of wheat proteins with safety for celiac disease patients. Nutrients 2014. https://doi.org/10.3390/nu6020575.

52. Penagini F, Dilillo D, Meneghin F, et al. Gluten-free diet in children: An approach to a nutritionally adequate and balanced diet. Nutrients 2013. https://doi.org/10.3390/nu5114553.

53. Thompson T. Thiamin, riboflavin, and niacin contents of the gluten-free diet: Is there cause for concern? J Am Diet Assoc 1999. https://doi.org/10.1016/S0002-8223(99)00205-9.

54. Thompson T. Folate, iron, and dietary fiber contents of the gluten-free diet. J Am Diet Assoc 2000. https://doi.org/10.1016/S0002-8223(00)00386-2.

55. Caruso R, Pallone F, Stasi E, et al. Appropriate nutrient supplementation in celiac disease. Ann Med 2013. https://doi.org/10.3109/07853890.2013.849383.

56. Shepherd SJ, Gibson PR. Nutritional inadequacies of the gluten-free diet in both recently-diagnosed and long-term patients with coeliac disease. J Hum Nutr Diet 2013. https://doi.org/10.1111/jhn.12018.

57. Paganizza S, Zanotti R, D'Odorico A, et al. Is adherence to a gluten-free diet by adult patients with celiac disease influenced by their knowledge of the gluten content of foods? Gastroenterol Nurs 2019;42(1):55–64.
58. White LE, Bannerman E, Gillett PM. Coeliac disease and the gluten-free diet: a review of the burdens; factors associated with adherence and impact on health-related quality of life, with specific focus on adolescence. J Hum Nutr Diet 2016. https://doi.org/10.1111/jhn.12375.
59. Silvester JA, Weiten D, Graff LA, et al. Living gluten-free: Adherence, knowledge, lifestyle adaptations and feelings towards a gluten-free diet. J Hum Nutr Diet 2016. https://doi.org/10.1111/jhn.12316.
60. Leffler DA, Edwards-George J, Dennis M, et al. Factors that influence adherence to a gluten-free diet in adults with celiac disease. Dig Dis Sci 2008. https://doi.org/10.1007/s10620-007-0055-3.
61. Moreno M de L, Rodríguez-Herrera A, Sousa C, et al. Biomarkers to monitor gluten-free diet compliance in celiac patients. Nutrients 2017;9(1). https://doi.org/10.3390/nu9010046.
62. Moreno MDL, Cebolla Á, Munõz-Suano A, et al. Detection of gluten immunogenic peptides in the urine of patients with coeliac disease reveals transgressions in the gluten-free diet and incomplete mucosal healing. Gut 2017;66(2):250–7.
63. Sharkey LM, Corbett G, Currie E, et al. Optimising delivery of care in coeliac disease - Comparison of the benefits of repeat biopsy and serological follow-up. Aliment Pharmacol Ther 2013. https://doi.org/10.1111/apt.12510.
64. Tursi A, Brandimarte G, Giorgetti GM. Lack of Usefulness of Anti-Transglutaminase Antibodies in Assessing Histologic Recovery After Gluten-Free Diet in Celiac Disease. J Clin Gastroenterol 2003. https://doi.org/10.1097/00004836-200311000-00007.
65. Rubio-Tapia A, Rahim MW, See JA, et al. Mucosal recovery and mortality in adults with celiac disease after treatment with a gluten-free diet. Am J Gastroenterol 2010. https://doi.org/10.1038/ajg.2010.10.
66. Slot IDB, van der Fels-Klerx HJ, Bremer MGEG, et al. Immunochemical Detection Methods for Gluten in Food Products: Where Do We Go from Here? Crit Rev Food Sci Nutr 2016;56(15):2455–66. https://doi.org/10.1080/10408398.2013.847817.
67. Rubio-Tapia A, Murray JA. Classification and management of refractory coeliac disease. Gut 2010. https://doi.org/10.1136/gut.2009.195131.
68. Zhang J, Portela SB, Horrell JB, et al. An integrated, accurate, rapid, and economical handheld consumer gluten detector. Food Chem 2019;275:446–56.
69. Home - Gluten Detective Home Gluten Test Kits. Available at: https://glutendetective.com/. Accessed February 12, 2020.
70. Lerner BA, Phan Vo LT, Yates S, et al. Detection of Gluten in Gluten-Free Labeled Restaurant Food: Analysis of Crowd-Sourced Data. Am J Gastroenterol 2019;114(5):792–7.

Gastrointestinal Food Allergies and Intolerances

Emily Hon, MD[a], Sandeep K. Gupta, MD[b,c],*

KEYWORDS

- Food allergy • Food intolerance • Anaphylaxis • Immunoglobulin G testing
- Allergy testing • Food protein-induced enterocolitis syndrome
- Irritable bowel syndrome • Oral allergy syndrome

KEY POINTS

- Differentiating between immunoglobulin E (IgE)-mediated food allergy, non-IgE-mediated food allergy, and food intolerances is important.
- In children, the most common allergens accounting for 85% of all pediatric food allergies are cow's milk protein, egg, peanut, soy, tree nuts, fish, shellfish, and wheat. Allergies to peanuts, tree nuts, and seafood tend to persist into adulthood, while the other childhood food allergies resolve in most cases.
- Detailed clinical history is extremely important in the diagnosis of food allergies and intolerances and should help guide appropriate testing if necessary.
- Atopy patch testing, serum immunoglobulin G testing, Alcat, and mediator-release testing have limited-to-no evidence of efficacy in effectively diagnosing food allergies and food intolerances.

INTRODUCTION

Adverse gastrointestinal (GI) reactions to food vary greatly in clinical presentation, severity, pathophysiology, diagnosis, and treatment. These reactions can be divided into 2 broad categories: immune-mediated and nonimmune-mediated.[1] (**Fig. 1**) Within immune-mediated disease are the food allergies (which are further subdivided into immunoglobulin E [IgE]-mediated, non-IgE-mediated, and mixed IgE- and non-IgE-mediated disorders) and celiac disease (primarily discussed in Chaudhry and

[a] Division of Pediatric Gastroenterology, Hepatology, and Nutrition, Riley Hospital for Children at IU Health, ROC 4210, 705 Riley Hospital Drive, Indianapolis, IN 46202, USA; [b] Community Health Network, 6626 E 75th Street, Suite 400, Indianapolis, IN 46250, USA; [c] Section of Pediatric Gastroenterology, Hepatology, Nutrition, Riley Hospital for Children at IU Health, Indiana University School of Medicine, ROC 4210, 705 Riley Hospital Drive, Indianapolis, IN 46202, USA
* Corresponding author. Section of Pediatric Gastroenterology, Hepatology, Nutrition, Riley Hospital for Children at IU Health, Indiana University School of Medicine, ROC 4210, 705 Riley Hospital Drive, Indianapolis, IN 46202, USA
E-mail address: sgupta@iu.edu

Gastroenterol Clin N Am 50 (2021) 41–57
https://doi.org/10.1016/j.gtc.2020.10.006
0889-8553/21/© 2020 Elsevier Inc. All rights reserved.

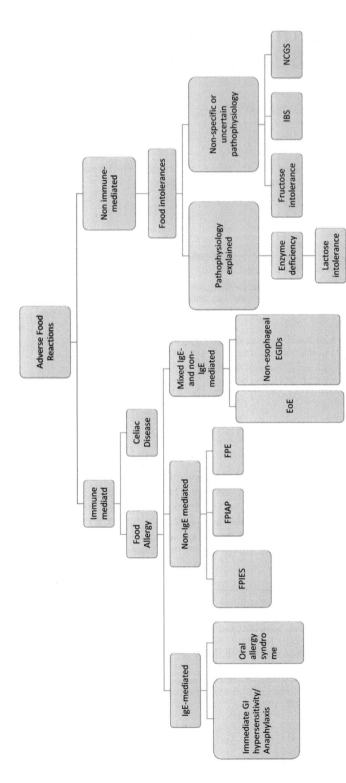

Fig. 1. Classification of adverse food reactions. IgE, immunoglobulin E; GI, gastrointestinal; FPIES, food protein-induced enterocolitis syndrome; FPIAP, food protein-induced allergic proctocolitis; FPE, food protein-induced enteropathy; EoE, eosinophilic esophagitis; EGIDs, eosinophilic gastrointestinal diseases; IBS, irritable bowel syndrome; NCGS, nonceliac gluten sensitivity.

Table 1
System-based symptoms encountered in acute immunoglobulin E-mediated food reactions

System Involved	Symptoms (Usual Onset Within Minutes to 1 to 2 Hours After Food Ingestion)
Cutaneous	Pruritis, flushing, urticaria, angioedema, atopic dermatitis flare
GI	Nausea, emesis, crampy abdominal pain, oral pruritis, angioedema (of lip, palate, pharynx)
Respiratory tract	Nasal congestion, pruritis, sneezing, laryngeal edema and hoarseness, cough, wheeze, chest tightness, dyspnea, cyanosis
Cardiovascular	Tachycardia, bradycardia, hypotension, cardiac arrest, dizziness
Neurologic	Sense of impending doom, syncope, dizziness

colleagues' article, "All things Gluten: A Review," in this issue).[2] Nonimmune disorders are generally referred to as food intolerances; some of these have known physiologic basis such as enzyme deficiency (eg, lactose intolerance), while others are of uncertain mechanisms (eg, irritable bowel syndrome [IBS]).[2] The toxic reactions to food contaminated by bacteria or reactions related to metabolic errors are not included in this review.

Although almost 20% of adults in the United States self-report food allergies, large cross-sectional survey studies show that the true prevalence is closer to 10% in adults[3] and 8% in children.[4] An incorrect diagnosis can have dramatic and needless effects on nutrition and/or quality of life if elimination diets are recommended for therapy.[5] Unwarranted elimination of foods based solely on allergy test results without taking into context the allergy history can actually lead to the loss of tolerance and increase the risk of an IgE-mediated reaction to a previously tolerated food.[6] The

Table 2
Common terminology in food allergies and sensitivities

Term	Characteristics
Food allergy	Immune IgE-mediated or non-IgE-mediated response to a particular food; symptoms should occur every time that food is ingested
Sensitization	Detection of specific IgE through skin prick or blood testing toward a specific food; predictable symptoms do not occur every time the food is ingested
IgE-mediated food allergy	When a food-specific IgE is formed, and attaches to the allergy cells throughout the body; every time the food is ingested, it causes immediate-onset symptoms, usually within minutes or up to 3 hours after ingestion (see **Table 1** for typical IgE-mediated symptoms); skin prick or blood-specific IgE testing is likely to be positive for that food
Anaphylaxis	Rapid onset, progressive, severe symptoms, involving more than 1 organ system that can occur with IgE-mediated food allergy
Non-IgE-mediated reaction	A non-IgE immune-mediated, delayed-onset reaction to a specific food; most common GI symptoms include vomiting, upset stomach, diarrhea, or blood in stool; skin prick or blood specific IgE testing is negative.
Sensitivity or intolerance	A nonimmunologic response to a certain food or foods; most often includes GI symptoms such as abdominal pain, bloating, diarrhea; does not include other systemic IgE reactions

authors write this article to serve as a tool to help the gastroenterologist evaluate GI adverse food reactions and refer to other specialists when appropriate. Additionally, the article is organized in subsections of clinical presentation, pathophysiology, diagnosis, and treatment.

FOOD ALLERGY

Food allergy is defined as "an adverse health effect arising from a specific immune response that occurs reproducibly on exposure to a given food."[1] Within food allergies are potential life-threatening reactions such as anaphylaxis, chronic disease such as eosinophilic esophagitis, and typically benign transient disorders such as food protein-induced allergic proctocolitis.[1]

Immunoglobulin E-Mediated Food Allergies

IgE antibodies, an important component of adaptive immune response to parasites, are increasingly recognized for their roles in IgE-mediated food allergies and other atopic disorders. Food protein is taken up by antigen-presenting cells that inappropriately trigger a T-helper 2 (TH2) predominant response leading to a Type 1 hypersensitivity and IgE-mediated food allergy.[2] The onset of these reactions is typically rapid, within minutes to hours of exposure of the offending food, and with reproducible effects on the skin, GI tract, and/or respiratory systems.[7] These reactions are mediated by products released from mast cell and basophil degranulation and include skin manifestations (eg, flushing, urticaria, or angioedema), GI manifestations (eg, emesis, diarrhea, or abdominal pain), and/or respiratory symptoms (eg, wheezing, shortness of breath, or hoarseness).[8] Progression to full-blown anaphylaxis with respiratory distress, hypotension, shock, or loss of consciousness and death can occur.[8] **Table 2** lists system-based symptoms encountered in acute IgE-mediated food reactions. The most common allergenic food proteins are water-soluble glycopeptides, with greater resistance to proteolytic enzymes, acid, and heat.[2] In children, the most common allergens, which account for 85% of all pediatric food allergies, are cow's milk protein, egg, peanut, soy, tree nuts, fish, shellfish, and wheat.[2] Allergies to peanuts, tree nuts, and seafood tend to persist into adulthood, while the other childhood food allergies resolve in most cases.[8]

Food-induced anaphylaxis is a systemic response in which the food protein binds to membrane-associated IgE on mast cells and basophils, leading to release of histamine, tryptase, and other inflammatory mediators. Unlike the cardiovascular collapse seen in anaphylaxis induced by drugs or venom, food-induced anaphylaxis is more likely to have GI and respiratory symptoms.[9] Death caused by food-induced

Table 3
Pollens (and latex) with their associated cross-reactive foods in patients with oral allergy syndrome

Pollen/ Plant	Fruit/Vegetable
Birch	Apple, cherry, apricot, carrot, potato, kiwi, hazelnut, celery, pear, peanut, soybean
Ragweed	Melon (eg, cantaloupe or honeydew), banana
Grass	Kiwi, tomato, watermelon, potato
Mugwort	Celery, fennel, carrot, parsley
Latex	Banana, avocado, chestnut, kiwi, fig, apple, cherry

anaphylaxis is fortunately quite rare, with 1.8 per million person-years in food-allergic individuals, with peanut being the most common trigger.[10]

Exercise-induced anaphylaxis is a rare disorder where allergic symptoms occur during or after exercise.[11] In one-third of cases, there is an associated food allergen that is ingested within 2 hours prior to the exercise and is termed *food dependent exerciseinduced anaphylaxis (FDEIA)*.[12] Symptoms include urticaria, angioedema, respiratory distress, GI symptoms, and anaphylactic shock. Shellfish and wheat are the most common triggers in children and adults.[12]

Oral allergy syndrome, also referred to as pollen-food allergy syndrome, is an IgE-mediated reaction localized to the oral mucosa and triggered by certain fresh fruits and vegetables.[13] These foods are usually well tolerated when cooked. The estimated prevalence is between 9% to 35% in the United States.[13] Patients complain of mild pruritis and/or angioedema of the mouth or throat without associated systemic reaction. This syndrome is common in patients with pollen sensitization (eg, environmental allergies) and is caused by heat-labile cross-reactive antigens present in plant and food antigens.[13] In fact, particular pollen allergies (birch, ragweed, mugwort, orchard grass, or timothy grass) are associated with a corresponding group of potential food allergens (**Table 3**), and symptoms are worse during times of high pollen counts. As latex is derived from rubber trees that have many cross-reactive foods; patients with latex allergy can also have an increased likelihood of having symptoms with banana, avocado, chestnut, kiwi, tomato, bell pepper, and other fruits.[14] Anaphylaxis to these cross-reactive fruits is rare, reported in around 2% of oral allergy syndrome cases.[15]

Nonimmunoglobulin E-Mediated Food Allergies

The individual pathophysiologies of non-IgE-mediated food allergies are not well-defined. These include FPIES, food protein-induced allergic protocolitis (FPIAP), and food protein-induced enteropathy (FPE). These often present in infancy, with symptoms isolated to the GI tract. Skin prick testing and food-specific serum IgE testing are usually negative.[16]

FPIES typically presents in the first year of life and can have acute or chronic presentation. It is rare for exclusively breastfed infants to develop FPIES.[17] The most common presentation is with the introduction of grains such as oat and rice. Other triggers include cow's milk protein, soy protein, egg, fish, fruits, and vegetables.[17,18] In older children and adults, seafood may be a trigger in patients who previously tolerated it.[19]

While the hallmark of acute FPIES is vomiting within 1 to 4 hours after ingestion of the suspected trigger without associated cutaneous or respiratory symptoms,[17] 3 or more minor criteria should also be met. These include 2 or more episodes of repetitive vomiting after eating the same suspected food trigger or repetitive vomiting after eating a different suspected food trigger, or any of the following suspected reactions

Extreme lethargy
Marked pallor
Need for emergency department visit
Need for parenteral fluid support
Diarrhea within 24 hours
Hypotension
Hypothermia[20]

Severe acute FPIES can lead to cyanosis, hypotension, metabolic acidosis, and methemoglobinemia. Symptoms should resolve within 24 hours. Infants should be growing and developing well in between these episodes.[17]

Chronic FPIES is more common in formula-fed infants with cow's milk or soy protein being the common triggers. Symptoms include frequent watery diarrhea that may have blood or mucous, progressively worsening emesis, and/or associated poor weight gain or weight loss.[21]

Food protein-induced allergic proctocolitis (FPIAP) is a transient benign condition presenting in early infancy with streaks of blood in watery or mucousy stools, benign remainder of history, and good weight gain.[16] This can occur with human milk or formula (cow's milk protein or soy-based) fed infants.[22] Cow's milk protein is the most common trigger, followed by soy and egg protein.[16] The long-term outcome of infants diagnosed with FPIAP is generally uneventful.[23,24]

Food protein-induced enteropathy (FPE) presents with diarrhea and malabsorption weeks to months after introduction of cow's milk protein (formula or milk), leading to small bowel villous injury and inflammation. The presentation can occur within a few hours of cow's milk ingestion to 4 weeks later.[16] Many of these patients can also have failure to thrive, vomiting, diarrhea, anemia, and hypoalbuminemia, but unlike chronic FPIES do not risk severe dehydration or metabolic acidosis with reintroduction of the food trigger.[25]

Mixed Immunoglobulin E- and Nonimmunoglobulin E-Mediated Food Allergy

Eosinophilic esophagitis (EoE) is a chronic, food antigen driven disease, localized to the esophagus with symptoms of esophageal dysfunction including dysphagia, vomiting, and food impactions.[26] EoE is more common in patients with atopic comorbidities,[27] but has also been associated with autoimmune[28] and connective tissue disorders.[29]

EoE is characterized by impaired epithelial barrier function with esophageal infiltration of activated eosinophils and mast cells.[30] Patients have higher rates of IgE food and aeroallergen sensitization than control populations[31] and can be induced with IgE-mediated oral or sublingual immunotherapy.[32] However, anti-IgE treatment has not been shown to be better than placebo in inducing EoE remission,[33] and elimination diets based on IgE-mediated testing have equivocal results.[34] EoE is considered a mixed IgE-, non-IgE mediated food antigen-driven hypersensitivity.

Nonesophageal eosinophilic gastrointestinal diseases (EGIDs) are comprised of eosinophilic gastritis, eosinophilic gastroenteritis, and eosinophilic colitis. Eosinophilic inflammation can be seen in the GI mucosa, muscular layers, or serosa.[35] The clinical presentations, diagnosis, and management of these varied and complex group of disorders are variable and depend on not only the depth of the eosinophilic inflammation but also the specific segment(s) of the GI tract involved. Eosinophilic gastritis presents with abdominal pain or vomiting, eosinophilic gastroenteritis with diarrhea, and anemia or hypoalbuminemia, and eosinophilic colitis can present with diarrhea or bloody stools. As such it often is important to map the GI tract in these patients using various diagnostic tools including imaging and endoscopic procedures.[36]

Celiac Disease

Celiac disease is a chronic immune-mediated adverse reaction to gluten in genetically susceptible individuals. Unlike a food allergy, the immune response is directed against one's own body (eg, autoimmune) rather than against foreign substances such as parasites or food antigen. Celiac enteropathy leads to malabsorption, causing similar symptoms as lactose intolerance and IBS in addition to potential extraintestinal symptoms.[37] Celiac disease will be discussed in more detail in Chaudhry and colleagues' article, "All things Gluten: A Review," in this issue.

Food Intolerances

Food intolerances are nonallergic, nonimmune-mediated undesirable reactions to food. Some involve a known pathophysiologic process such as lactose intolerance, while the mechanisms of other food intolerances such as in IBS and in nonceliac gluten sensitivity (NCGS) are not known.

Lactose intolerance is a syndrome in which lactose ingestion causes abdominal pain, bloating, flatulence, nausea, or diarrhea because of lactase deficiency. Lactase is an intestinal brush border enzyme that hydrolyzes the disaccharide lactose to monosaccharides glucose and galactose. Congenital lactase deficiency is extremely rare and presents in infants with severe life-threatening diarrhea and dehydration and resolves with lactose-free age-appropriate formula. In children and adults, lactose intolerance is caused by reduced production of lactase (eg, lactase nonpersistence), and is more common in Asian[38] and African[39] populations. Symptoms within 1 to 2 hours of ingestion are caused by malabsorbed lactose that reaches the colon and undergoes bacterial fermentation.[40] Most people with lactase nonpersistence retain some lactase activity and can tolerate limited dietary lactose. For example, they can often tolerate yogurt or certain cheeses but have symptoms with cow's milk or ice cream beyond a certain quantity.[40]

Symptoms of *fructose intolerance* are similar to lactose intolerance and are attributed to the presence of unabsorbed fructose in colonic lumen with resultant bacterial fermentation and osmotic diarrhea.[41] Fructose is a monosaccharide naturally present in certain fruits, vegetables, and honey. In many diets, fructose is present primarily as high fructose corn syrup (HFCS) found in processed foods, sweeteners, and soft drinks. Fructose is mainly absorbed through carrier-mediated facilitative diffusion and active GLUT-5 transporter.[41] Studies have shown no difference in expression of GLUT-5 transporters in fructose-tolerant versus -intolerant patients, so pathophysiology of fructose intolerance is unclear.[42]

Sucrose-isomaltase deficiency has also been found in 11 of 31 (35%) patients with a presumed diagnosis of IBS (diarrhea and mixed subtypes).[43]

Nonceliac gluten sensitivity (NCGS) will be discussed in Chaudhry and colleagues' article, "All things Gluten: A Review," in this issue.

IBS is a chronic functional GI disorder defined in Rome IV criteria as recurrent abdominal pain on average at least 1 day per week in the last 3 month and onset at least 6 months prior. Symptoms are also associated with 2 or more of the following: related to defecation, associated with a change in frequency of stool, and/or associated with a change in form (appearance of stool).[44] It is likely multifactorial in etiology, with contributions from gut-brain dysfunction, genetic factors, postinfectious changes, abnormalities in serotonin metabolism, gut dysmotility, mucosal inflammation, and intestinal microbiota playing roles.[45] Symptoms often worsen postprandially, leading many patients to first investigate food allergy or other food intolerances. Common triggers include fatty foods, caffeine, alcohol, spices, and foods rich in carbohydrates, which lead to abdominal cramps with constipation or diarrhea. Some theorize that the cramping and urge to defecate may be an exaggerated gastrocolic response; manometric studies show caffeine precipitates rectosigmoid contractions within minutes.[46]

COMMON DIAGNOSTIC TESTS FOR FOOD ALLERGY: UTILITY AND LIMITATIONS

The diagnosis of food allergy can be challenging, with available testing having significant weaknesses. Correctly diagnosing food allergies is important to prevent the symptoms and potentially life-threatening reactions that can occur; however, overdiagnosis of food allergies can also be harmful when patients eliminate entire food groups unnecessarily. This can dramatically impair their quality of life, affect social interactions, be burdensome financially, and can lead to loss of tolerance.[6,47,48]

Diagnosis of IgE-mediated food allergy starts with a detailed history to help guide testing.[1]

As most IgE-mediated testing is sensitive, but not specific, indiscriminate or panel testing can lead to false-positive results. Prior to any testing, it is essential to obtain the following

1. A description of typical symptoms of IgE-mediated allergy (see **Table 1**)
2. Timing of symptoms about the food ingestion (usually within minutes to 1–2 hours)
3. Reproducibility of symptoms with subsequent food ingestion
4. The form of food (raw, cooked, processed)
5. The amount of food ingested
6. Frequency of ingestion of the food in question

Atopic patients are at higher risk of food allergies. Associated cofactors such as febrile illness, asthma exacerbation, exercise, alcohol ingestion, drugs that increase gastric pH and nonsteroidal anti-inflammatory drugs (NSAIDs) can worsen the severity of allergic reaction and should be assessed.[2]

Several testing modalities are universally accepted by expert consensus panels on the diagnosis of IgE-mediated food allergy.[1,7]

Immunoglobulin E-Mediated Testing

Oral food challenges
The double-blind, placebo-controlled food challenge (DBPCFC) is the gold standard for diagnosis of food allergy[7] but can be labor- and time-intensive. DBPCFC involves a strict protocol of ingesting increasing amounts of the suspected allergen or placebo for a day while monitoring for symptoms in a controlled health care setting. The test is then repeated hours or days later using the placebo or allergen not used for the first test. As the name suggests, both clinicians and patients are blinded. Given the significant risk of anaphylaxis, these tests should be carried out in facilities that are prepared to monitor and emergently treat anaphylaxis. Open oral food challenge is most often used in the clinical setting but carries risk of bias.

Food-specific serum immunoglobulin E
Food-specific serum immunoglobulin E (sIgE) testing is widely available and easy to perform. The assay involves a surface-fixed allergen that is incubated with the patient's serum. sIgE antibody from the serum binds the allergen and the complex measured by binding of labeled anti-IgE. It is extremely important to take these results into context with a patient's clinical history. The presence of food antigen-specific IgE in the serum is called sensitization and by itself does not confirm the diagnosis of food allergy. Although sIgE levels correlate with the likelihood of a clinically significant reaction, these do not inform likely severity of reaction.[49] sIgE levels may be preferred over skin prick testing in patients who are unable to cooperate with skin testing, those with extensive skin disease, or in patients unable to discontinue oral antihistamines. In general, sIgE has high sensitivity but low specificity for food allergy. Panels to a large number of foods have become increasingly popular, especially among primary care providers.[50] Testing in this manner often leads to overdiagnosis of food allergy and unnecessary elimination diets with additional emotional and financial burden for patients and families.[5] In patients with convincing stories for IgE-mediated allergy, but negative sIgE testing, OFC is recommended.[51] The basophil activation test, a functional test

that measures the ability of IgE to induce activation of basophils in the presence of an allergen, is felt to reproduce IgE-mediated reactions in vitro. It is currently used in research to study allergic reactions but may help support diagnosis of IgE-mediated allergic conditions in the future.[52]

Skin prick tests

In skin prick tests (SPTs), the skin surface is pricked with allergen extract to assess the allergen-specific IgE bound to cutaneous mast cells. A wheal and flare response is measured within 20 minutes. Dermatographism can lead to false-positives, and recent use of systemic antihistamines can lead to false-negative results.[1] Wheal sizes vary with age, body site used for testing (usually greater on back than forearms), device used, extract potency, and whether commercial extract or fresh food is used. A positive SPT response indicates the presence of IgE specific to the antigen in question and represents an observable physiologic response to that allergen. SPTs have high sensitivity and low specificity, so should be correlated with the patient's history to determine clinical relevance.[2] Similar to sIgE testing, positive tests are considered sensitization and are not sufficient to diagnose a food allergy without appropriate clinical context. The negative predictive value (NPV) of SPT is greater than 90%, and the test is useful to help exclude food allergy in the absence of a convincing clinical history.[53] The positive predictive value (PPV) of SPTs depends on the patient's age and food allergen and can differ with the SPT method used and presence of atopy.[53] SPTs should be performed by trained personnel in a facility capable of managing anaphylaxis, which can rarely be triggered by an SPT.[7]

Nonimmunoglobuin E-Mediated Food Allergy Testing

Elimination diets with the removal of suspected food triggers have a diagnostic and therapeutic role in non-IgE mediated food allergy disorders. In FPIES, FPIAP, and FPE, improvement in symptoms with removal of suspected antigens helps support the diagnosis. In eosinophilic esophagitis, removing of the suspected food trigger for 6 to 8 weeks with follow-up endoscopy and histology is important.

Limited or Unclear Utility for Gastrointestinal Food Allergies and Intolerances

In a 2006 study of patients surveyed at a food allergy conference and a pediatric allergy clinic, over 20% of patients previously diagnosed with food allergies had previously undergone unproven diagnostic testing.[54] Inappropriate testing can lead to incorrect diagnoses, unnecessary elimination diets, and drastic changes in patient and family quality of life. Therefore, it is important for providers to understand the methodology and research (or lack thereof) between proven and unproven techniques and to counsel patients appropriately. Several tests have not been studied in rigorous trials and/or have conflicting data regarding their roles in evaluation of *food allergies and intolerances*.

Atopy patch testing (APT) is a diagnostic procedure intended for delayed hypersensitivity reactions commonly used in the diagnosis of contact dermatitis. Intact protein allergens are mounted on tape for 48 hours to the skin with evaluation of the test reaction after 48 to 72 hours.[55] Unfortunately, the lack of standardization of methods and interpretation has made using this test difficult.[56] APT has limited utility in the evaluation of patients with eosinophilic esophagitis or other clinical presentations such as anaphylaxis, eczema, urticaria, and proctocolitis.[57,58]

Studies have shown that the presence of food-specific serum immunoglobulin G (sIgG) is the body's natural response to a regularly ingested food;[59,60] therefore positive *food-specific serum IgG testing* is unlikely to an indication of pathology. sIgG to cow's milk protein can be detected in 98% of healthy children by 2 years of age.[61] There are no established, standardized reference values for sIgG specific for foods. However, several panel assays are easily available to providers with promotion, suggesting that they are helpful in diagnosing food-mediated disease such as IBS, chronic fatigue, and migraines. A widely cited article by Atkinson and colleagues[62] enrolled 150 patients with IBS into a randomized controlled trial where they received diet based on elevated IgG values versus a sham diet. Those who eliminated foods based on IgG values had a 10% higher reduction in symptom score when compared with subjects on the sham diet.

Foods that were most commonly eliminated in the IgG test-based diet included yeast, milk, whole egg, and wheat. The sham diet involved eliminating foods to which the patient had not formed antibodies, so they usually did not exclude yeast, milk, whole egg, and/or wheat. Wheat- and dairy-containing foods are often IBS triggers and may have improved patients' symptoms irrespective of their IgG status; therefore, the slight improvement in symptoms with patients on this diet is not surprising. Lack of further supportive evidence for specific IgG testing in the literature leads one to question if this result is reproducible or meaningful.

As described in the Cell Science System Alcat Scientific Dossier, the *Alcat test* measures a change in the volume and shape of neutrophils after exposure to the test substance, which can include over 450 individual items including, foods, medicinal herbs, additives, colorings, and pharmaceutical agents. It is recommended for chronic GI disorders, skin diseases, neurologic and psychological disorders, respiratory problems, metabolic diseases, endocrine disorders, musculoskeletal disorders, immune disorders, and periodontal diseases. In a parallel-group double-blind, randomized controlled trial of 58 adults with IBS, Ali and colleagues[63] saw greater improvement in IBS Global Improvement Scale scores (but not in Adequate Relief or Quality of Life scores) in patients treated with Alcat-based diets versus sham diets. Further studies are needed.

Mediator release testing (MRT) is a widely available diagnostic test and is stated to be "the most reliable and clinically useful food sensitivity test that exists" on the Web site nowleap.com. The authors were unable to find any literature or evidence to support its use at the time of this article.

Diagnosis of Nonimmunoglobulin E-Mediated Food Allergies

IgE-mediated testing in the non-IgE mediated diseases (FPIES, FPIAP, and FPE) is not helpful and would typically be negative. These diagnoses are primarily based on presenting features and resolution of symptoms after removal of the offending protein or reoccurrence of symptoms with reintroduction.[16]

For acute FPIES, an OFC can be considered for a definitive diagnosis but is usually not needed; 5% to 30% of patients may have low IgE against their food triggers, which is associated with persistent FPIES.[64] Chronic FPIES can be difficult to diagnose, and there are no specific diagnostic criteria. When the offending food (typically cow's milk protein or soy) is removed, the symptoms usually resolve within 3 to 10 days. If the food trigger is reintroduced after a period of avoidance, severe acute FPIES reaction can occur, and, as such, these trials need to be conducted in adequately staffed and supported health care settings under guidance of appropriately trained medical professionals. Ruling out other disorders is important in chronic FPIES. The differential diagnosis includes food poisoning, metabolic disorders, cyclic vomiting, GI obstruction, necrotizing enterocolitis, severe gastroesophageal reflux disease (GERD), inflammatory bowel disease (IBD), eosinophilic gastrointestinal disease (EGID), celiac disease, and anatomic abnormalities. The correct diagnosis is often delayed after several reactions or months after presentation because of the broad differential and high index of suspicion needed for diagnosis.[65,66] Laboratory findings are often nonspecific and can include neutrophilia, eosinophilia, and thrombocytosis.[17,67]

In FPIAP, biopsies are typically not obtained, but eosinophils have been seen in colonic or rectal biopsies. Allergy testing is not indicated, but IgE testing is usually negative. Of course, other more serious causes of bloody stools in infants should be considered such as volvulus, necrotizing enterocolitis, infectious colitis, anal fissures, GI obstruction, and coagulopathy.

In FPE, small bowel villous injury and increased intraepithelial lymphocytes can be seen similar to celiac disease's enteropathy.[68] SPT or food-specific IgE levels are not useful in diagnosing FPE.[16]

Diagnosis of Mixed Immunoglobulin E- and Nonimmunoglobulin E-Mediated Food Allergy

For EoE, diagnosis requires symptoms of esophageal dysfunction and esophageal biopsies with greater than 14 eosinophils per high powered field.[69]

Diagnosis of non-esophageal EGIDs can be challenging, as the diseases have variable clinical presentation, may be segmental in location, and may be outside the reach of endoscopically obtained biopsies. Endoscopy can be grossly normal or have mucosal erythema, edema, ulcerations, nodularity, or polypoid lesions. Diagnosis is usually based on prominent eosinophilia on biopsies in the appropriate clinical setting. Other histologic findings can include eosinophil degranulation, cryptitis, crypt abscess, and/or chronic architectural changes.[36]

Diagnosis of Food Intolerances and Irritable Bowel Syndrome

Diagnosis of food intolerances
Diagnoses of lactose and fructose intolerance are most often made based on history and response to appropriate dietary changes. If needed, diagnosis of lactose intolerance can be confirmed with lactose tolerance test, lactose breath hydrogen test, intestinal biopsies to measure lactase, or genetic testing for 13910C > T polymorphism.[40] Fructose breath test provides the best objective evidence for fructose intolerance when needed.[41]

Diagnosis of irritable bowel syndrome
Patients who meet Rome Criteria without alarm features do not require excessive testing.[70] There is no evidence that IgE-mediated testing is helpful in IBS or food sensitivity and insufficient evidence that IgG testing, Alcat, or MRT is useful.

TREATMENT
Treatment of Immunoglobulin E-Mediated Food Allergy

For patients with food anaphylaxis, a clinician must be ready to advise with appropriate dietary treatment. In addition to avoidance of the established food trigger, one must also be familiar with known allergic associations. For example, patients with peanut allergy may need to be evaluated for tree nut and sesame allergy. Patients should be advised how to eliminate these foods, check food labels, and discern whether baked forms may be tolerated or trialed in a challenge. This typically requires trained allergist and registered dietitian assistance. Elimination of food groups can be restrictive in specific nutrients, and supplementation or replacement with other foods may be needed. Patients should be prepared for accidental exposure with an alert bracelet, an epinephrine autoinjector, and an exposure action plan that describes features of reactions and how to inject epinephrine.

If a responsible food allergen is identified in FDEIA, it should be avoided 4 to 6 hours before exercise and for a period after exercise. If no food allergen is identified, exercise should be terminated immediately if allergic symptoms develop. Prophylaxis with antihistamine, leukotriene antagonists, and mast cell degranulation inhibitors may be helpful. Some recommend avoiding all foods and other known FDEIA provocations such as NSAIDs, aspirin, and alcohol prior to exercise. Patients with FDEIA must still carry epinephrine injectors with exercise activities and be advised not to exercise alone.[12]

Management of oral allergy syndrome involves avoidance of raw trigger foods and treatment of associated allergic rhinitis. Because most of the immunogenic proteins are found within the fruit/vegetable skin, peeling or cooking should diminish the reaction. Patients with only mild oral symptoms may choose to continue consuming trigger foods. As mentioned previously, anaphylaxis is rare in OAS; therefore, most do not need epinephrine autoinjector pens.

Food allergen-specific immunotherapy (food IT) is an approach to food mediated allergies with a similar concept to the aeroallergen subcutaneous immunotherapy commonly known as allergy shots. Food IT has been studied with various delivery methods, including subcutaneous, oral, sublingual, and epicutaneous. Oral immunotherapy (OIT) is the best studied option for IgE-mediated food allergies and can reduce the severity of reactions to accidental exposures in most patients, but there are many safety concerns because of the potential for significant reactions.[71] Currently, there is one US Food and Drug Administration-approved OIT product, Palforzia, for peanut allergy. Other OIT is usually done using foods found at the grocery store. Benefits of OIT include partial desensitization and improvement in quality of life. Drawbacks include the risks of anaphylaxis, the potential development of EoE, and the significant time and schedule commitments.[72]

Treatment for Nonimmunoglobulin E-Mediated Food Allergy

FPIES management relies on supportive care in cases of accidental exposures. Long-term management of FPIES requires avoidance of food triggers and periodic re-evaluations with an allergist and supervised OFCs to monitor for resolution.[17] Treatment of *FPIAP*[73] is typically maternal elimination of cow's milk protein and soy (if breastfed) or transition to protein-hydrolysate formula; sometimes an amino acid-based formula is necessary. Patients with FPIAP can usually reintroduce milk and soy into the diet safely at 1 to 2 years of age without recurrence of bloody stools.[73] For *FPE*, symptoms resolve within 3 days to 3 weeks of food elimination. At 1 to 3 years of age, foods can gradually be reintroduced at home after a safe period. If symptoms recur, the food is often removed, and reintroduction attempted every 6 to 12 months thereafter.[16]

Treatment of Mixed Immunoglobulin E- Nonimmunoglobulin E-Mediated Food Allergy

Treatment of *EoE* currently includes high-dose proton pump inhibition, swallowed topical glucocorticoids, empiric or allergy testing-based elimination diet, and/or esophageal dilation.[74] Treatment of *EG, EGE, and EC* is challenging as current data are limited to case series. Treatment has included systemic steroids, topical steroids such as enteral budesonide, elimination diets, and mast cell agents.[75,76] Vedolizumab has led to improvement in a small number of cases.[76]

Treatment of Food Intolerances and Irritable Bowel Syndrome

Food intolerances are treated by avoidance of food at a level that prevents the symptoms, typically of abdominal pain, bloating, or diarrhea. There is no immune reaction, so if small amounts are ingested without symptoms, there is no harm or sequela. Treatment of IBS is diverse and multifactorial, often including lifestyle modification, changes in diet, and/or symptom-based pharmacotherapy.[70]

SUMMARY

GI symptoms such as abdominal pain, diarrhea and bloating, are often triggered by food, and it is common for patients and their providers to look to food as a cause of these symptoms. There is a broad spectrum of food allergies from immediate life-threatening symptoms to chronic inflammatory diseases with delayed presentation after prolonged exposure to the offending agent. Most food-related GI symptoms are likely not allergy-related and may represent an intolerance or other GI etiology such as celiac disease, IBD, or IBS. As described previously, there are various food allergy/sensitivity testing, with varying degrees of usefulness. The clinician needs to consider food allergies and intolerances with food-related symptoms, be comfortable with obtaining appropriate history to target testing, and know when to refer to an allergist.

ACKNOWLEDGEMENTS

Special thanks to McKenzi Sidor for her valuable administrative support and to Girish Vitalpur for his valuable Allergy-related insights for this article.

DISCLOSURE

E. Hon has no conflict of interest to disclose. S. Gupta is a consultant for Adare, Abbott, Allakos, Gossamer Bio, Receptos, and Medscape; royalties UpToDate; research support Shire.

CLINICS CARE POINTS

- Correctly diagnosing food allergies is important to prevent the symptoms and potentially life-threatening reactions that can occur. However, overdiagnosis of food allergies can also be harmful when patients eliminate entire food groups unnecessarily.
- Food intolerances are nonallergic, nonimmune mediated undesirable reactions to food. Treatment is with avoidance of food at a level that prevents the adverse symptoms, typically abdominal pain, bloating, or diarrhea.
- Symptoms of the eosinophilic gastrointestinal diseases depend on the segment of GI tract involved and depth of eosinophilic inflammation.

REFERENCES

1. Boyce JA, Assa'ad A, Burks AW, et al. Guidelines for the diagnosis and management of food allergy in the United States: Summary of the NIAID-Sponsored Expert Panel Report. J Allergy Clin Immunol 2010;126(6):1105–18.
2. Turnbull JL, Adams HN, Gorard DA. Review article: the diagnosis and management of food allergy and food intolerances. Aliment Pharmacol Ther 2015; 41(1):3–25.

3. Gupta RS, Warren CM, Smith BM, et al. Prevalence and severity of food allergies among US Adults. JAMA Netw Open 2019;2(1):e185630.
4. Gupta RS, Springston EE, Warrier MR, et al. The prevalence, severity, and distribution of childhood food allergy in the United States. Pediatrics 2011;128(1): e9–17.
5. Bird JA, Crain M, Varshney P. Food allergen panel testing often results in misdiagnosis of food allergy. J Pediatr 2015;166(1):97–100.
6. Eapen AA, Kloepfer KM, Leickly FE, et al. Oral food challenge failures among foods restricted because of atopic dermatitis. Ann Allergy Asthma Immunol 2019;122(2):193–7.
7. Sicherer SH, Sampson HA. Food allergy: a review and update on epidemiology, pathogenesis, diagnosis, prevention, and management. J Allergy Clin Immunol 2018;141(1):41–58.
8. Sampson HA, O'Mahony L, Burks AW, et al. Mechanisms of food allergy. J Allergy Clin Immunol 2018;141(1):11–9.
9. Keet CA, Wood RA. Food allergy and anaphylaxis. Immunol Allergy Clin North Am 2007;27(2):193–212, vi.
10. Umasunthar T, Leonardi-Bee J, Hodes M, et al. Incidence of fatal food anaphylaxis in people with food allergy: a systematic review and meta-analysis. Clin Exp Allergy 2013;43(12):1333–41.
11. Giannetti MP. Exercise-induced anaphylaxis: literature review and recent updates. Curr Allergy Asthma Rep 2018;18(12):72.
12. Beaudouin E, Renaudin JM, Morisset M, et al. Food-dependent exercise-induced anaphylaxis–update and current data. Eur Ann Allergy Clin Immunol 2006;38(2): 45–51.
13. Carlson G, Coop C. Pollen food allergy syndrome (PFAS): A review of current available literature. Ann Allergy Asthma Immunol 2019;123(4):359–65.
14. Blanco C. Latex-fruit syndrome. Curr Allergy Asthma Rep 2003;3(1):47–53.
15. Ma S, Sicherer SH, Nowak-Wegrzyn A. A survey on the management of pollen-food allergy syndrome in allergy practices. J Allergy Clin Immunol 2003;112(4): 784–8.
16. Leonard SA. Non-IgE-mediated Adverse Food Reactions. Curr Allergy Asthma Rep 2017;17(12):84.
17. Nowak-Wegrzyn A, Berin MC, Mehr S. Food protein-induced enterocolitis syndrome. J Allergy Clin Immunol Pract 2020;8(1):24–35.
18. Blackman AC, Anvari S, Davis CM, et al. Emerging triggers of food protein-induced enterocolitis syndrome: Lessons from a pediatric cohort of 74 children in the United States. Ann Allergy Asthma Immunol 2019;122(4):407–11.
19. Gonzalez-Delgado P, Caparros E, Moreno MV, et al. Food protein-induced enterocolitis-like syndrome in a population of adolescents and adults caused by seafood. J Allergy Clin Immunol Pract 2019;7(2):670–2.
20. Nowak-Wegrzyn A, Chehade M, Groetch ME, et al. International consensus guidelines for the diagnosis and management of food protein-induced enterocolitis syndrome: executive summary-workgroup report of the Adverse Reactions to Foods Committee, American Academy of Allergy, Asthma & Immunology. J Allergy Clin Immunol 2017;139(4):1111–26.e4.
21. Weinberger T, Feuille E, Thompson C, et al. Chronic food protein-induced enterocolitis syndrome: characterization of clinical phenotype and literature review. Ann Allergy Asthma Immunol 2016;117(3):227–33.
22. Elizur A, Cohen M, Goldberg MR, et al. Cow's milk associated rectal bleeding: a population based prospective study. Pediatr Allergy Immunol 2012;23(8):766–70.

23. Xanthakos SA, Schwimmer JB, Melin-Aldana H, et al. Prevalence and outcome of allergic colitis in healthy infants with rectal bleeding: a prospective cohort study. J Pediatr Gastroenterol Nutr 2005;41(1):16–22.

24. Molnár K, Pintér P, Győrffy H, et al. Characteristics of allergic colitis in breast-fed infants in the absence of cow's milk allergy. World J Gastroenterol 2013;19(24): 3824–30.

25. Nowak-Wegrzyn A, Katz Y, Mehr SS, et al. Non-IgE-mediated gastrointestinal food allergy. J Allergy Clin Immunol 2015;135(5):1114–24.

26. Dellon ES, Hirano I. Epidemiology and natural history of eosinophilic esophagitis. Gastroenterology 2018;154(2):319–32.e3.

27. Capucilli P, Hill DA. Allergic comorbidity in eosinophilic esophagitis: mechanistic relevance and clinical implications. Clin Rev Allergy Immunol 2019;57(1):111–27.

28. Peterson K, Firszt R, Fang J, et al. Risk of autoimmunity in EoE and families: a population-based cohort study. Am J Gastroenterol 2016;111(7):926–32.

29. Abonia JP, Wen T, Stucke EM, et al. High prevalence of eosinophilic esophagitis in patients with inherited connective tissue disorders. J Allergy Clin Immunol 2013;132(2):378–86.

30. O'Shea KM, Aceves SS, Dellon ES, et al. Pathophysiology of Eosinophilic Esophagitis. Gastroenterology 2018;154(2):333–45.

31. Jyonouchi S, Brown-Whitehorn TA, Spergel JM. Association of eosinophilic gastrointestinal disorders with other atopic disorders. Immunol Allergy Clin North Am 2009;29(1):85–97, x.

32. Cafone J, Capucilli P, Hill DA, et al. Eosinophilic esophagitis during sublingual and oral allergen immunotherapy. Curr Opin Allergy Clin Immunol 2019;19(4): 350–7.

33. Loizou D, Enav B, Komlodi-Pasztor E, et al. A pilot study of omalizumab in eosinophilic esophagitis. PLoS One 2015;10(3):e0113483.

34. Henderson CJ, Abonia JP, King EC, et al. Comparative dietary therapy effectiveness in remission of pediatric eosinophilic esophagitis. J Allergy Clin Immunol 2012;129(6):1570–8.

35. Rothenberg ME. Eosinophilic gastrointestinal disorders (EGID). J Allergy Clin Immunol 2004;113(1):11–28 [quiz: 29].

36. Naramore S, Gupta SK. Nonesophageal eosinophilic gastrointestinal disorders: clinical care and future directions. J Pediatr Gastroenterol Nutr 2018;67(3): 318–21.

37. Verdu EF, Armstrong D, Murray JA. Between celiac disease and irritable bowel syndrome: the "no man's land" of gluten sensitivity. Am J Gastroenterol 2009; 104(6):1587–94.

38. Vandenplas Y. Lactose intolerance. Asia Pac J Clin Nutr 2015;24(Suppl 1):S9–13.

39. Bayless TM, Rosensweig NS. A racial difference in incidence of lactase deficiency. A survey of milk intolerance and lactase deficiency in healthy adult males. JAMA 1966;197(12):968–72.

40. Micic D, Rao VL, Rubin DT. Clinical approach to lactose intolerance. JAMA 2019. https://doi.org/10.1001/jama.2019.14740.

41. Fedewa A, Rao SS. Dietary fructose intolerance, fructan intolerance and FODMAPs. Curr Gastroenterol Rep 2014;16(1):370.

42. Wilder-Smith CH, Li X, Ho SS, et al. Fructose transporters GLUT5 and GLUT2 expression in adult patients with fructose intolerance. United European Gastroenterol J 2014;2(1):14–21.

43. Kim SB, Calmet FH, Garrido J, et al. Sucrase-isomaltase deficiency as a potential masquerader in irritable bowel syndrome. Dig Dis Sci 2020;65(2):534–40.

44. Mearin F, Lacy BE, Chang L, et al. Bowel disorders. Gastroenterology 2016; 150(6):p1393–407.
45. Holtmann GJ, Ford AC, Talley NJ. Pathophysiology of irritable bowel syndrome. Lancet Gastroenterol Hepatol 2016;1(2):133–46.
46. Brown SR, Cann PA, Read NW. Effect of coffee on distal colon function. Gut 1990; 31(4):450–3.
47. Feng C, Kim JH. Beyond avoidance: the psychosocial impact of food allergies. Clin Rev Allergy Immunol 2019;57(1):74–82.
48. Jackson KD, Howie LD, Akinbami LJ. Trends in allergic conditions among children: United States, 1997-2011. NCHS Data Brief 2013;(121):1–8.
49. Perry TT, Matsui EC, Kay Conover-Walker M, et al. The relationship of allergen-specific IgE levels and oral food challenge outcome. J Allergy Clin Immunol 2004;114(1):144–9.
50. Stukus DR, Kempe E, Leber A, et al. Use of food allergy panels by pediatric care providers compared with allergists. Pediatrics 2016;138(6):e20161602.
51. Sampson HA. Utility of food-specific IgE concentrations in predicting symptomatic food allergy. J Allergy Clin Immunol 2001;107(5):891–6.
52. Hemmings O, Kwok M, McKendry R, et al. Basophil activation test: old and new applications in allergy. Curr Allergy Asthma Rep 2018;18(12):77.
53. Sicherer SH, Sampson HA. Food allergy: Epidemiology, pathogenesis, diagnosis, and treatment. J Allergy Clin Immunol 2014;133(2):291–307 [quiz: 308].
54. Ko J, Lee JI, Munoz-Furlong A, et al. Use of complementary and alternative medicine by food-allergic patients. Ann Allergy Asthma Immunol 2006;97(3):365–9.
55. Wollenberg A, Vogel S. Patch testing for noncontact dermatitis: the atopy patch test for food and inhalants. Curr Allergy Asthma Rep 2013;13(5):539–44.
56. Hammond C, Lieberman JA. Unproven diagnostic tests for food allergy. Immunol Allergy Clin North Am 2018;38(1):153–63.
57. Caglayan Sozmen S, Povesi Dascola C, Gioia E, et al. Diagnostic accuracy of patch test in children with food allergy. Pediatr Allergy Immunol 2015;26(5): 416–22.
58. Mehl A, Rolinck-Werninghaus C, Staden U, et al. The atopy patch test in the diagnostic workup of suspected food-related symptoms in children. J Allergy Clin Immunol 2006;118(4):923–9.
59. Host A, Husby S, Gjesing B, et al. Prospective estimation of IgG, IgG subclass and IgE antibodies to dietary proteins in infants with cow milk allergy. Levels of antibodies to whole milk protein, BLG and ovalbumin in relation to repeated milk challenge and clinical course of cow milk allergy. Allergy 1992;47(3):218–29.
60. Keller KM, Burgin-Wolff A, Lippold R, et al. The diagnostic significance of IgG cow's milk protein antibodies re-evaluated. Eur J Pediatr 1996;155(4):331–7.
61. Martins TB, Bandhauer ME, Wilcock DM, et al. Specific immunoglobulin (Ig) G reference intervals for common food, insect, and mold allergens. Ann Clin Lab Sci 2016;46(6):635–8.
62. Atkinson W, Sheldon TA, Shaath N, et al. Food elimination based on IgG antibodies in irritable bowel syndrome: a randomised controlled trial. Gut 2004; 53(10):1459–64.
63. Ali A, Weiss TR, McKee D, et al. Efficacy of individualised diets in patients with irritable bowel syndrome: a randomised controlled trial. BMJ Open Gastroenterol 2017;4(1):e000164.
64. Caubet JC, Ford LS, Sickles L, et al. Clinical features and resolution of food protein-induced enterocolitis syndrome: 10-year experience. J Allergy Clin Immunol 2014;134(2):382–9.

65. Sopo SM, Giorgio V, Dello Iacono I, et al. A multicentre retrospective study of 66 Italian children with food protein-induced enterocolitis syndrome: different management for different phenotypes. Clin Exp Allergy 2012;42(8):1257–65.

66. Ludman S, Harmon M, Whiting D, et al. Clinical presentation and referral characteristics of food protein-induced enterocolitis syndrome in the United Kingdom. Ann Allergy Asthma Immunol 2014;113(3):290–4.

67. Kimura M, Shimomura M, Morishita H, et al. Eosinophilia in infants with food protein-induced enterocolitis syndrome in Japan. Allergol Int 2017;66(2):310–6.

68. Berin MC. Immunopathophysiology of food protein-induced enterocolitis syndrome. J Allergy Clin Immunol 2015;135(5):1108–13.

69. Dellon ES, Liacouras CA, Molina-Infante J, et al. Updated international consensus diagnostic criteria for eosinophilic esophagitis: proceedings of the AGREE conference. Gastroenterology 2018;155(4):1022–33.e10.

70. Chey WD, Kurlander J, Eswaran S. Irritable bowel syndrome: a clinical review. JAMA 2015;313(9):949–58.

71. Kim EH, Burks AW. Food allergy immunotherapy: OIT and EPIT. Allergy 2020; 75(6):p1337–46.

72. Chan ES, Dinakar C, Gonzales-Reyes E, et al. Unmet needs of children with peanut allergy: Aligning the risks and the evidence. Ann Allergy Asthma Immunol 2020;124(5):479–86.

73. Erdem SB, Nacaroglu HT, Karaman S, et al. Tolerance development in food protein-induced allergic proctocolitis: Single centre experience. Allergol Immunopathol (Madr) 2017;45(3):212–9.

74. Hirano I, Chan ES, Rank MA, et al. AGA Institute and the Joint Task Force on Allergy-Immunology Practice Parameters Clinical Guidelines for the Management of Eosinophilic Esophagitis. Gastroenterology 2020;158(6):1776–86.

75. Reed C, Woosley JT, Dellon ES. Clinical characteristics, treatment outcomes, and resource utilization in children and adults with eosinophilic gastroenteritis. Dig Liver Dis 2015;47(3):197–201.

76. Grandinetti T, Biedermann L, Bussmann C, et al. Eosinophilic gastroenteritis: clinical manifestation, natural course, and evaluation of treatment with corticosteroids and vedolizumab. Dig Dis Sci 2019;64(8):2231–41.

Dietary Management of Eosinophilic Esophagitis

Man Versus Food or Food Versus Man?

Joy W. Chang, MD, MS[a],*, Emily Haller, MS, RDN[a],
Evan S. Dellon, MD, MPH[b]

KEYWORDS

- Eosinophilic esophagitis • Food antigens • Diet elimination • Treatment

KEY POINTS

- An elimination diet is an effective first-line treatment for the long-term management of eosinophilic esophagitis and offers patients a nonpharmacologic alternative to disease control.
- Empiric elimination approaches are favored over allergy test-based approaches.
- Partnering with a dietitian or nutritionist is important to maximize adherence to and success of this treatment modality.

INTRODUCTION: FOOD VERSUS MAN

Eosinophilic esophagitis (EoE) is a recently recognized chronic inflammatory disease of both children and adults, characterized by symptoms of esophageal dysfunction and eosinophilia, which can lead to sequelae of fibrosis and strictures.[1-3] Since EoE was first described nearly 30 years ago, the prevalence and incidence have rapidly increased to as many as 1 case per 1000 people and up to 12.8 per 100,000 new cases per year, respectively.[4-6] EoE is now one of the most common causes of dysphagia, diagnosed in up to one-half of adults with an esophageal food impaction, up to 23% undergoing endoscopy for dysphagia, and up to 8% for the indication of reflux.[7-9] The clinical presentation in children can vary and include feeding difficulties, failure to thrive, vomiting, abdominal pain, and more typical reflux symptoms. Epidemiologic studies suggest that there are environmental and early life risk factors

[a] Division of Gastroenterology and Hepatology, Department of Internal Medicine, University of Michigan, 3912 Taubman Center, 1500 E. Medical Center Drive, SPC 5362, Ann Arbor, MI 48109, USA; [b] Division of Gastroenterology and Hepatology, Department of Internal Medicine, Center for Esophageal Diseases and Swallowing, University of North Carolina School of Medicine, CB #7080, Bioinformatics Building, 130 Mason Farm Road, Chapel Hill, NC 27599, USA
* Corresponding author.
E-mail address: chjoy@med.umich.edu
Twitter: @JoyWChang (J.W.C.)

Gastroenterol Clin N Am 50 (2021) 59–75
https://doi.org/10.1016/j.gtc.2020.10.009
0889-8553/21/© 2020 Elsevier Inc. All rights reserved.

Table 1
Pooled response rates for various diet therapy strategies

	Pediatrics	Adults
Elemental diet	90%	94%
6-food empiric elimination diet	73%	71%
4-food empiric elimination diet	60%	46%
2-food empiric elimination diet	43%	
1-food empiric elimination diet (milk only)	66%	100%
Targeted diet	48%	32%

Data from Arias A, Gonzalez-Cervera J, Tenias JM, et al. Efficacy of dietary interventions for inducing histologic remission in patients with eosinophilic esophagitis: a systematic review and meta-analysis. Gastroenterology 2014;146:1639-48 and Molina-Infante J, Arias A, Alcedo J, et al. Step-up empiric elimination diet for pediatric and adult eosinophilic esophagitis: The 2-4-6 study. J Allergy Clin Immunol 2018;141:1365-1372.

including aeroallergens, Cesarean delivery, prematurity, antibiotics, and formula feeding.[10,11] Similar to trends in other allergic disorders, the recent increase in EoE prevalence and incidence may also be related to changes in food processing. EoE is frequently associated with other atopic diseases including allergic rhinitis, asthma, eczema, and food allergies, suggesting common disease mechanisms.[12] EoE is a Th2-mediated response to food allergens, but does not seem to be IgE mediated.[13]

Current first-line treatments for EoE include diet elimination or medications (eg, proton pump inhibitors [PPI] and topical corticosteroids), with therapeutic goals of histologic, endoscopic, and symptomatic improvement.[14] Because the eosinophil-predominant inflammation is precipitated by food antigens (ie, food vs man), a dietary approach to treatment involving the avoidance of food triggers (ie, man vs food) has become an effective and acceptable long-term therapy for EoE. Since this concept was first validated in a landmark study reporting complete resolution of esophageal eosinophilia on an allergen-free formula, several prospective studies demonstrate the success of dietary elimination. The goal of EoE diet therapy is to induce disease remission by removing a set of foods from the diet, then systematically reintroducing single foods or food groups to identify which triggers to avoid in the long term (**Fig. 1**). Ideally, a smaller number of foods are initially eliminated, thus minimizing the amount of restrictions. Depending on a patients' individual values, attitudes, preferences, resources, and motivation, diet therapy can be an appealing option over pharmacologic treatments. The three dietary strategies for EoE include elemental diet, empiric elimination diet, and targeted elimination diet (**Table 1**).

TREATMENT OPTIONS: MAN VERSUS FOOD
Elemental Diet

As the first proof of concept that food antigens play a role in the pathogenesis of EoE, hypoallergenic amino acid–based elemental formula was shown to induce clinical and histologic remission in children.[15] This finding was validated by additional pediatric studies reporting histologic remission in up to 96%.[16,17] Later studies in adults also demonstrated significant improvement in esophageal eosinophilia and symptoms in up to 72% of patients.[18,19] A meta-analysis by Arias and colleagues[20] found a pooled histologic response rate to elemental formula of 91%. However, notable challenges in applying this diet include the need for an enteric feeding tube, poor palatability of the formula, and high financial cost because these feeds are often not covered by insurance. Additionally, food reintroduction is challenging because all foods have been

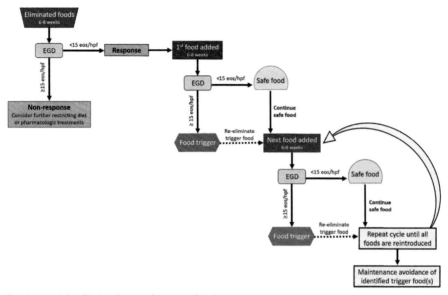

Fig. 1. Empiric elimination and reintroduction strategy.

eliminated, and thus must be sequentially added back. Although there are no standardized guidelines for the use of an elemental diet, we recommend gradual food reintroduction and identification of potential food triggers once histologic remission is demonstrated on an exclusively elemental diet for 4 to 6 weeks. In this setting, food groups that are thought to have a low trigger potential (ie, nonlegume vegetables, fruits, rice) can be added sequentially before an endoscopy, leaving more allergenic foods (ie, legumes, milk, egg, soy, wheat, nuts, meat, fish and shellfish, and corn) to be individually added last.[21]

Empiric Elimination Diets: Elimination, Reintroduction, and Maintenance

Six-food elimination diet

In contrast with the highly restrictive elemental formula approach, a more attractive and feasible option is empiric elimination. This approach focuses on inducing disease remission by removing the most common food triggers, systematic food reintroduction, and ultimately, avoidance of only the specific trigger(s) to maintain long-term disease control. The 6-food elimination diet (SFED) with avoidance of dairy, wheat, soy, eggs, nuts, and seafood is the prototypical empiric elimination diet in the United States (**Fig. 2**). In Spain, investigators using the SFED further eliminate cereal grains (eg, wheat, barley, rye, oats, rice, corn) and legumes. Kagalwalla and colleagues[22] first demonstrated a response rate of 74% with SFED (vs 88% on elemental diet) in children. Since then, success in attaining histologic remission on the SFED has been validated in children (ranging from 50% to 81%) and adults (ranging from 52% to 73%),[17,23–25] with a pooled rate of 72%.[20] Once patients have demonstrated resolution of eosinophilic inflammation and symptom improvement on the full elimination diet, each food group is sequentially added back beginning with the least allergenic, followed by endoscopy with biopsy to monitor response to food reintroduction. Ultimately, the goal of the elimination diet is to identify the particular food triggers that a patient should avoid to achieve long-term disease and symptom control. Guidance with a licensed dietitian is instrumental in providing education and practical tips to succeed and is recommended during all phases of diet therapy. Although the elimination diet is an effective strategy to attain drug-free disease control, downsides include

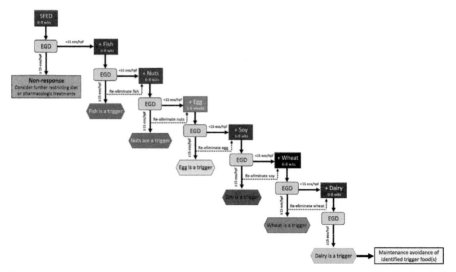

Fig. 2. Empiric SFED protocol. (*Adapted from* Kagalwalla AF, Wechsler JB, Amsden K, et al. Efficacy of a 4-Food Elimination Diet for Children With Eosinophilic Esophagitis. Clin Gastroenterol Hepatol 2017;15:1698-1707.)

adherence to a strict diet initially, at least 7 endoscopies to determine treatment response and food triggers, and long-term compliance with dietary trigger avoidance.

Four-food elimination diet

Since the introduction of the SFED, milk and wheat have been identified in food reintroduction studies as the most common EoE triggers and less commonly, nuts and fish/shellfish.[26] As a result, the 4-food elimination diet (4FED), which removes dairy, wheat, egg, and soy, was developed as an effective alternative with less dietary restrictions and fewer endoscopies to identify potential food triggers. Success with 47% histologic response ($\leq$5 eos/hpf, 60% with $\leq$10 eos/hpf) and 40% symptom improvement was achieved in a clinical study of children and adults undergoing 4FED.[27] A prospective study of adult Spanish patients with EoE avoiding milk, wheat, eggs, and legumes reported 54% clinicopathologic response and among those, milk was identified as the trigger in one-half of the participants.[28] In parallel, a prospective study of American children on the 4FED avoiding milk, wheat, egg, and soy demonstrated 64% response rates for histologic remission and symptom improvement in 91%.[29] Among these children, reintroduction phases showed that milk was the most common trigger in 85%, followed by egg (35%) and wheat (33%).

The 2-4-6 step-up diet

In an attempt to make EoE dietary elimination more patient-friendly, the Spanish group developed a "step-up" approach, beginning with elimination of milk and wheat or "2-food" elimination. This approach allows patients to avoid the most common food triggers first, and only move to additional restriction if there is nonresponse. In a prospective study of Spanish adults and children, 2-food elimination of milk, wheat, and gluten yielded a 43% clinical and histologic response rate.[30] Nonresponders were stepped up to increasingly restrictive diets (4FED and SFED) and subsequent remission rates were 54% for 4FED, and 79% for SFED. compared with starting with empiric SFED, this step-up strategy improves the time and number of endoscopies required by 20% to 30% and offers an efficient option for patients electing diet therapy. It is important to note, however, that at each step-up in restriction a proportion of patients opted to not continue with the protocol and sought out other treatments. Therefore, the response rates in the 4FED and 6FED groups are reflective of highly motivated and adherent patients.

Milk elimination

Because milk is the most common EoE trigger, dairy exclusion or a 1-food elimination diet (1FED) is also a reasonable approach in diet therapy. An early retrospective study of pediatric patients with EoE undergoing cow's milk elimination reported histologic and clinical remission in 65%.[31] This finding was further validated by prospective pediatric studies showing histologic response rates ranging from 43% to 64% to cow's milk elimination, presenting the possibility for an even more abbreviated and less burdensome option to diet therapy.[32–34] A recent multisite prospective randomized clinical trial of children undergoing 12 weeks of 1FED versus 4FED reported that, although symptom improvement was found to be greater in the 4FED, the histologic response rates were similar between the 2 diets (44% for 1FED, 41% for 4FED). Furthermore, quality of life was improved with 1FED compared with 4FED.[35] Success with exclusive milk elimination was also reported in a recent retrospective study of pediatric patients attaining histologic remission in 57% with 1FED compared with 52% with SFED.[36] For adults, a multisite randomized clinical trial of 1FED versus SFED is currently underway (NCT02778867) and may further highlight dairy elimination as a reasonable first treatment option in EoE. Finally, there has been one modeling study that attempted to clarify an optimal empiric elimination approach based on published food trigger data.[37] This study suggested that a "1 to 3" diet, where dairy is eliminated first and then wheat and eggs are additionally eliminated if there is no response to dairy, and a "1-4-8" diet, which steps up from dairy, to 4FED, and then to an additional elimination of corn, chicken, beef, and pork, are optimal depending on the treatment goal (most effective response, which is 1-4-8, or least number of endoscopies, which is 1–3). However, these strategies have yet to be tested clinically.

Concomitant Proton Pump Inhibitor Therapy

For patients who prefer a medication-free approach to treatment, the empiric elimination diet is often prescribed without concurrent pharmacologic therapies. PPIs are also a first-line treatment and estimated to be effective in up to half of patients with EoE.[38] In a recent Australian multisite clinical trial, histologic remission was higher in pediatric patients receiving PPI plus 4FED (88%) versus PPI alone (45%).[39] Similarly, children who received PPI with a dairy-free diet demonstrated higher histologic response rates (61%) compared with those treated with dairy-free diet alone (25%).[36] This result suggests there might be a synergistic effect between diet and PPI treatment, but the mechanism of this effect is not known.

Targeted Elimination Diet

In contrast with empiric elimination of common EoE food triggers, targeted elimination diet is avoidance of foods identified by traditional allergy testing such as a skin prick test, atopy patch test, or serum-specific IgE testing. This would seem to make intuitive sense; if EoE is a food-triggered disease, then allergy tests should identify the food trigger. Indeed, initial studies in children demonstrated response rates ranging from 53% to 72% using a skin prick test and an atopy patch test.[17,40] In contrast, more recent data showing low responses from 12% to 37% to an atopy patch test in children with EoE has put the benefit of allergy testing for EoE in question.[41–43] Adult studies also showed poor concordance (13%) between the skin prick test and identified EoE trigger foods.[24,25,44,45] In the meta-analysis by Arias and colleagues,[20] the pooled response rate to targeted elimination was 46%, lower that either elemental formula or SFED. As a result of these findings suggesting that conventional allergy testing is unreliable to identify EoE triggers, this process is no longer recommended as a dietary approach to EoE treatment and may be detrimental if patients are prescribed strict or overly restrictive diets based on testing.

CHALLENGES OF DIETARY THERAPY: FOOD VERSUS MAN

Although diet therapy is an effective means of maintaining disease control by addressing the root cause of food antigens in EoE, several challenges in adopting this treatment strategy are worth mentioning. Practical downsides to elimination diets include adherence to a strict diet and frequent endoscopies initially, financial costs and burden of a special diet, long-term compliance with dietary trigger avoidance, and potential losses in quality of life.

Cost and Burden

For the long-term management of celiac disease, the increased cost of commercially available gluten-free products is estimated to range from 183% to 242% more expensive compared with regular foods.[46,47] Along similar lines, the empiric elimination diet for EoE includes the exclusion of ubiquitous and commonly consumed food groups and purchase of specialty foods, resulting in significant financial costs and burden to patients. From a payer perspective, the SFED is reported to be more cost effective than topical corticosteroids, likely owing to the high cost of long-term medication use. However, this factor does not account for patient-level food costs not covered by insurance or decrements in quality of life.[48,49] Perhaps more impactful, a study of real-world patient-level costs using grocery store prices showed that adherence to an SFED costs $650 per year more than an unrestricted diet.[50] Additionally, purchasing foods for an SFED required visiting more than one grocery or specialty store, increasing the shopping burden for patients and families. Other notable but less observed costs include days of missed work or school for both patients and caregivers, as well as increased insurance costs.[51]

Because clinical symptoms do not correlate well with esophageal inflammation and underlying disease activity, endoscopy with esophageal biopsies is recommended to guide decisions about treatment.[52,53] The empiric elimination diet and systematic food reintroduction requires frequent endoscopies to monitor response and determination of food triggers. Patients undergoing SFED ought to expect a minimum of six endoscopies over one year's time, but this process can be prolonged with more procedures if food triggers are identified during reintroduction, reflecting a significant burden on time and convenience on both patients and their families.

Nonresponse to Diet Therapy

Although diet therapy can be an effective treatment for EoE for many, several factors may impact either symptomatic or histologic response and should be considered in the nonresponsive patient. Nonadherence to the diet is perhaps the most obvious cause, which may be due to the increased financial cost of dietary alternatives, lack of knowledge and support, lack of positive results, or a desire to consume trigger foods. Cross-contamination can also occur and may be prevented or minimized with guidance from a dietitian. Finally, because current treatment end points include improvement of symptoms, endoscopic findings, and histology, persistent fibrostenotic disease and stricture management with endoscopic dilation should be considered in the setting of ongoing symptoms despite histologic remission. Conversely, in patients who report subjective symptom improvement but fail to attain histologic remission, a detailed history about recent dilation and modified eating behaviors should be further investigated. Finally, there is one report that some patients with initial symptomatic and endoscopic, but no histologic, improvement may benefit from an extended course of dietary elimination, and ultimately achieve remission after at least 12 weeks of dietary adherence.[54]

Adherence and Long-Term Effectiveness

Despite the effectiveness of diet therapy, long-term avoidance of food triggers can be burdensome, resulting in nonadherence and recurrence of disease activity. The short-term effectiveness of diet exclusion is well-established, but response rates may wane owing to decreased adherence. Studies of long-term follow-up outcomes of the SFED in up to three years report that less than one-half of patients sustain histologic response owing to nonadherence to the diet,[24,55–57] although one study does report excellent long-term remission rates.[25] Factors impacting adherence to diet therapy include treatment effectiveness, limitations of social situations, and anxiety related to the diet.[57]

Quality of Life

Patients with EoE experience impaired quality of life, not only from symptoms, but also around eating, social, and emotional impacts, as well as anxiety around their disease and choking.[58–60] Treatments significantly improve quality of life, but the burdens of the treatments themselves are often overlooked. Although initial study of adults undergoing SFED showed increase in overall quality of life as measured with the Short Form-36, individual mental well-being scores decreased.[24] Similarly, the mental component score of the Short Form-36 assessment was lower in adult patients with EoE undergoing empiric elimination diet.[61] In a prospective study of adult Spanish patients with EoE, emotional impact was significantly worse in those undergoing dietary restriction, but the overall quality of life scores were not significantly worse compared with those without restriction and undergoing pharmacologic therapies.[62] In the pediatric population, children treated with diet reported lower quality of life scores,[63,64] highlighting realistic psychosocial concerns about initiating restrictive diets in young patients.

Access to Other Support

Because implementing diet therapy can be challenging for both patients and clinicians, we recommend that all patients attempting an elimination diet do so with the support of a dietitian. Dietitian support is critical, not only to improve diet adherence during the elimination phase, but also to provide personalized education and practical guidance on how to maintain a nutritionally balanced and palatable diet. Despite increasing interest in dietary interventions for several gastrointestinal diseases, such as irritable bowel syndrome, inflammatory bowel disease, and gastroesophageal reflux disease, many patients and providers realistically may not have access to a dietitian or nutrition resources, and many gastroenterology providers (especially those caring for adults) may not have had adequate training in nutrition and face time constraints during clinic visits to provide patient support. In a recent provider survey, only 65% of respondents reported having readily available support with a licensed dietitian when recommending diet therapy.[65] In parallel, only 36% patients with eosinophilic gastrointestinal disorders reported having easy access to a dietitian or nutritionist who understood the challenges of eosinophilic gastrointestinal disorders.[66]

Although the use of allergy testing to guide elimination diets has been supplanted by empiric elimination diets, clinical support by an allergist for patients with concomitant atopic disorders is very helpful in the management of EoE. This is particularly true given the high prevalence of atopy in children and adults with EoE including allergic rhinitis, asthma, and atopic dermatitis. Additionally, a multidisciplinary approach between the gastroenterologist and allergist may be advantageous for concomitant IgE mediated food reactions and potentially in unique cases of nonresponse to the empiric elimination diet.

PRACTICAL TIPS AND CONSIDERATIONS FOR STARTING DIET THERAPY

When considering starting treatment for EoE, all options including diet, pharmacologic therapy (e.g. PPI, topical corticosteroids), and endoscopic dilation ought to be presented to the patient. Success with an elimination diet depends on both patient selection and ability execute the avoidance and food reintroduction phases.

Considerations in patient selection for diet therapy
• Patient's desire and motivation to undergo diet therapy
• Personal preferences and values
• Patient's age, life stage, living situation, lifestyle (e.g. ability to adhere to a strict diet)
• Patient's willingness to have frequent endoscopies and travel
• Patient's finances and insurance coverage (e.g. high deductibles for procedures)

Practical Aspects of Applying Diet Therapy for Initial and Maintenance Treatment

When working with a registered dietitian, commonly addressed patient concerns include ensuring the diet is healthy and meets nutrient needs, travel and dining out tips, what foods are allowed and specific product options, cross-contamination, and nutrition label reading.

Navigating the supermarket
• Where to shop, specific to patient location and access
• Use of online ordering/shopping for specialty items if or as desired
• Food labels: education on the Food Allergen Labeling and Consumer Protection Act, which mandates that companies list foods containing major allergens including milk, wheat, eggs, fish, shellfish, peanuts, tree nuts, and soy in plain language.
• Review of precautionary labeling (i.e. May contain [fish]; Manufactured in a facility that uses [egg] ingredients; Manufactured in a facility which processes [egg])
Dining out and social events
• Doerfler's "Dining Out Checklist"[67]
• Bring a dish or appetizer of safe foods
• Shift the focus away from food and toward an activity
Nutritional implications of diet therapy
• Ensure macronutrient and micronutrient needs are met
• Provide hypoallergenic multivitamin recommendations, potential use of vitamin D and/or calcium supplements
Diet "holidays"
• During the diet therapy trial there may be times after a patient completes a reintroduction that they need a break or "diet holiday" and may need to lift their diet restrictions. If this happens, endoscopy must be scheduled 6 to 8 weeks out from when they resume the diet.
• If the patient is responsive to both diet therapy and medications, they may also elect to switch between the 2 treatment modalities for periods of time depending on life events and situation (e.g. around traveling or holidays if known food allergens may be consumed).

What to expect during dietitian-guided EoE diet therapy

Initial visit with dietitian consists of (1-hour visit)

1. Thorough diet history including a patient's food preferences, eating habits, known food allergies and intolerances, a diet recall of typical a weekday and weekends, symptoms (i.e. dysphagia), vitamin/mineral and supplement use.
2. Nutrition education
   - Comprehensive review of avoiding food allergens (e.g. 2-, 4-,SFED) that will need to be avoided and individualized dietary advice. Recommendations of what to eat should be customized to a patient's food preferences, cooking knowledge and skills, as well as local food availability and access.
   - Meal and snack ideas and preparation tips, creating a balanced plate
   - Review of common sources of cross-contamination at home, dining out, and in the grocery store (i.e. cooking equipment and surfaces, shared sponges, shared condiments, bulk bins, deli slicers, salad bars); review of high-risk foods and situations.
   - Resources provided
     ○ Sample menu of meal, snack, and beverage ideas (**Box 1**)
     ○ List of "allowed foods" (**Table 2**)
     ○ Groetch's "Cooking without Common Allergens"[68]
     ○ FARE "Tips for Avoiding Your Allergen"[69]
     ○ Computer and phone resources available (Pinterest board, Yummly.com and phone applications)
     ○ Cookbook recommendations

Follow-up nutrition reassessment during food reintroduction (telephone visit, 30 minutes)

- Assess how the patient feels (i.e. their energy, weight maintenance, how they are dealing with life on the diet, any questions and/or concerns)
- Screening for any potential deficiencies and diet recall
- Review of food reintroduction
- Recommend eating the challenge food daily or every other day, providing examples of what foods to use, and reinforcing checking all nutrition labels and ingredients for other allergens. For example, during soy challenge, a patient could use soymilk, soy yogurt, edamame, tofu, and soy sauce that must be labeled as gluten free, reinforcing that regular soy sauce contains wheat.

Box 1
Six-food elimination diet sample menu

Breakfast
- Gluten-free oatmeal with ½ cup fresh berries, topped with ground flaxseed or chia seeds, rice milk

Lunch
- Corn quesadilla or tacos with chicken or black beans, vegan cheese products (soy free)[a] like Daiya Cheddar Style Shreds, salsa, avocado

Dinner
- Gluten-free pasta[a] or spaghetti squash with ground turkey/beef or lentils, allowed marinara sauce,[a] broccoli; side salad with homemade or bottled dressing[a]

Snack ideas
- Popcorn
- Corn tortilla chips and salsa or guacamole[a]
- Hummus[a] with vegetables (baby carrots, cucumber, bell pepper, broccoli, etc)
- Fruit and small handful pumpkin/sunflower seeds
- Apple or banana with Sunbutter

[a] Read ingredients on all packaged foods for dairy (milk), wheat, egg, soy, fish, and nuts.

Table 2
Six-food elimination diet "allowed foods" list

Dairy Group	Proteins	Grains and Starches Group	Fats and Oils	Beverages	Fruits and Vegetables
Coconut milk/yogurt/ice cream	All nonprocessed meats:	Corn and Rice Chex[a]	Avocado	Coffee (with dairy free creamer)	All fresh fruits and vegetables Processed fruits and vegetables[a]
Flax milk	Beef	Corn tortillas[a]	Dairy and soy-free margarine	Fruit juice	
Hemp milk	Chicken	Corn flour	Oil, any type	Rice/coconut/flax/hemp milk	
Oat milk (must be from gluten free oats)	Lamb	Gluten-free breads/cereals/baked goods[a]	Seeds	Soft drinks	
Pea milk	Pork	Gluten-free crackers[a]	Sunflower seed butter	Tea[a]	
Rice milk/ice cream[a]	Turkey	Gluten-free flour/baking mixes[a]	Vegan mayo (ie, Veganaise)	Water	
Vegan cheese products (soy-free)[a]	Venison	Gluten-free pasta: rice, quinoa, corn, lentil/black bean[a]		Alcohol: wine, gluten-free beer, plain distilled liquors	
	Legumes (other than soybeans)	Grits			
	Processed meats[a]	Gluten-free oatmeal[a]			
	Protein powders: rice, hemp, pea, quinoa[a]	Popcorn[a]			
		Potato			
		Potato chips[a]			
		Quinoa			
		Rice			
		Rice/popcorn cakes[a]			
		Soba noodles (buckwheat)[a]			
		Tortilla chips[a]			
		Sweet potato			

[a] Please be careful to read all labels for dairy (milk), wheat, egg, soy (soy oil and soy lecithin is ok), nuts, and fish/shellfish. This eliminates many of the common foods in the typical US diet.

NOVEL TESTING AND FUTURE DIRECTIONS: MAN VERSUS FOOD

With advancements in refining dietary approaches for EoE, several unanswered questions arise around better identifying food triggers, developing less invasive testing for the reintroduction phases, quantifying how much allergen must be avoided for disease remission, and assessing how much time is required to induce disease activity with food or conversely, to washout an allergen.

Given recent data to support the role of food-specific IgG4 in EoE,[70] a recent novel allergen-specific signature testing approach to identify triggers using lymphocyte proliferation assays and esophageal IgG4 levels demonstrated accuracy rates approaching 53% to 75%, outperforming traditional allergy testing.[71] In this pilot work, histologic, endoscopic, and symptomatic improvements were observed, and on average, only two to three trigger foods were necessary to eliminate. However, the histologic response rate was only 25% among diet-compliant subjects.[71] Another novel approach to identifying food triggers is the esophageal prick test in which allergen extracts are endoscopically injected into the esophageal mucosa.[72] In response to wheat, soy, milk, and other allergens, acute and delayed responses were observed in patients with EoE, but not controls. Based on successfully epicutaneous immunotherapy desensitization for IgE-mediated milk and peanut reactions, a recent pilot study demonstrated histologic response in 47% of milk-induced patients with EoE in a per-protocol analysis.[73] Although these approaches are not ready for clinical use, they highlight the need for personalized approaches to guide and simplify dietary restrictions.

During the food reintroduction phase, serial endoscopy is currently required to identify trigger foods. This comes at the cost of several endoscopies, burdens of time and convenience, and risks associated with sedation. These are all limitations to patient acceptability of the dietary elimination approach. Less invasive alternatives to traditional endoscopy are needed and include unsedated transnasal endoscopy, Cytosponge, and the Esophageal String Test. Unsedated transnasal endoscopy with collection of esophageal biopsies can be easily and safely performed in the outpatient setting, is well-tolerated by adult and pediatric patients, and significantly reduced costs compared with sedated esophagogastroduodenoscopy.[74–79] The novel Cytosponge device is a swallowed capsule with an attached string, which expands into a mesh sponge and collects esophageal epithelial specimens when pulled back through the mouth, was initially developed for Barrett's esophagus screening and has an excellent safety profile.[80,81] The Cytosponge has now been shown to be a safe and accurate method to not only assess histologic activity in EoE, but also in pilot data to direct food reintroduction after 6-food elimination, offering an alternative test for monitoring of EoE.[82,83] Additionally, compared with traditional endoscopy with biopsies, this method was found to be considerably less expensive. The Esophageal String Test (EST) is a similarly ingestible capsule attached to a string, which unravels and absorbs esophageal inflammatory samples when withdrawn. In a prospective, multisite study of pediatric and adult patients with EoE, EST accurately identified active versus inactive disease and eosinophil-associated biomarkers obtained from EST correlated with endoscopic severity scores and peak eosinophil counts.[84] Although these minimally alternatives are not currently available for clinical use, they offer promise for techniques in the near-future to streamline diet therapy.

For many patients electing diet therapy, a commonly asked question is how strictly to avoid food triggers. For celiac disease, absolute adherence to a gluten-free diet is supported as the only treatment and tolerable gluten contamination is recommended to be less than 50 miligram per day.[85,86] These thresholds for EoE food triggers and the dose responses to food antigens remain unknown, and may be key factors in understanding patient adherence and long-term effectiveness of the elimination diet. Additionally, a 6- to 8-week time interval is currently recommended between food reintroductions, but the time to histologic, symptomatic, and endoscopic recovery is unclear.

SUMMARY

Diet therapy can be an effective, feasible, and durable means of controlling both the symptoms and eosinophilic inflammation in EoE. As an alternative to pharmacologic therapies, this first-line treatment strategy is ideally directed at the allergic basis of EoE by avoiding food antigen triggers; it is a "man versus food" approach. The elemental diet devoid of food allergens yields the best response, but a formula-based diet without solid foods and prolonged food reintroduction can be unpalatable and onerous. In contrast to an allergen-free diet, a targeted elimination approach is limited by poor predictive values of allergy testing to identify EoE food triggers. As a result, allergy testing is not recommended to guide EoE diet therapy in children or adults. The empiric elimination diet involving removal of the most common food triggers and systemic reintroduction is a more acceptable and recommended approach to identifying which foods should be avoided to maintain long-term disease control. However, implementation of the diet is often faced with challenges such as financial cost, inconvenience, patient adherence, cross-contamination, quality of life, and access to resources including nutritional support and endoscopic procedures. Success on diet therapy and long-term adherence relies not only on patient motivation, but can be augmented by partnering with a dietitian who can provide education, feedback, and personalized nutritional treatment plans. Acknowledging these potential barriers and patient preferences, pharmacologic treatments are also reasonable options to maintain disease control in patients who do not respond to dietary restriction, need respite from food avoidance, or struggle with diet adherence. Future directions for EoE dietary therapy include the use of minimally invasive diagnostic tools to simplify food reintroduction and optimizing testing to identify individualized food triggers.

CLINICS CARE POINTS

- Diet therapy is effective at inducing and maintaining disease remission and is an alternative to pharmacologic therapies.
- Empiric elimination and elemental diets are effective in in 43-91% of patients with eosinophilic esophagitis and offers advantages over allergy-test targeted diets.
- The six-food elimination diet meets USDA dietary guidelines for adults.
- Patient-level barriers to the effectiveness of diet therapy include compliance to a restrictive diet, contamination, and education.
- Identifying strategies to maximize patient quality of life and adherence are crucial to successful implementation of diet therapy.

DISCLOSURE

This work was supported in part by NIH award number R01 DK101856.

REFERENCES

1. Furuta GT, Liacouras CA, Collins MH, et al. Eosinophilic esophagitis in children and adults: a systematic review and consensus recommendations for diagnosis and treatment. Gastroenterology 2007;133:1342–63.

2. Liacouras CA, Furuta GT, Hirano I, et al. Eosinophilic esophagitis: updated consensus recommendations for children and adults. J Allergy Clin Immunol 2011;128:3–20.

3. Dellon ES, Gonsalves N, Hirano I, et al. ACG clinical guideline: evidenced based approach to the diagnosis and management of esophageal eosinophilia and eosinophilic esophagitis (EoE). Am J Gastroenterol 2013;108:679–92.

4. Dellon ES. Epidemiology of eosinophilic esophagitis. Gastroenterol Clin North Am 2014;43:201–18.

5. Dellon ES, Erichsen R, Baron JA, et al. The increasing incidence and prevalence of eosinophilic oesophagitis outpaces changes in endoscopic and biopsy practice: national population-based estimates from Denmark. Aliment Pharmacol Ther 2015;41:662–70.

6. Dellon ES, Hirano I. Epidemiology and natural history of eosinophilic esophagitis. Gastroenterology 2018;154:319–32.

7. Prasad GA, Talley NJ, Romero Y, et al. Prevalence and predictive factors of eosinophilic esophagitis in patients presenting with dysphagia: a prospective study. Am J Gastroenterol 2007;102:2627–32.

8. Veerappan GR, Perry JL, Duncan TJ, et al. Prevalence of eosinophilic esophagitis in an adult population undergoing upper endoscopy: a prospective study. Clin Gastroenterol Hepatol 2009;7:420–6.

9. Dellon ES, Speck O, Woodward K, et al. Clinical and endoscopic characteristics do not reliably differentiate PPI-responsive esophageal eosinophilia and eosinophilic esophagitis in patients undergoing upper endoscopy: a prospective cohort study. Am J Gastroenterol 2013;108:1854–60.

10. Jensen ET, Kappelman MD, Kim HP, et al. Early life exposures as risk factors for pediatric eosinophilic esophagitis. J Pediatr Gastroenterol Nutr 2013;57:67–71.

11. Jensen ET, Kuhl JT, Martin LJ, et al. Prenatal, intrapartum, and postnatal factors are associated with pediatric eosinophilic esophagitis. J Allergy Clin Immunol 2018;141:214–22.

12. Jyonouchi S, Brown-Whitehorn TA, Spergel JM. Association of eosinophilic gastrointestinal disorders with other atopic disorders. Immunol Allergy Clin North Am 2009;29:85–97.

13. Simon D, Marti H, Heer P, et al. Eosinophilic esophagitis is frequently associated with IgE-mediated allergic airway diseases. J Allergy Clin Immunol 2005;115:1090–2.

14. Dellon ES, Gupta SK. A conceptual approach to understanding treatment response in eosinophilic esophagitis. Clin Gastroenterol Hepatol 2019;17:2149–60.

15. Kelly KJ, Lazenby AJ, Rowe PC, et al. Eosinophilic esophagitis attributed to gastroesophageal reflux: improvement with an amino acid-based formula. Gastroenterology 1995;109:1503–12.

16. Markowitz JE, Spergel JM, Ruchelli E, et al. Elemental diet is an effective treatment for eosinophilic esophagitis in children and adolescents. Am J Gastroenterol 2003;98:777–82.

17. Spergel JM, Brown-Whitehorn TF, Cianferoni A, et al. Identification of causative foods in children with eosinophilic esophagitis treated with an elimination diet. J Allergy Clin Immunol 2012;130:461–7.

18. Peterson KA, Byrne KR, Vinson LA, et al. Elemental diet induces histologic response in adult eosinophilic esophagitis. Am J Gastroenterol 2013;108:759–66.

19. Warners MJ, Vlieg-Boerstra BJ, Verheij J, et al. Elemental diet decreases inflammation and improves symptoms in adult eosinophilic oesophagitis patients. Aliment Pharmacol Ther 2017;45:777–87.

20. Arias A, Gonzalez-Cervera J, Tenias JM, et al. Efficacy of dietary interventions for inducing histologic remission in patients with eosinophilic esophagitis: a systematic review and meta-analysis. Gastroenterology 2014;146:1639–48.

21. Dellon ES, Liacouras CA. Advances in clinical management of eosinophilic esophagitis. Gastroenterology 2014;147:1238–54.

22. Kagalwalla AF, Sentongo TA, Ritz S, et al. Effect of six-food elimination diet on clinical and histologic outcomes in eosinophilic esophagitis. Clin Gastroenterol Hepatol 2006;4:1097–102.

23. Henderson CJ, Abonia JP, King EC, et al. Comparative dietary therapy effectiveness in remission of pediatric eosinophilic esophagitis. J Allergy Clin Immunol 2012;129:1570–8.

24. Gonsalves N, Yang GY, Doerfler B, et al. Elimination diet effectively treats eosinophilic esophagitis in adults; food reintroduction identifies causative factors. Gastroenterology 2012;142:1451–9.

25. Lucendo AJ, Arias A, Gonzalez-Cervera J, et al. Empiric 6-food elimination diet induced and maintained prolonged remission in patients with adult eosinophilic esophagitis: a prospective study on the food cause of the disease. J Allergy Clin Immunol 2013;131:797–804.

26. Kagalwalla AF, Shah A, Li BU, et al. Identification of specific foods responsible for inflammation in children with eosinophilic esophagitis successfully treated with empiric elimination diet. J Pediatr Gastroenterol Nutr 2011;53:145–9.

27. Gonsalves N, Doerfler B, Schwartz S, et al. Prospective trial of four food elimination diet demonstrates comparable effectiveness in the treatment of adult and pediatric eosinophilic esophagitis. Gastroenterology 2013;144:S-1–54.

28. Molina-Infante J, Arias A, Barrio J, et al. Four-food group elimination diet for adult eosinophilic esophagitis: a prospective multicenter study. J Allergy Clin Immunol 2014;134:1093–9.

29. Kagalwalla AF, Wechsler JB, Amsden K, et al. Efficacy of a 4-food elimination diet for children with eosinophilic esophagitis. Clin Gastroenterol Hepatol 2017;15: 1698–707.

30. Molina-Infante J, Arias A, Alcedo J, et al. Step-up empiric elimination diet for pediatric and adult eosinophilic esophagitis: the 2-4-6 study. J Allergy Clin Immunol 2018;141:1365–72.

31. Kagalwalla AF, Amsden K, Shah A, et al. Cow's milk elimination: a novel dietary approach to treat eosinophilic esophagitis. J Pediatr Gastroenterol Nutr 2012; 55:711–6.

32. Kruszewski PG, Russo JM, Franciosi JP, et al. Prospective, comparative effectiveness trial of cow's milk elimination and swallowed fluticasone for pediatric eosinophilic esophagitis. Dis Esophagus 2016;29:377–84.

33. Wechsler JB, Schwartz S, Ross JN, et al. Cow's milk elimination for treatment of eosinophilic esophagitis: a prospective pediatric study. Gastroenterology 2017; 152:S855.

34. Teoh T, Mill C, Chan E, et al. Liberalized versus strict cow's milk elimination for the treatment of children with eosinophilic esophagitis. J Can Assoc Gastroenterol 2019;2:81–5.

35. Kliewer K, Aceves S, Atkins D, et al. Efficacy of 1-food and 4-food elimination diets for pediatric eosinophilic esophagitis in a randomized multi-site study. Gastroenterology 2019;156. S-172-S-173.

36. Wong J, Goodine S, Samela K, et al. Efficacy of dairy free diet and 6-food elimination diet as initial therapy for pediatric eosinophilic esophagitis: a retrospective single-center study. Pediatr Gastroenterol Hepatol Nutr 2020;23:79–88.
37. Zhan T, Ali A, Choi JG, et al. Model to determine the optimal dietary elimination strategy for treatment of eosinophilic esophagitis. Clin Gastroenterol Hepatol 2018;16:1730–7.
38. Lucendo AJ, Arias A, Molina-Infante J. Efficacy of proton pump inhibitor drugs for inducing clinical and histologic remission in patients with symptomatic esophageal eosinophilia: a systematic review and meta-analysis. Clin Gastroenterol Hepatol 2016;14:13–22.
39. Heine RG, Peters R, Cameron DJ, et al. Effect of a 4-food elimination diet and omeprazole in children with eosinophilic esophagitis – a randomized, controlled trial. J Allergy Clin Immunol 2019;143:AB309.
40. Spergel JM, Andrews T, Brown-Whitehorn TF, et al. Treatment of eosinophilic esophagitis with specific food elimination diet directed by a combination of skin prick and patch tests. Ann Allergy Asthma Immunol 2005;95:336–43.
41. Assa'ad AH, Putnam PE, Collins MH, et al. Pediatric patients with eosinophilic esophagitis: an 8-year follow-up. J Allergy Clin Immunol 2007;119:731–8.
42. Rizo Pascual JM, De La Hoz Caballer B, Redondo Verge C, et al. Allergy assessment in children with eosinophilic esophagitis. J Investig Allergol Clin Immunol 2011;21:59–65.
43. Paquet B, Begin P, Paradis L, et al. Variable yield of allergy patch testing in children with eosinophilic esophagitis. J Allergy Clin Immunol 2013;131:613.
44. Philpott H, Nandurkar S, Royce SG, et al. Allergy tests do not predict food triggers in adult patients with eosinophilic oesophagitis. A comprehensive prospective study using five modalities. Aliment Pharmacol Ther 2016;44:223–33.
45. Eckmann JD, Ravi K, Katzka DA, et al. Efficacy of atopy patch testing in directed dietary therapy of eosinophilic esophagitis: a pilot study. Dig Dis Sci 2018;63:694–702.
46. Stevens L, Rashid M. Gluten-free and regular foods: a cost comparison. Can J Diet Pract Res 2008;69:147–50.
47. Lee AR, Wolf RL, Lebwohl B, et al. Persistent economic burden of the gluten free diet. Nutrients 2019;11:399.
48. Schneider Y, Saumoy M, Otaki F, et al. A cost-effectiveness analysis of treatment options for adult eosinophilic esophagitis utilizing a Markov model. Am J Gastroenterol 2016;111:S213–24.
49. Cotton CC, Erim D, Eluri S, et al. Cost utility analysis of topical steroids compared with dietary elimination for treatment of eosinophilic esophagitis. Clin Gastroenterol Hepatol 2017;15:841–9.
50. Wolf WA, Huang KZ, Durban R, et al. The six-food elimination diet for eosinophilic esophagitis increases grocery shopping cost and complexity. Dysphagia 2016;31:765–70.
51. Leiman DA, Kochar B, Posner S, et al. A diagnosis of eosinophilic esophagitis is associated with increased life insurance premiums. Dis Esophagus 2018;31:doy008.
52. Pentiuk S, Putnam PE, Collins MH, et al. Dissociation between symptoms and histological severity in pediatric eosinophilic esophagitis. J Pediatr Gastroenterol Nutr 2009;48:152–60.
53. Dellon ES, Woodward K, Speck O, et al. Symptoms do not correlate with histologic response in eosinophilic esophagitis. Gastroenterology 2012;142:S-432.

54. Philpott H, Dellon E. Histologic improvement after 6 weeks of dietary elimination for eosinophilic esophagitis may be insufficient to determine efficacy. Asia Pac Allergy 2018;8:e20.

55. Philpott H, Nandurkar S, Royce SG, et al. A prospective open clinical trial of a proton pump inhibitor, elimination diet and/or budesonide for eosinophilic oesophagitis. Aliment Pharmacol Ther 2016;43:985–93.

56. Reed CC, Fan C, Koutlas NT, et al. Food elimination diets are effective for long-term treatment of adults with eosinophilic oesophagitis. Aliment Pharmacol Ther 2017;46:836–44.

57. Wang R, Hirano I, Doerfler B, et al. Assessing adherence and barriers to long-term elimination diet therapy in adults with eosinophilic esophagitis. Dig Dis Sci 2018;63:1756–62.

58. Taft TH, Kern E, Keefer L, et al. Qualitative assessment of patient-reported outcomes in adults with eosinophilic esophagitis. J Clin Gastroenterol 2011;45: 769–74.

59. Safroneeva E, Coslovsky M, Kuehni CE, et al. Eosinophilic oesophagitis: relationship of quality of life with clinical, endoscopic and histological activity. Aliment Pharmacol Ther 2015;42:1000–10.

60. Mukkada V, Falk GW, Eichinger CS, et al. Health-related quality of life and costs associated with eosinophilic esophagitis: a systematic review. Clin Gastroenterol Hepatol 2018;16:495–503.

61. Chang N, Raja S, Betancourt R, et al. Impact of eosinophilic esophagitis disease activity on quality of life: results from a prospective patient registry. Gastroenterology. 2020 May;158(6):S-831–S832.

62. Lucendo AJ, Arias-Gonzalez L, Molina-Infante J, et al. Determinant factors of quality of life in adult patients with eosinophilic esophagitis. United European Gastroenterol J 2018;6:38–45.

63. Franciosi JP, Hommel KA, Bendo CB, et al. PedsQL eosinophilic esophagitis module: feasibility, reliability, and validity. J Pediatr Gastroenterol Nutr 2013;57: 57–66.

64. Menard-Katcher P, Marks KL, Liacouras CA, et al. The natural history of eosinophilic oesophagitis in the transition from childhood to adulthood. Aliment Pharmacol Ther 2013;37:114–21.

65. Chang JW, Saini SD, Mellinger JL, et al. Management of eosinophilic esophagitis is often discordant with guidelines and not patient-centered: results of a survey of gastroenterologists. Dis Esophagus 2019;32:doy133.

66. Hiremath G, Kodroff E, Strobel MJ, et al. Individuals affected by eosinophilic gastrointestinal disorders have complex unmet needs and frequently experience unique barriers to care. Clin Res Hepatol Gastroenterol 2018;42:483–93.

67. Doerfler B, Bryce P, Hirano I, et al. Practical approach to implementing dietary therapy in adults with eosinophilic esophagitis: the Chicago experience. Dis Esophagus 2015;28:42–58.

68. Groetch M, Venter C, Skypala I, et al. Dietary therapy and nutrition management of eosinophilic esophagitis: a work group report of the American Academy of Allergy, Asthma, and Immunology. J Allergy Clin Immunol Pract 2017;5:312–24.

69. Food Allergy Research and Education. Tips for avoiding your allergen. McLean (VA): Your Food Allergy Field Guide; 2018. p. 13–4.

70. Wright BL, Kulis M, Guo R, et al. Food-specific IgG4 is associated with eosinophilic esophagitis. J Allergy Clin Immunol 2016;138:1190–2.

71. Dellon ES, Guo R, McGee SJ, et al. A novel allergen-specific immune signature-directed approach to dietary elimination in eosinophilic esophagitis. Clin Transl Gastroenterol 2019;10:e00099.
72. Warners MJ, Terreehorst I, van den Wijngaard RM, et al. Abnormal responses to local esophageal food allergen injections in adult patients with eosinophilic esophagitis. Gastroenterology 2018;154:57–60.
73. Spergel JM, Elci OU, Muir AB, et al. Efficacy of epicutaneous immunotherapy in children with milk-induced eosinophilic esophagitis. Clin Gastroenterol Hepatol 2020;18:328–36.
74. Jobe BA, Hunter JG, Chang EY, et al. Office-based unsedated small-caliber endoscopy is equivalent to conventional sedated endoscopy in screening and surveillance for Barrett's esophagus: a randomized and blinded comparison. Am J Gastroenterol 2006;101:2693–703.
75. Sami SS, Subramanian V, Ortiz-Fernandez-Sordo J, et al. Performance characteristics of unsedated ultrathin video endoscopy in the assessment of the upper GI tract: systematic review and meta-analysis. Gastrointest Endosc 2015;82:782–92.
76. Friedlander JA, DeBoer EM, Soden JS, et al. Unsedated transnasal esophagoscopy for monitoring therapy in pediatric eosinophilic esophagitis. Gastrointest Endosc 2016;83:299–306.
77. Philpott H, Nandurkar S, Royce SG, et al. Ultrathin unsedated transnasal gastroscopy in monitoring eosinophilic esophagitis. J Gastroenterol Hepatol 2016;31:590–4.
78. Nguyen N, Lavery WJ, Capocelli KE, et al. Transnasal endoscopy in unsedated children with eosinophilic esophagitis using virtual reality video goggles. Clin Gastroenterol Hepatol 2019;17:2455–62.
79. Honing J, Kievit W, Bookelaar J, et al. Endosheath ultrathin transnasal endoscopy is a cost-effective method for screening for Barrett's esophagus in patients with GERD symptoms. Gastrointest Endosc 2019;89:712–22.
80. Ross-Innes CS, Chettouh H, Achilleos A, et al. Risk stratification of Barrett's oesophagus using a non-endoscopic sampling method coupled with a biomarker panel: a cohort study. Lancet Gastroenterol Hepatol 2017;2:23–31.
81. Januszewicz W, Tan WK, Lehovsky K, et al. Safety and acceptability of esophageal cytosponge cell collection device in a pooled analysis of data from individual patients. Clin Gastroenterol Hepatol 2019;17:647–56.
82. Katzka DA, Smyrk TC, Alexander JA, et al. Accuracy and safety of the cytosponge for assessing histologic activity in eosinophilic esophagitis: a two-center study. Am J Gastroenterol 2017;112:1538–44.
83. Alexander JA, Katzka DA, Ravi K, et al. Efficacy of cytosponge directed food elimination diet in eosinophilic esophagitis: a pilot trial. Gastroenterology 2018;154:S76.
84. Ackerman SJ, Kagalwalla AF, Hirano I, et al. One-hour esophageal string test: a nonendoscopic minimally invasive test that accurately detects disease activity in eosinophilic esophagitis. Am J Gastroenterol 2019;114:1614–25.
85. Hischenhuber C, Crevel R, Jarry B, et al. Review article: safe amounts of gluten for patients with wheat allergy or coeliac disease. Aliment Pharmacol Ther 2006;23:559–75.
86. Catassi C, Fabiani E, Iacono G, et al. A prospective, double-blind, placebo-controlled trial to establish a safe gluten threshold for patients with celiac disease. Am J Clin Nutr 2007;85:160–6.

The Life-Long Role of Nutrition on the Gut Microbiome and Gastrointestinal Disease

Joann Romano-Keeler, MD, MS[a], Jilei Zhang, PhD[b], Jun Sun, PhD[b,c],*

KEYWORDS

- Cancer • Dysbiosis • Gut-brain axis • Inflammation • Infant • Nutrition
- Microbiome • Micronutrients

KEY POINTS

- Diet is a key extrinsic factor that impacts the gut microbiome, particularly during the dynamic colonization process that occurs in the first several years of life.
- An imbalance in the complex gut ecosystem referred to as a dysbiosis can have short- and long-term effects on immune system development and impart life-long health complications on an individual in intestine and extraintestine (eg, breast).
- New research suggests effects of microbiome on the central nervous system. The "gut-brain-microbiome axis" may have a significant role on brain development and the pathogenesis of neuropsychiatric disorders.
- Poor macronutrient and micronutrient intake contribute to a dysbiosis. However, supplementation with specific prebiotics and probiotics might modulate the microbiome and restore host homeostasis.

INTRODUCTION

The human body is composed of a vast population of microbes, including bacteria, viruses, fungi, and phages, that outnumber human cells 1.3 to 1.0 based on recent calculations and estimates.[1,2] The densest community of these microbes, which are referred to as the human microbiota, resides in the gut. The microbiome refers

Funding Support: This work was supported by the U.S. National Institutes of Health grant NIDDK R01 DK105118, R01DK114126, DOD BC160450P1, and the UIC Cancer Center support (J. Sun).
^a Division of Neonatology, Department of Pediatrics, University of Illinois at Chicago, 840 South Wood Street, MC 856, Suite 1252, Chicago, IL 60612, USA; ^b Division of Gastroenterology and Hepatology, Department of Medicine, University of Illinois at Chicago, 840 South Wood Street, Room 704 CSB, MC716, Chicago, IL 60612, USA; ^c University of Illinois Cancer Center, 818 South Wolcott Avenue, Chicago, IL 60612, USA
* Corresponding author. 840 South Wood Street, Room 704 CSB, MC716, Chicago, IL 60612.
E-mail address: junsun7@uic.edu

Gastroenterol Clin N Am 50 (2021) 77–100
https://doi.org/10.1016/j.gtc.2020.10.008
0889-8553/21/© 2020 Elsevier Inc. All rights reserved.

gastro.theclinics.com

to the collective genomes of these microbial communities and each niche of the human body has a distinct microbiome responsible for key biologic functions. Since the advent of the US National Institutes of Health Human Microbiome Project, European Metagenomics Human Intestinal Tract project, and multiple worldwide population-based studies more than a decade ago, scientists have cataloged up to 2000 resident gut microbes composed of 100 trillion cells that express a greater number of unique genes than their host's genome.[3–5] An individual's microbiome, which is affected by both intrinsic (ie, genetics, age) and extrinsic (ie, diet, medications) factors, is critical for development of mucosal immunity and is a key driver of human health and disease.[6]

Homeostasis of the intestinal microbiota, often referred to as eubiosis, fosters interactions between the gut microbiome and the host that promote effective innate and adaptive immunity, including pathogen recognition, self-tolerance, and identification of beneficial commensals.[6] Disruptions in the gut microbiome or dysbiosis can lead to misdirected immune responses to environmental or self-antigens that may result in atopic disorders, autoimmune diseases, and inflammatory conditions (**Fig. 1**). A well-balanced intestinal microbiome is also responsible for harvesting energy from food sources, producing short chain fatty acids (SCFAs) from indigestible carbohydrates, and synthesizing vitamins and amino acids for maintenance of gut barrier function.[7] Dysbiosis can affect any of these critical processes and increase an individual's risk of developing chronic diseases, for example, obesity and other metabolic comorbidities.[8]

Diet is recognized as one of the key, modifiable environmental factors and may account for 20% and 50% of microbial structural variations in humans and mice, respectively.[9,10] Recent population-based studies demonstrate that effects of diet on the gut microbiome and long-term health outcomes may dominate over host genetics.[11]

The purpose of this review is to highlight how diet affects microbial community composition and the development of gastrointestinal (GI) disease from early life to adulthood. We describe how nutrition during pregnancy, including maternal obesity and gestational diabetes, may contribute to adult onset of diseases. We discuss postnatal nutrition (micronutrients, prebiotics, and probiotics) and bacterial colonization, including the role of breast milk on necrotizing enterocolitis. We highlight how diet impacts adult GI diseases, such as gastric pathologies, intestinal disorders (inflammatory bowel disease [IBD], celiac disease [CD], and irritable bowel syndrome [IBS]), obesity, and colorectal cancer (CRC). Finally, we provide a brief overview of how cross-talk between the gut microbiome and other organ systems may drive extraintestinal disorders.

MICROBIOME IN PREGNANCY AND EARLY NUTRITIONAL PROGRAMMING OF THE NEWBORN

Dietary intake is most influential on microbial colonization during the first 2 to 3 years of life when the dynamic and nascent gut microbiome is in its early stages of assembly.[2] As an infant's diet expands from breast milk or formula to solid foods, α-diversity (bacterial diversity in one specific region of the body) increases and β-diversity (regional differences in bacterial composition in different parts of the body), which is initially highest at birth, gradually decreases. However, as the gut microbiome stabilizes in adulthood, individuals separate into clusters or "enterotypes," which are classified based on proportions of major taxa.[12] Environmental factors, including medications, malnutrition, and infections, which can cause large shifts in bacterial composition and the relative abundance of some taxonomic groups.[13] Although adults are likely to return to their baseline enterotypes, infants may have permanent shifts in their

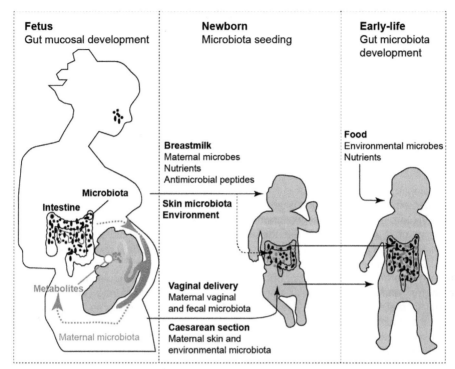

Fig. 1. Role of diet on establishing intestinal eubiosis or dysbiosis. Intestinal homeostasis or eubiosis, which is established through a healthy diet including breast milk, foods rich in fiber and low in fat, and prebiotics, imparts health benefits on an individual by promoting normal microbial colonization, a functional intestinal barrier, and a milieu favoring anti-inflammatory cytokines. However, derangements in the gut microbiome, also referred to as a dysbiosis, result from an unhealthy diet composed mainly of commercial formula and foods high in fat and low in fiber. Shifts in bacterial abundance, decreased microbial diversity, increased inflammatory mediators, and increased intestinal permeability are consequences of this type of diet and subsequently increase an individual's risk for a host of gastrointestinal pathologies.

gut flora owing to these acute or chronic perturbations that occur during a critical window of intestinal development.

The microbiome during pregnancy is dynamic, with shifts in both composition and bacterial load unique to each trimester.[14,15] Environmental factors, primarily diet, along with prepregnancy body mass index (BMI) and maternal weight gain during pregnancy, may significantly influence offspring's gut microbiome and increase their risk of obesity and metabolic syndrome as children and adults.[16] The microbiome of pregnant women was evaluated during the first and second trimester in overweight women (BMI >30) and compared with normal weight individuals (BMI <25). Overweight pregnant women had significantly higher levels of *Bacteroides* and *Staphylococcus* compared with controls.[15] Other studies of microbiota shifts during pregnancy in obese women versus controls found a decrease in *Bifidobacterium* and *Bacteroides*, findings similar to those in nonpregnant obese individuals.[17]

Maternal prepregnancy BMI impacts outcomes for mothers and infants postnatally. Excessive weight gain during pregnancy is a known risk factor for maternal preeclampsia and gestational diabetes, along with an increased risk of diabetes and cardiovascular disease later in life. Infants of mothers who are overweight or obese have a higher likelihood of being macrosomic, whereas infants of mothers who are underweight have a higher likelihood of delivering prematurely and being small for gestational age.[18] Health outcomes of these infants later in life may also be affected. A study of 935 mother–infant dyads found that infants of obese or overweight mothers had a 3-fold increased risk of being obese at 1 year of age.[19]

Controversy still exists over whether the fetus develops in a sterile in utero environment or is colonized by microbes during pregnancy. In a number of human and murine studies well-controlled for environmental contaminants, microbial DNA was detected in humans and mice, which most closely resembled maternal microbiomes of the oral cavity.[20,21] These novel studies suggest a role for modulation of maternal diet, including use of prebiotics and probiotics to improve the microbiota of offspring and decrease the risk of adult onset disease. The effect of early life nutritional stimuli, both in utero and postnatally, on infant and adult health is intriguing and evolving areas of research (**Fig. 2**). Barker's decades-old hypothesis, now recoined as the developmental origins of health and disease, explores how nutritional programming during fetal development can drive one's lifelong health status and adult-onset of cardiometabolic disorders.[22,23] Maternal noncommunicable diseases, including obesity, type 2 diabetes, and high cholesterol, can result from malnutrition during pregnancy and result in maternal dysbiosis that perturbs the newborn microbiome. Offspring are also at an increased risk to have noncommunicable diseases as adults if subsequently exposed to postnatal factors (neonatal intensive care unit hospitalization, antibiotic exposure, formula feeds) known to interfere with normal bacterial colonization.[24]

NEWBORN MICROBIOME AND NECROTIZING ENTEROCOLITIS

Normal newborn colonization commences when a healthy bolus of vaginal flora is imparted to the infant during delivery, followed by the introduction of breast milk. Breast milk is rich in nondigestible oligosaccharides that serve as prebiotics to promote the growth of beneficial bacteria, including *Lactobacillus acidophilus*, *Bacteroides fragilis*, and *Bifidobacterium infantis*.[25] These commensal bacteria promote the fermentation of oligosaccharides into SCFAs. A symbiotic relationship evolves between the infant and colonizing bacteria as microbes begin to interact with the developing mucosal immune system. Although newborns are also rapidly colonized by a variety of environmental factors (eg, maternal oral and skin flora, household, or hospital organism), the most important environmental factor, much like with adults, is diet whether it be breast milk or formula. Deviations from this normal colonization occur secondary to preterm delivery, cesarean section, antibiotics, and formula feeds. Any of these variables affect the infant microbiome, including sparse and inadequate colonization and the delay of final microbiome assembly until 4 to 6 years of age, increasing these individuals' susceptibility to infections and immune-mediated diseases.

Necrotizing enterocolitis, the most common GI emergencies in newborn infants, occurs in 1% to 5% of patients admitted to the neonatal intensive care unit.[26,27] The etiology of necrotizing enterocolitis is complex, but is attributed to the triad of an aberrant intestinal microbiome, an immature mucosal immune system, and an exaggerated inflammatory response aggravated by "stressors," including the introduction of formula-based feeds.[28] A single organism or group of organisms responsible for necrotizing enterocolitis remains enigmatic despite a myriad of studies using both traditional and culture-independent techniques.[29] However, the majority of studies have been

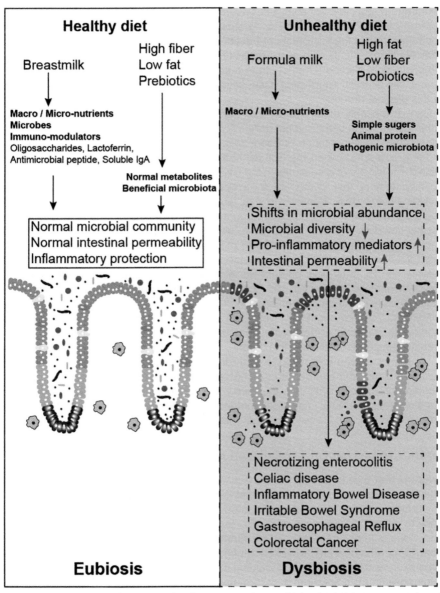

Fig. 2. Early life mucosal immune development and microbial colonization. Maternal oral and intestinal microbial flora and bacterial metabolites may be introduced to the growing fetus through the placenta. Mode of delivery (vaginal or caesarean section), diet (breast milk or commercial formula), and environmental factors, including mom's oral and skin flora, are key contributing factors to the developing infant microbiome and mucosal immune system. Early life influences on infant's colonization include the infant's diet and environmental exposures. Introduction of solid foods during this window is associated with the most robust expansion of a child's microbiome, which will reach a steady state by approximately 3 years of life.

restricted to stool sample analyses, which are collected distal to the ileum, the most common area affected in necrotizing enterocolitis. As such, stool samples may not accurately reflect the microbiota at the actual site of injury. Studies in intestinal tissue samples from patients with necrotizing enterocolitis and from patients with noninfectious intestinal disorders demonstrate a tissue-level gut microbiome unique to each area of the GI tract, suggesting tissue-level bacterial communities as the key drivers of this disease process.[20]

One of the only dietary strategies that has proven preventative for necrotizing enterocolitis is the use of breast milk.[30,31] The importance of this strategy has led to widespread implementation of donor breast milk programs at institutions for infants at the greatest risk when the optimal choice of expressed maternal milk is unavailable.[26,32] Delivery of breast milk to the newborn infant transfers a host of immunomodulating factors that contribute to a decreased risk of necrotizing enterocolitis, including human milk oligosaccharides, lactoferrin, antimicrobial peptide, and soluble IgA.[33,34] Transmission of bacteria through breast milk is also critical to promote a normal newborn intestinal microbiome, which demonstrates derangements early on secondary to prematurity, exposure to medications, and the intensive care environment itself, including decreased populations of commensal bacteria and increased colonization by potentially pathogenic microorganisms.[35] Infants fed directly at the breast have the added benefit of direct contact with the mother's skin, increasing bacterial diversity of the gut microbiome.[36]

Mechanisms that might be involved in the protective role of breast milk include indole-3-lactic acid, a metabolite from breast milk tryptophan, which acts as an anti-inflammatory molecule.[37] In a recent study, indole-3-lactic acid decreased the inflammatory cytokine IL-8 response after IL-1β stimulus by interacting with the transcription factor aryl hydrocarbon receptor and by preventing transcription of IL-8. Human milk oligosaccharides, the third most abundant component of human milk not present in formula, may also contribute to the lower incidence of necrotizing enterocolitis in infants receiving breast milk.[38,39]

INFANCY TO CHILDHOOD: ESTABLISHING AN ADULT-LIKE MICROBIOTA

Over the first 3 years of life, infants transition from an immature gut microbiome to one that can function with the same metabolic capacity as an adult.[40] One of the major turning points in this maturation is cessation of breast milk with shifts in infant flora to adult microbes, including *Bacteroides*, *Bilophila*, *Roseburia*, *Clostridium*, and *Anaerostipes*. Interestingly, in infants who continue consuming breast milk past 12 months, this shift toward adult flora is delayed and colonization with organisms expressed in breast milk, including *Bifidobacterium* species, persists.[41] During this transition from breast milk or formula to a solid food diet, α-diversity increases dramatically. The final transition to a stable, adult microbiome occurs from 18 to 36 months of age, and diet has a major effect on its composition, including establishing the balance of *Bacteroidetes* to *Firmicutes*. SCFAs, especially butyrate levels, increase dramatically, along with functional changes that allow for the breakdown of complex carbohydrates, starch, and xenobiotic degradation, as well as vitamin production.[2] Although a more adult-like bacterial profile is associated with an increase in stability and a landscape less likely to experience major shifts in composition, significant insults (eg, malnutrition, use of antibiotics, and acute illnesses) can still disrupt the newly laid foundation of the gut microbiome and increase an individual's risk of adulthood diseases and lifelong health complications, including those discussed elsewhere in this article.

MICROBIOTA OF GASTRIC PATHOLOGIES: ESOPHAGEAL ADENOCARCINOMA, BARRETT'S ESOPHAGUS, AND GASTROESOPHAGEAL REFLUX

Over the last 40 years, a dramatic increase in the incidence of esophageal adenocarcinoma (EAC) has been observed more than with any other malignancy or growth.[42] Although not all individuals with Barrett's esophagus (BE) develop EAC, the metaplastic changes of the distal esophageal mucosa observed with BE are often precursors to malignancy.[43] Gastroesophageal reflux disease (GERD), which produces inflammation at the gastroesophageal junction, can lead to the transformation of the mucosal lining from squamous to metaplastic columnar epithelial cells. Thus, individuals with GERD are at an increased risk of BE and the development of EAC.

Cross-talk between one's diet and gastric and esophageal microbiomes drives these malignant transformations. Patients with GERD and BE have lower esophageal tract microbiomes that are high in gram negative organisms, including *Proteobacteria*, *Fusobacteria*, and *Spirochaetes*.[44] *Helicobacter pylori* and *Escherichia coli* are present in BE and EAC, likely secondary to the highly acidic environment generated by GERD.[45] High-fiber and low-fat diets support a gut microbiome robust with commensals that stimulate normal metabolism, nutrient and vitamin absorption, and elimination of pathogenic bacteria and toxins. Conversely, diets rich in fat and processed foods (simple sugars, animal proteins) are associated with chronic inflammation of the esophagus and a dysbiosis that contributes to BE and EAC.

Dietary differences contributing to perturbations of the microbiota at the gastroesophageal junction and esophageal and gastric pathologies have been observed in rural versus urban populations. Individuals in rural areas, who are more likely to have balanced diets with adequate fiber intake, have microbiomes high in *Prevotella*, *Treponema*, and *Succinovibrio*. These organisms assist with the digestion of fiber-rich foods and polysaccharides. People in urban areas, who are more likely to consume diets high in fat and processed foods, have a gut microbiota with increased levels of *Bacteroidetes* and decreased amounts of *Firmicutes*.[46]

MICROBIOTA, DIETARY TRIGGERS, AND THE PATHOGENESIS OF CELIAC DISEASE

CD is a classic example of a diet-sensitive chronic immune disorder that occurs in predisposed individuals in the setting of a microbial imbalance.[47] The old adage that CD was solely a sequela of a person's genotype and interactions with environmental triggers was debunked when discordance in the penetrance of CD between monozygotic twins was observed.[48] In addition, although the introduction of gluten occurs during childhood, disease onset can occur at any point in a person's lifetime. These observations suggest that other factors could contribute to the pathogenesis of CD, including interactions between the intestinal immune system and the gut microbiota.

One hypothesis behind CD is that an intestinal dysbiosis occurs during critical windows of early life immune development in genetically susceptible individuals.[49] The integrity of the intestinal epithelium depends on the stimulation of T regulatory cells (Tregs) and activation of intestinal epithelial cells[5] by the gut microbiota. Tregs stimulation of immune cells by gut bacteria referred to as microbial programming, can be disrupted in certain individuals, and in the setting of defunct immune programming, gut permeability increases even before onset of gluten-induced inflammation.

CD may also be a product of defects in transmembrane proteins and intestinal tight junctions in individuals who have an abnormal gut microbiome and are predisposed to CD. Zonulin is a transmembrane protein responsible for tight junction disassembly that reversibly regulates intestinal permeability to luminal antigens.[50]

Expression of zonulin is upregulated by enteric bacteria and gliadin, a key component of gluten to triggers proinflammatory cytokine release. This process results in increased epithelial permeability and exposure of the submucosa to an even higher antigen load.

The multifactorial nature of CD–microbial imbalance, increased intestinal permeability, and proinflammatory response to gluten exposure makes treatment of this disease more complex than simple adherence to a gluten free diet. Recent studies are evaluating the role of prebiotics, probiotics, and fermentable oligosaccharides, disaccharides, monosaccharides and, polyols (FODMAP) as potential therapies for CD.[51] In CD patients, it is suspected that levels of *Bifidobacteria* and *Lactobacilli* are decreased, and probiotics that target these strains might be beneficial.[52] Other effective strains in patients with CD might be those that produce enzymes capable of degrading gliadin peptides and inducing anti-inflammatory effects.[53]

INFLAMMATORY BOWEL DISEASES

IBD, including CD and ulcerative colitis, typically occurs during early adulthood and is followed by periods of remission and relapses, which are often responsive to immunomodulatory, immunosuppressive, and dietary interventions.[54–56] In individuals predisposed to IBD, poor nutrition has detrimental effects on the intestinal microbiome, including the production of proinflammatory mediators, disruption of the GI tract's protective mucus layer, and increased intestinal permeability, making diet a key environmental factor in IBD pathogenesis.[57,58]

A Western diet, characterized by excessive consumption of refined sugars, salt, and saturated fat, low consumption of dietary fiber, and limited food diversity, is associated with an increased risk of IBD.[59] Such a diet promotes the production of bacterial metabolites with adverse effects on the gut microbiota and the intestinal immune system. Conversely, a diet rich in fiber in individuals predisposed to IBD promotes fiber fermentation and stimulates SCFA producing bacteria. SCFAs, notably acetate, propionate, and butyrate, have a variety of anti-inflammatory properties in T cells, specifically Tregs. They can be used as an energy source in intestinal epithelial cells and are vital to maintaining normal intestinal barrier function, including a protective mucus layer.

A swing from breast milk to artificial formula use in the first year of life often accompanies a shift to a Westernized diet.[60] Breast milk, which is considered to be protective against IBD, contains *Lactobacillus rhamnosus*, *Lactobacillus gasseri*, *Lactococcus lactic*, *Leuconostoc mesenteroides*, and *Bifidobacteria* which promote immune tolerance and strengthens the intestinal epithelial barrier. Human milk oligosaccharides contained in breast milk can block adhesion to intestinal epithelial cells by pathogenic organisms, including *E coli*, *Vibrio cholera*, and *Salmonella fyris*.[61] In the absence of human milk oligosaccharides, these pathobionts can adhere to the intestinal epithelium, where they can invade and drive inflammatory cascades.

Commercial formula use and Western diets, more frequently consumed by urban populations and developed countries with easy access to ultraprocessed foods, are also associated with decreased intestinal bacterial diversity.[62,63] Regardless of exposure to a Western diet, individuals with IBD consistently have decreased biodiversity, specifically a decrease in α-diversity and species richness when compared with controls.[64] Metagenomic studies of patients with IBD have also demonstrated imbalances in other bacterial species related to dietary intake, including a decrease in *Clostridium leptum*, a member of the Firmicutes phylum, many of whom have anti-inflammatory effects.[65,66]

IRRITABLE BOWEL SYNDROME

With approximately 11% of the population diagnosed worldwide, IBS is the most widespread functional gut disorder, characterized by recurrent abdominal pain, bloating, and stool inconsistency.[67,68] Although it is unclear what specific aspects of an affected individual's gut microbiome are "abnormal" or "unhealthy," recent studies examining interactions between host and microbial metabolites have informed our design of nutrition therapies for IBS. Bile acids, SCFAs, vitamins, and amino acids are some of the key host- and microbial-derived metabolites that may be effective treatments.[69,70]

For example, patients with IBS have aberrant levels of primary bile acids (host metabolites synthesized by the liver from cholesterol) and secondary bile acids (bacterial metabolites produced by colonic microorganisms).[71] Patients with diarrhea-predominant IBS have elevated levels of primary bile acids in feces, which may be consistent with bile acid malabsorption that drives diarrheal symptoms.[72,73] Other variations in primary and secondary bile acid levels are also observed in constipation-predominant IBS. However, in both cases, it is difficult to understand how such alterations in primary and secondary bile acid metabolism drive disease pathogenesis.

OBESITY AND THE GUT MICROBIOME

The interplay between diet and the gut microbiota and its effect on obesity have been a focal area of research since the inception of microbiome research. It is now hypothesized that the microbiota interacts with diet to (1) increase energy extraction from food sources, (2) increase intestinal epithelial permeability resulting in chronic inflammation, and (3) decrease angiopoietin-like protein expression and lipoprotein lipase–mediated fatty acid uptake.[74] Early studies demonstrated that genetically obese mice, when compared with lean subjects, had lower community diversity along with a 50% decrease in *Bacteroidetes* and a corresponding increase in *Firmicutes*.[75,76] Additional studies in which germ-free mice were inoculated with bacteria from obese donors revealed an increased fat mass in recipient mice when compared with those receiving bacteria from lean donors.[77] These studies suggest that a shift in the *Bacteroidetes:-Firmicutes* ratio occurs with obesity and that the microbiome alone could drive changes in body.

Although caloric intake is a major driver of obesity, an individual's gut microbiota and its capacity to harvest energy from food sources are key contributors to an individual's risk of developing obesity. For example, gut microbiota are capable of fermenting soluble fibers to produce SCFAs, a major energy source for colonocytes, that promote commensal organisms' growth and limit pathogenic bacteria overgrowth. SCFAs also decrease adipose storage, improve insulin sensitivity, and decrease local and systemic inflammation. Conversely, insoluble fibers that cannot be metabolized will not provide these robust health benefits.[78]

MICROBIOME AND DIETARY ASSOCIATIONS WITH COLORECTAL CANCER

CRC, the third most common cancer and the leading cause of cancer deaths in the United States among men and women is strongly influenced by dietary risk factors that affect the intestinal microbiome.[79,80] In fact, up to 60% of CRC cases are attributable to modifiable risk factors, including BMI, physical activity, and diet.[81] Specific dietary factors, including fiber and red and processed meat, and mechanisms for how they drive inflammation and risk of CRC are discussed elsewhere in this article and reviewed in **Fig. 3**.

Studies on the effects of fiber intake on the intestinal microbiome and CRC risk have demonstrated varied results. No linear association was found between fiber intake and CRC risk in a meta-analysis of 21 prospective studies in the United States.[82] In addition, results from a series of 64 randomized controlled trials summarized in a 2018 meta-analysis where healthy adults received supplementation with fiber or related prebiotics demonstrated how fiber supplementation increased the abundance of *Bifidobacterium* and *Lactobacillus* species with no effect on SCFA-producing bacteria.[83] Conversely, data from the European Prospective Investigation into Cancer and Nutrition have consistently demonstrated an association between fiber intake and a decreased risk of CRC.[84,85] Differences in the findings between these 2 populations are hypothesized to be due to the dietary sources of fiber, which in the United States is typically whole grains and in Europe is mainly fruits and vegetables, as well as the relatively low amounts of fiber consumed by individuals in US study cohorts.[86]

One of the hypotheses for how fiber affects the intestinal microbiome and reduces CRC risk includes fermentation of fiber by intestinal bacteria into SCFAs. In several studies, SCFAs and SCFA-producing bacteria, including *Eubacterium rectale*, *Roseburia* species, and *F prausnitzii*, were enriched in the feces of individuals with higher fiber intake.[87,88] Individuals who consumed less dietary fiber had decreased abundance of SCFA-producing bacteria (*Bacteroidetes*, *Firmicutes*) and bacterial metabolites, including propionate, acetate, butyrate, and lactate which decreased energy metabolism within the intestines and shifted the balance from anti-inflammatory to proinflammatory mediators. Macrophages and other immune cells in the submucosa were then activated to increase IL-6 and tumor necrosis factor-α production. As a result, nuclear factor-κB and STAT-3 signaling were further stimulated, promoting inflammation both within the intestines and in downstream extraintestinal tissue locations.

Red and processed meats may also be implicated in the pathogenesis of CRC. Specifically, the high content of choline and carnitine in red meat can serve as precursors for the production of trimethylamine and trimethylamine *N*-oxide (TMAO) by the gut microbiota now with pathologic enrichment of gram-negative organisms including Prevotella, Bacteroides, and bacteria from the Teneriticutes and Deferribacteres phyla.[89] Several meta-analyses of fecal shotgun metagenomic studies supporting the choline–TMAO pathway in the development of CRC have found that CRC patients have higher levels of 2 bacterial genes that regulate TMA synthesis.[90] One outcome of TMAO synthesis is decreased intestinal epithelial barrier function secondary to DNA mutagenesis and intestinal dysplasia. Macrophage expression of proatherogenic scavenger receptors, CD36, and SRA, is also increased to generate local and systemic inflammation.

Another mechanism through which processed, red meat may increase CRC risk is by the bacterial production of hydrogen sulfide from inorganic sulfur, routinely used as a preservative for red meats. Bacteria driving these hydrogen sulfide–producing pathways, which are known to be increased in metabolomic analyses of fecal samples from CRC patients, include gram-negative Proteobacteria *Bilophila wadsworthia* and *Desulfovibrio* spp and *Fusobacterium nucleatum*, an oral commensal with this surprising link to a GI malignancy. These shifts in bacteria-driven hydrogen sulfide activity trigger increased activity of Tregs and oversuppression of effector T cells, without which tumorigenic activity proceeds unopposed.[91,92]

Finally, secondary bile acids produced by bacteria after red meat consumption might also increase CRC risk through a number of downstream pathways that affect antimicrobial peptide expression and the occurrence of intestinal dysplasia. High

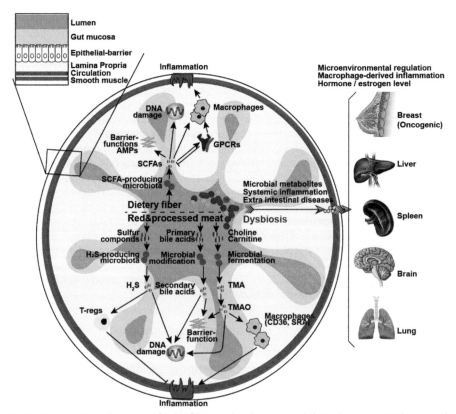

Fig. 3. Proposed mechanisms of how fiber and red meat modulate the gut microbiota and the risk of colorectal cancer (CRC). Lack of dietary fiber decreases abundance of SCFA-producing bacteria, mainly from the Bacteroidetes and Firmicutes phyla. Decreased SCFAs in the intestinal lumen disrupt signaling of cell surface G-protein coupled receptors (GPCRs) to activate macrophages and increase proinflammatory cytokines, including tumor necrosis factor-α, IL-17, and IL-6. These key cytokines upregulate NF-κB and STAT3 signaling pathways to generate inflammation. A reduction in SCFA-producing bacteria disrupts epithelial barrier integrity by blunting antimicrobial peptide (AMP) synthesis and promoting proliferation of dysplastic intestinal epithelial cells. Extraintestinal effects may also ensue secondary to bacterial and estrogen metabolites produced by increased populations of *Clostridia*, *Enterobacterium*, *Lactobacillus*, *Bacteroides*, and *E coli*. Red and processed meat contain choline and carnitine, which are metabolized to trimethylamine (TMA) and TMAO by commensal gut bacteria, which can increase macrophage expression of proatherogenic scavenger receptors, CD36 and SRA, to generate inflammation. TMA and TMAO also increase DNA mutations in proliferating intestinal epithelial cells and decrease barrier function. Meat is also high in sulfur-containing amino acids and processed meats are often packaged with sulfur-containing preservatives. Microbes, including *Bilophila wadsworthia*, *Fusobacterium nucleatum*, and *Desulfovibrio* spp, generate hydrogen sulfide from these compounds, which upregulates Tregs suppression of effector T cells. This impairment of T-cell responses decreased immunity against tumorigenesis. Finally, meat intake increases the risk of colorectal cancer through bacterial fermentation of primary bile acids into secondary bile acids, including deoxycholic acid (DCA), which can cause DNA damage and intestinal dysplasia. Systemic inflammatory mediators generated through all of these pathways may also contribute to extraintestinal diseases.

quantities of fat from red meat enhance the regular activity of colonic organisms, including a cadre of gram-positive bacteria (*Clostridium*, *Enterococcus*, *Bifidobacterium*, and *Lactobacillus*) that express bile salt hydrolases and are capable of metabolizing primary bile acids to secondary bile acids.[93] The significance of this shift in an individual's bile acid profile is still poorly understood, however, these secondary bile acids are all hypothesized to coalesce on pathways that change interactions with nuclear and G-coupled protein receptors and expression of antimicrobial peptides.[94] The change in bile acid metabolism also results in DNA mutation and reduced ability to undergo apoptosis to correct these deleterious cellular changes.[95]

Another aspect of microorganisms and mucosal immune system cross-talk, which may be a part of CRC development, involve the 3 major bacteria that populate the colon—*E coli*, *Enterococcus Faecalis*, and *Bacteroides Fragilis*. Although typically symbionts, these species can assume a pathogenic role and induce carcinogenic changes within the colon. For example, *E coli* can release cell death toxins to cause epithelial proliferation, adenoma formation, and malignant transformation of cells. *Enterococcus faecalis* can be responsible for DNA destruction via free radical production.[96] *B fragilis* carcinogenicity impacts the colon when colonic integrity is disrupted through the release of *B fragilis* toxin, which cleaves tumor suppressor protein, E-cadherin to incite procarcinogenic effects of E-cadherin Wnt signaling, including colonic epithelial cell proliferation, and epithelial barrier dysfunction.[97]

IMPACT OF DIET AND ABNORMAL MICROBIAL COLONIZATION ON EXTRAINTESTINAL ORGANS

Interestingly, patients with breast cancer have similar alterations in their gut microbiome, including enrichment of *Clostridia*, *Enterobacterium*, *Lactobacillus*, *Bacteroides*, and *E coli*.[98] In a mouse model with commensal bacterial dysbiosis secondary to administration of systemic antibiotics, hormone receptor positive breast cancer cells had increased dissemination to distal sites, including lungs, peripheral blood, and axillary lymph nodes receptor.[99] The dysbiosis also affected mammary tissue homeostasis with an increased presence of macrophage-derived inflammatory cytokines (granulocyte macrophage colony stimulating factor, CCL2, and CXLC2).[100] Another mechanism for how the microbiome can influence the development of breast cancer is through the regulation of steroid hormone metabolism by GI bacteria. The "estrobolome" or collection of enteric bacterial genes responsible for estrogen metabolism may directly mitigate the pathogenesis of estrogen receptor-positive breast cancer.[101] Bacterial expression of β-glucuronidase and β-glucosidase and their subsequent deconjugation of estrogen control circulating levels of this hormone, which is a well-known risk factor for breast cancer. Conversely, the gut microbiome breaks down indigestible dietary phytoestrogens to synthesize estrogen-like compounds, which can act on the estrogen receptor to effect steroid metabolites and reduce circulating estrogen levels, decreasing the risk of breast cancer.[102]

Western diets are identified as a risk factor for developing breast cancer.[103] Western diets are rich in refined starches, sugar, red and processed meats, and saturated and trans fats, and low in fruits, vegetables, and whole grains. Processed food, which composes one-half of the calories in Western diets, are also correlated with this increased risk.[104,105] Conversely, more plant-based Mediterranean diets, which include soluble fibers and lignans, found in whole grains, soy, fruits, and vegetables, may decrease the risk of breast cancer.[106,107] This risk reduction is attributed to the ability of Mediterranean diets to promote intestinal bacterial diversity and increase the growth of *Firmicutes*. Products of lignans metabolism by *Firmicutes* are enterolignans, enterolactone, and enterodiol, which may act as selective modulators of estrogen signaling and may be associated with lowering the risk of breast cancer.[108]

More recent research suggests the effects of enteric organisms on the central nervous system, now referred to as the "gut–brain axis,", ay have a significant role on the pathogenesis of neuropsychiatric disorders, including schizophrenia and autism spectrum disorder.[109,110] Meta-analyses of studies to date in autistic children report dysbiotic profiles when compared with neurotypical children, including an increased abundance of harmful bacteria, specifically the proinflammatory genus *Clostridium*, and a lesser abundance of protective bacteria such as *Bifidobacterium*.[111,112] These changes in the gut microbiome can contribute not only to comorbid GI problems observed in the majority of patients with autism spectrum disorder, but also the severity of autistic symptomatology. Higher levels of bacterial metabolites (SCFAs, gamma-aminobutyric acid, serotonin, and catecholamines) accompany this shift in microbial composition and likely contribute to the pathogenesis of autism, which further supports the intricate, bidirectional communication between the gut microbiome and the central nervous system.[113–115] Nutritional interventions have shown some promise in their ability to alter the dysbiosis observed with autism spectrum disorder and to correct imbalances in signaling molecules negatively impacting brain function. Some of these interventions include casein and gluten-free diets, ketogenic diets, and consumption of simple monosaccharides versus complex carbohydrates.[116–118] However, many of these dietary strategies have been more thoroughly researched in patients with IBD, and the effects in patients with autism spectrum disorder have only recently become the subject of further investigations.

ROLE OF DIET AND MICRONUTRIENTS IN MICROBIOME AND DISEASE PREVENTION

Dietary interventions that may modulate the gut microbiome and be protective or therapeutic for GI diseases now include not only macronutrients (fat, carbohydrates, protein), but micronutrients (vitamins, minerals, trace elements) and novel prebiotics and probiotics. All micronutrients and prebiotics and probiotics are unable to be synthesized by the body and are solely derived from the diet, making an individual's nutritional status critical in the prevention of their deficiencies.[119] The goal in modulating the gut microbiome through the ingestion of these dietary components would be to either correct a dysbiosis or generate a healthier gut flora, thus, improving microbiota-driven immune development and function. Micronutrient, prebiotic, and probiotic modulation of the gut microbiome has proven most promising during the first 1000 days of life when nascent communities of microbes are still establishing their niches.[120]

Vitamin D, which can come from diet or from sunlight exposure, is one of the micronutrients recently identified to have a major impact on chronic intestinal inflammation, including IBD.[121,122] Novel studies in intestinal epithelial vitamin D receptor knockout mice demonstrated exaggerated intestinal colitis owing to activation of the nuclear factor-κB pathway and shifts in the gut microbiome toward increased *E coli* and decreased *Lactobacillus* and butyrate-producing bacteria.[123] Vitamin D receptor knock out mice also had fewer Paneth cells and decreased Paneth cell function, including decreased ileal secretion of antimicrobial peptides, which is a well-recognized mechanism behind IBD. Vitamin D deficiency, common in patients with IBD owing to intestinal malabsorption, was associated with a greater risk of clinical relapse.[124] In the recent Nurses' Health Study Cohort which included 72,219 individuals, women with predicted highest vitamin D levels had a significantly lower incidence of Crohn's disease.[125]

Other fat-soluble vitamins that may have a role in maintaining homeostasis of the gut microbiota include vitamins A and E. In one study, children with infectious diarrhea, who were also found to be vitamin A deficient, had a decrease in butyrate-producing bacteria (*E coli*, *Clostridium butyricum*), an increase in opportunistic pathogens (*Enterococcus*), and an overall decreased bacterial diversity.[126] Vitamin A may also have a role in modulating the microbiome of children with autism spectrum disorder and in improving behavioral symptoms by restoring *Bacteroidetes* and *Bacteroidales* populations and reducing the *Firmicutes/Bacteroidetes* ratios.[127] Vitamin E, a well-recognized antioxidant, may have an anti-inflammatory role in the gut microbiome by scavenging for excess free radicals and protecting against mucosal immune damage. These beneficial properties may be attributed to the ability of vitamin E to increase *Bacteroidetes*, decrease *Firmicutes*, and increase α-diversity.[128] Water-soluble vitamins, including vitamin C and the eight B-group vitamins, are likely just as essential in gut microbiota homeostasis. Vitamin C, which is exclusively obtained from dietary sources, has antioxidant properties similar to vitamin E and may support the gut microbiota by increasing intestinal populations of *Lactobacillus* and *Bifidobacterium* populations while decreasing *E coli*.[129] In contrast, B vitamins, which are essential cofactors for a cadre of cellular reactions, may have multiple effects on bacterial activities including promoting bacterial growth, enhancing bacterial virulence, and engaging in pathogen interactions through modification of the host defense system.[130]

Queuine (q), a precursor of sugar is nucleotide queuosine (Q) and an essential factor for tRNA modification, is a micronutrient with an enigmatic role in the human body and is the subject of several recent studies. Both queuosine and its precursor, queuine, are exclusively obtained from dietary sources and from the gut microbiota in animals and humans.[131,132] A large number of neoplastic tissues and cancer cell lines have decreased Q-modification of $tRNA_{GUN}$, exploiting the ability of *E coli* TGT (transglycosylase) to insert radiolabeled guanine into unmodified $TRNA_{GUN}$.[133–138] Specifically, tRNA-guanine transglycosylase is absent in human colonic adenocarcinoma cell lines and Q-deficient tRNA is found in 2 of 13 carcinomas. In this same study, the colon adenocarcinoma-derived cell line had a complete deficiency of Q-modification compared with control cell cultures, attributed to defective queuine-insertase activity.[139] Proposed etiologies for Q-tRNA deficiencies include decreased uptake of queuine owing to inhibition of transporters or low bioavailability, and deregulation of translation owing to queuine depletion.[131] Because Q is a micronutrient obtained from food and the gut microbiota, the intestinal microbiome plays an important role in Q metabolism, and Q deficiency caused cancer, including CRC. However, the function of Q in mammals, especially in the intestines, remains poorly understood owing to limitations in experimental models.

Trace elements, including zinc and iron, have demonstrated important roles modulating host immune–bacteria interactions and GI disease pathogenesis.[140] Zinc supplementation may promote growth of beneficial bacteria and limit replication of pathogenic organisms. This has been demonstrated best in animal models, including broiler chickens. In chickens infected with *Salmonella typhimurium*, zinc supplementation increased *Lactobacillus* growth and decreased pathogenic bacterial populations, including *Salmonella*. However, human studies on zinc deficiency are limited impairing our ability to provide guidance on appropriate dietary supplementation.[141] Iron deficiency is the most common micronutrient deficiency and studies have demonstrated how poor dietary iron during early life assembly of the microbiome has profound and permanent impact on microbial composition, which may be linked with numerous inflammatory diseases.[142,143] One of the mechanisms underlying an iron deficiency dysbiosis may be expansion of pathogenic organisms and diminished colonization by beneficial organisms.[144] For example, one study in colitis-resistant and colitis-susceptible mice highlighted how luminal iron deficiency mediated a reduction of numerous taxa of Firmicutes but an expansion of pathogenic *Enterobacteriaceae*, including *E coli*.[143] Iron supplementation, however, has not proven to be straightforward, and depending on the specific iron formulation, may also be associated with a bloom of Enterobacteriaceae and subsequent intestinal inflammation.[145]

PREBIOTIC AND PROBIOTIC MODULATION OF THE MICROBIOME IN DISEASES

Prebiotics are dietary oligosaccharides degraded by intestinal bacteria into byproducts that may support normal gut colonization or restore intestinal homeostasis after specific GI insults.[146] Although health benefits were initially attributed to the ability of prebiotics to stimulate growth of *Bifidobacterium*, more expansive activities have been identified including SCFA and vitamin production, metabolism of primary to secondary bile salts, regulation of GI transit time, activation stem cells and increased enterocyte regeneration, and neutralization of carcinogens.[147,148] More specific immunomodulatory mechanisms of human milk oligosaccharides contained in breast milk may be protective against necrotizing enterocolitis, including their ability to interfere with pathogen adhesion to the intestinal epithelium and expand anti-inflammatory Th-2 immune responses.[149] A limited number of studies suggest anticarcinogenic properties of prebiotics in the prevention of CRC, including downregulation of cyclo-oxygenase 2, inducible nitric oxide synthase, nuclear factor-κB, and GI glutathione peroxidase.[150]

Probiotics, defined as live bacteria beneficial to the host, are promising therapeutics for promoting eubiosis and manipulating the gut microbiome to restore disordered metabolic machinery.[151] However, variability in strains that are used in clinical trials has interfered with the broader application of study results to patients. This is particularly the case with probiotics in preterm infants for the prevention of necrotizing enterocolitis. Although many studies, most of which use strains of *Bifidobacteria* or *Lactobacilli*, have had promising results, including improvements in feeding intolerance and decreased incidence of necrotizing enterocolitis, studies have not consistently used the same type and number of live bacteria. As such, limited data are available for each strain and, when analyzed collectively, there is insufficient evidence to support the supplementation of neonates with a specific bacterial strain. However, probiotics may have a role in modulating the maternal microbiome during pregnancy or in other disease pathologies, including IBD and CRC. In addition, a larger number of studies have been conducted in these populations who are more likely to be immunocompetent with a decreased risk of sepsis from the probiotic or a contaminated probiotic preparation. Growing interest is in synbiotics, which is a preparation of a prebiotic substrate that selectively favors the probiotic organism. Such a preparation might improve survival of the probiotic as it passes through the highly acidic upper GI tract and provide synergistic benefits to an individual's health.[152]

SUMMARY AND FUTURE DIRECTIONS

Diet and the gut microbiome have an intricate, mainly symbiotic relationship with the human host that is responsible for a cadre of health outcomes. This relationship starts early in life, perhaps as early as gestation, when maternal nutrition and intestinal flora seed the microbiota of the fetus and stimulate immune cell development in utero. A dysbiosis from early life insults, including malnutrition and infection, establish the basis for chronic GI disorders as described elsewhere in this article. As evidence mounts to support the important role of diet and the gut microbiome on GI disorders, research has shifted to include how these two factors affect extraintestinal organs. Systemic effects of the gut microbiome can be mediated by microbiota-derived molecules (endotoxin or lipopolysaccharide) or metabolites (SCFAs, bile acids) that interact with distal organs either directly or through intestinal neural networks or gut-synthesized hormones.[74,153] This bidirectional communication offers exciting opportunities for dietary therapeutics of diseases traditionally not thought to be connected with GI health.

Genetics contributes to the composition of the gut microbiome as evidenced by several inheritable bacterial taxa and associations between single nucleotide polymorphisms and individual bacterial communities and pathways.[154,155] We have contributed to identifying the first human gene *Vdr* that shapes the diversity of gut microbiome.[156] However, the precise role of the human genome in modulating the gut microbiome remains elusive.[157] Tissue-specific strategies for mechanisms and well-designed clinical studies on microbiome and metabolites are needed for the future research.[158–160]

The complex interplay among nutrients, the microbiome, and mucosal immune function makes the GI tract a major nidus for disease pathogenesis and therapeutic interventions. Over the last two decades, studies have mapped the bacterial landscape within the intestines, including identifying dietary substrates for these microorganisms, and are now outlining functional roles of bacteria in both the GI tract and more distal organs. Future studies will need to include other major players in this diverse ecosystem, including viruses and fungi, to fully understand how the gut microbiome processes nutrients, shapes immune development, and impacts human health.

CLINICS CARE POINTS

- Derangements in the neonatal microbiome due to excessive maternal weight gain during pregnancy has been shown to drive adverse outcomes in newborns including obesity, heart disease, and diabetes.
- Breastmilk is the only proven strategy for protection against necrotizing enterocolitis, which is the most common gastrointestinal emergency in newborns.
- Recent evidences supports how gastrointestinal disorders, including celiac disease and inflammatory bowel disease, are not just a sequelae of an individual's genotype and environmental triggers, but are also a product of interactions between the gut microbiome and the host immune system.
- Systemic effects of the gut microbiome are mediated by microbiota-derived molecules or metabolites interacting directly or indirectly through intestinal neural networks or gut-synthesized hormones.

DISCLOSURE

None of the authors have actual or potential conflict of interest in relationship to this publication.

REFERENCES

1. Sender R, Fuchs S, Milo R. Revised Estimates for the Number of Human and Bacteria Cells in the Body. PLoS Biol 2016;14(8):e1002533.
2. Koenig JE, Spor A, Scalfone N, et al. Succession of microbial consortia in the developing infant gut microbiome. Proc Natl Acad Sci U S A 2011;108(Suppl 1):4578–85.

3. Turnbaugh PJ, Ley RE, Hamady M, et al. The human microbiome project. Nature 2007;449(7164):804–10.
4. Almeida A, Mitchell AL, Boland M, et al. A new genomic blueprint of the human gut microbiota. Nature 2019;568(7753):499–504.
5. Le Chatelier E, Nielsen T, Qin J, et al. Richness of human gut microbiome correlates with metabolic markers. Nature 2013;500(7464):541–6.
6. Belkaid Y, Harrison OJ. Homeostatic Immunity and the Microbiota. Immunity 2017;46(4):562–76.
7. Oliphant K, Allen-Vercoe E. Macronutrient metabolism by the human gut microbiome: major fermentation by-products and their impact on host health. Microbiome 2019;7(1):91.
8. Cuevas-Sierra A, Ramos-Lopez O, Riezu-Boj JI, et al. Diet, gut microbiota, and obesity: links with host genetics and epigenetics and potential applications. Adv Nutr 2019;10(suppl_1):S17–30.
9. Zhang C, Zhang M, Wang S, et al. Interactions between gut microbiota, host genetics and diet relevant to development of metabolic syndromes in mice. ISME J 2010;4(2):232–41.
10. Zhernakova A, Kurilshikov A, Bonder MJ, et al. Population-based metagenomics analysis reveals markers for gut microbiome composition and diversity. Science 2016;352(6285):565–9.
11. Rothschild D, Weissbrod O, Barkan E, et al. Environment dominates over host genetics in shaping human gut microbiota. Nature 2018;555(7695):210–5.
12. Costea PI, Hildebrand F, Arumugam M, et al. Enterotypes in the landscape of gut microbial community composition. Nat Microbiol 2018;3(1):8–16.
13. Maier L, Typas A. Systematically investigating the impact of medication on the gut microbiome. Curr Opin Microbiol 2017;39:128–35.
14. Koren O, Goodrich JK, Cullender TC, et al. Host remodeling of the gut microbiome and metabolic changes during pregnancy. Cell 2012;150(3):470–80.
15. Collado MC, Isolauri E, Laitinen K, et al. Distinct composition of gut microbiota during pregnancy in overweight and normal-weight women. Am J Clin Nutr 2008;88(4):894–9.
16. Sridhar SB, Darbinian J, Ehrlich SF, et al. Maternal gestational weight gain and offspring risk for childhood overweight or obesity. Am J Obstet Gynecol 2014; 211(3):259.e1-8.
17. Santacruz A, Collado MC, Garcia-Valdes L, et al. Gut microbiota composition is associated with body weight, weight gain and biochemical parameters in pregnant women. Br J Nutr 2010;104(1):83–92.
18. Liu P, Xu L, Wang Y, et al. Association between perinatal outcomes and maternal pre-pregnancy body mass index. Obes Rev 2016;17(11):1091–102.
19. Tun HM, Bridgman SL, Chari R, et al. Roles of Birth Mode and Infant Gut Microbiota in Intergenerational Transmission of Overweight and Obesity From Mother to Offspring. JAMA Pediatr 2018;172(4):368–77.
20. Romano-Keeler J, Moore DJ, Wang C, et al. Early life establishment of site-specific microbial communities in the gut. Gut Microbes 2014;5(2):192–201.
21. Younge N, McCann JR, Ballard J, et al. Fetal exposure to the maternal microbiota in humans and mice. JCI Insight 2019;4(19):e127806.
22. Barker DJ. The fetal and infant origins of disease. Eur J Clin Invest 1995;25(7): 457–63.
23. Hanson M. The birth and future health of DOHaD. J Dev Orig Health Dis 2015; 6(5):434–7.

24. Heidari-Beni M. Early Life Nutrition and Non Communicable Disease. Adv Exp Med Biol 2019;1121:33–40.
25. Walker WA. Initial intestinal colonization in the human infant and immune homeostasis. Ann Nutr Metab 2013;63(Suppl 2):8–15.
26. Battersby C, Marciano Alves Mousinho R, Longford N, et al, UK Neonatal Collaborative Necrotising (UKNC-NEC) Study Group. Use of pasteurised human donor milk across neonatal networks in England. Early Hum Dev 2018;118:32–6.
27. Lin PW, Stoll BJ. Necrotising enterocolitis. Lancet 2006;368(9543):1271–83.
28. Neu J, Pammi M. Pathogenesis of NEC: impact of an altered intestinal microbiome. Semin Perinatol 2017;41(1):29–35.
29. Neu J, Walker WA. Necrotizing enterocolitis. N Engl J Med 2011;364(3):255–64.
30. Sullivan S, Schanler RJ, Kim JH, et al. An exclusively human milk-based diet is associated with a lower rate of necrotizing enterocolitis than a diet of human milk and bovine milk-based products. J Pediatr 2010;156(4):562–7.e1.
31. Cristofalo EA, Schanler RJ, Blanco CL, et al. Randomized trial of exclusive human milk versus preterm formula diets in extremely premature infants. J Pediatr 2013;163(6):1592–5.e1.
32. Sharpe J, Way M, Koorts PJ, et al. The availability of probiotics and donor human milk is associated with improved survival in very preterm infants. World J Pediatr 2018;14(5):492–7.
33. Trend S, Strunk T, Lloyd ML, et al. Levels of innate immune factors in preterm and term mothers' breast milk during the 1st month postpartum. Br J Nutr 2016;115(7):1178–93.
34. Rogier EW, Frantz AL, Bruno ME, et al. Secretory antibodies in breast milk promote long-term intestinal homeostasis by regulating the gut microbiota and host gene expression. Proc Natl Acad Sci U S A 2014;111(8):3074–9.
35. Warner BB, Tarr PI. Necrotizing enterocolitis and preterm infant gut bacteria. Semin Fetal Neonatal Med 2016;21(6):394–9.
36. Timmerman HM, Rutten N, Boekhorst J, et al. Intestinal colonisation patterns in breastfed and formula-fed infants during the first 12 weeks of life reveal sequential microbiota signatures. Sci Rep 2017;7(1):8327.
37. Meng D, Sommella E, Salviati E, et al. Indole-3-lactic acid, a metabolite of tryptophan, secreted by Bifidobacterium longum subspecies infantis is anti-inflammatory in the immature intestine. Pediatr Res 2020;88(2):209–17.
38. Kunz C, Rudloff S, Baier W, et al. Oligosaccharides in human milk: structural, functional, and metabolic aspects. Annu Rev Nutr 2000;20:699–722.
39. Moukarzel S, Bode L. Human milk oligosaccharides and the preterm infant: a journey in sickness and in health. Clin Perinatol 2017;44(1):193–207.
40. Palmer C, Bik EM, DiGiulio DB, et al. Development of the human infant intestinal microbiota. PLoS Biol 2007;5(7):e177.
41. Backhed F, Roswall J, Peng Y, et al. Dynamics and Stabilization of the Human Gut Microbiome during the First Year of Life. Cell Host Microbe 2015;17(6):852.
42. Chen Z, Ren Y, Du XL, et al. Incidence and survival differences in esophageal cancer among ethnic groups in the United States. Oncotarget 2017;8(29):47037–51.
43. Hvid-Jensen F, Pedersen L, Drewes AM, et al. Incidence of adenocarcinoma among patients with Barrett's esophagus. N Engl J Med 2011;365(15):1375–83.
44. Nardone G, Compare D, Rocco A. A microbiota-centric view of diseases of the upper gastrointestinal tract. Lancet Gastroenterol Hepatol 2017;2(4):298–312.
45. Yang L, Chaudhary N, Baghdadi J, et al. Microbiome in reflux disorders and esophageal adenocarcinoma. Cancer J 2014;20(3):207–10.

46. Martin JC, Moran LJ, Teede HJ, et al. Exploring Diet Quality between Urban and Rural Dwelling Women of Reproductive Age. Nutrients 2017;9(6):586.
47. Kabi A, Nickerson KP, Homer CR, et al. Digesting the genetics of inflammatory bowel disease: insights from studies of autophagy risk genes. Inflamm Bowel Dis 2012;18(4):782–92.
48. Greco L, Romino R, Coto I, et al. The first large population based twin study of coeliac disease. Gut 2002;50(5):624–8.
49. Valitutti F, Fasano A. Breaking down barriers: how understanding celiac disease pathogenesis informed the development of novel treatments. Dig Dis Sci 2019; 64(7):1748–58.
50. Drago S, El Asmar R, Di Pierro M, et al. Gliadin, zonulin and gut permeability: effects on celiac and non-celiac intestinal mucosa and intestinal cell lines. Scand J Gastroenterol 2006;41(4):408–19.
51. Bascunan KA, Elli L, Pellegrini N, et al. Impact of FODMAP Content Restrictions on the Quality of Diet for Patients with Celiac Disease on a Gluten-Free Diet. Nutrients 2019;11(9):2220.
52. de Sousa Moraes LF, Grzeskowiak LM, de Sales Teixeira TF, et al. Intestinal microbiota and probiotics in celiac disease. Clin Microbiol Rev 2014;27(3):482–9.
53. Francavilla R, De Angelis M, Rizzello CG, et al. Selected Probiotic Lactobacilli Have the Capacity To Hydrolyze Gluten Peptides during Simulated Gastrointestinal Digestion. Appl Environ Microbiol 2017;83(14):e00376-17.
54. Lloyd-Price J, Arze C, Ananthakrishnan AN, et al. Multi-omics of the gut microbial ecosystem in inflammatory bowel diseases. Nature 2019;569(7758):655–62.
55. Loftus EV Jr. Clinical epidemiology of inflammatory bowel disease: incidence, prevalence, and environmental influences. Gastroenterology 2004;126(6): 1504–17.
56. Cosnes J, Gower-Rousseau C, Seksik P, et al. Epidemiology and natural history of inflammatory bowel diseases. Gastroenterology 2011;140(6):1785–94.
57. Albenberg LG, Lewis JD, Wu GD. Food and the gut microbiota in inflammatory bowel diseases: a critical connection. Curr Opin Gastroenterol 2012;28(4): 314–20.
58. Lewis JD, Abreu MT. Diet as a Trigger or Therapy for Inflammatory Bowel Diseases. Gastroenterology 2017;152(2):398–414.e6.
59. Myles IA. Fast food fever: reviewing the impacts of the Western diet on immunity. Nutr J 2014;13:61.
60. Xu L, Lochhead P, Ko Y, et al. Systematic review with meta-analysis: breastfeeding and the risk of Crohn's disease and ulcerative colitis. Aliment Pharmacol Ther 2017;46(9):780–9.
61. Coppa GV, Facinelli B, Magi G, et al. Human milk glycosaminoglycans inhibit in vitro the adhesion of Escherichia coli and Salmonella fyris to human intestinal cells. Pediatr Res 2016;79(4):603–7.
62. Broussard JL, Devkota S. The changing microbial landscape of Western society: diet, dwellings and discordance. Mol Metab 2016;5(9):737–42.
63. Segata N. Gut microbiome: westernization and the disappearance of intestinal diversity. Curr Biol 2015;25(14):R611–3.
64. Manichanh C, Rigottier-Gois L, Bonnaud E, et al. Reduced diversity of faecal microbiota in Crohn's disease revealed by a metagenomic approach. Gut 2006; 55(2):205–11.
65. Sokol H, Seksik P. The intestinal microbiota in inflammatory bowel diseases: time to connect with the host. Curr Opin Gastroenterol 2010;26(4):327–31.

66. David LA, Maurice CF, Carmody RN, et al. Diet rapidly and reproducibly alters the human gut microbiome. Nature 2014;505(7484):559–63.

67. Hsu BB, Gibson TE, Yeliseyev V, et al. Dynamic Modulation of the Gut Microbiota and Metabolome by Bacteriophages in a Mouse Model. Cell Host Microbe 2019; 25(6):803–14.e5.

68. Mearin F, Lacy BE, Chang L, et al. Bowel Disorders. Gastroenterology. 2016 Feb 18:S0016-5085(16)00222-5. http://doi.org/10.1053/j.gastro.2016.02.031

69. Barbachano A, Fernandez-Barral A, Ferrer-Mayorga G, et al. The endocrine vitamin D system in the gut. Mol Cell Endocrinol 2017;453:79–87.

70. Vernocchi P, Del Chierico F, Putignani L. Gut microbiota profiling: metabolomics based approach to unravel compounds affecting human health. Front Microbiol 2016;7:1144.

71. Long SL, Gahan CGM, Joyce SA. Interactions between gut bacteria and bile in health and disease. Mol Aspects Med 2017;56:54–65.

72. Dior M, Delagreverie H, Duboc H, et al. Interplay between bile acid metabolism and microbiota in irritable bowel syndrome. Neurogastroenterol Motil 2016; 28(9):1330–40.

73. Duboc H, Dior M, Coffin B. Irritable bowel syndrome: new pathophysiological hypotheses and practical issues. Rev Med Interne 2016;37(8):536–43 [in French].

74. Cani PD, Amar J, Iglesias MA, et al. Metabolic endotoxemia initiates obesity and insulin resistance. Diabetes 2007;56(7):1761–72.

75. Ley RE, Backhed F, Turnbaugh P, et al. Obesity alters gut microbial ecology. Proc Natl Acad Sci U S A 2005;102(31):11070–5.

76. Turnbaugh PJ, Ley RE, Mahowald MA, et al. An obesity-associated gut micro-biome with increased capacity for energy harvest. Nature 2006;444(7122): 1027–31.

77. Turnbaugh PJ, Backhed F, Fulton L, et al. Diet-induced obesity is linked to marked but reversible alterations in the mouse distal gut microbiome. Cell Host Microbe 2008;3(4):213–23.

78. den Besten G, van Eunen K, Groen AK, et al. The role of short-chain fatty acids in the interplay between diet, gut microbiota, and host energy metabolism. J Lipid Res 2013;54(9):2325–40.

79. Siegel RL, Miller KD, Jemal A. Cancer statistics, 2020. CA Cancer J Clin 2020; 70(1):7–30.

80. Song M, Chan AT, Sun J. Influence of the Gut Microbiome, Diet, and Environ-ment on Risk of Colorectal Cancer. Gastroenterology 2020;158(2):322–40.

81. Islami F, Goding Sauer A, Miller KD, et al. Proportion and number of cancer cases and deaths attributable to potentially modifiable risk factors in the United States. CA Cancer J Clin 2018;68(1):31–54.

82. World Cancer Research Fund International/ American Institute for Cancer Research. Continuous Update Project Report: Diet, Nutrition, Physical activity and Colorectal Cancer. 2017. Available at: https://wwwwcrforg/sites/default/files/Colorectal-Cancer-2017-Reportpdf.

83. So D, Whelan K, Rossi M, et al. Dietary fiber intervention on gut microbiota composition in healthy adults: a systematic review and meta-analysis. Am J Clin Nutr 2018;107(6):965–83.

84. Murphy N, Norat T, Ferrari P, et al. Dietary fibre intake and risks of cancers of the colon and rectum in the European prospective investigation into cancer and nutrition (EPIC). PLoS One 2012;7(6):e39361.

85. Bingham SA, Day NE, Luben R, et al. Dietary fibre in food and protection against colorectal cancer in the European Prospective Investigation into Cancer and Nutrition (EPIC): an observational study. Lancet 2003;361(9368):1496–501.

86. Song M, Garrett WS, Chan AT. Nutrients, foods, and colorectal cancer prevention. Gastroenterology 2015;148(6):1244–60.e6.

87. O'Keefe SJ, Li JV, Lahti L, et al. Fat, fibre and cancer risk in African Americans and rural Africans. Nat Commun 2015;6:6342.

88. Chen HM, Yu YN, Wang JL, et al. Decreased dietary fiber intake and structural alteration of gut microbiota in patients with advanced colorectal adenoma. Am J Clin Nutr 2013;97(5):1044–52.

89. Tanji N, Ross MD, Cara A, et al. Effect of tissue processing on the ability to recover nucleic acid from specific renal tissue compartments by laser capture microdissection. Exp Nephrol 2001;9(3):229–34.

90. Wirbel J, Pyl PT, Kartal E, et al. Meta-analysis of fecal metagenomes reveals global microbial signatures that are specific for colorectal cancer. Nat Med 2019;25(4):679–89.

91. Yachida S, Mizutani S, Shiroma H, et al. Metagenomic and metabolomic analyses reveal distinct stage-specific phenotypes of the gut microbiota in colorectal cancer. Nat Med 2019;25(6):968–76.

92. Kanazawa K, Konishi F, Mitsuoka T, et al. Factors influencing the development of sigmoid colon cancer. Bacteriologic and biochemical studies. Cancer 1996; 77(8 Suppl):1701–6.

93. Ridlon JM, Harris SC, Bhowmik S, et al. Consequences of bile salt biotransformations by intestinal bacteria. Gut Microbes 2016;7(1):22–39.

94. Swann JR, Want EJ, Geier FM, et al. Systemic gut microbial modulation of bile acid metabolism in host tissue compartments. Proc Natl Acad Sci U S A 2011;108(Suppl 1):4523–30.

95. Bernstein H, Bernstein C, Payne CM, et al. Bile acids as endogenous etiologic agents in gastrointestinal cancer. World J Gastroenterol 2009;15(27):3329–40.

96. Gagniere J, Raisch J, Veziant J, et al. Gut microbiota imbalance and colorectal cancer. World J Gastroenterol 2016;22(2):501–18.

97. Chung L, Orberg ET, Geis AL, et al. Bacteroides fragilis Toxin Coordinates a Procarcinogenic Inflammatory Cascade via Targeting of Colonic Epithelial Cells. Cell Host Microbe 2018;23(3):421.

98. Zhu J, Liao M, Yao Z, et al. Breast cancer in postmenopausal women is associated with an altered gut metagenome. Microbiome 2018;6(1):136.

99. Adolph TE, Tomczak MF, Niederreiter L, et al. Paneth cells as a site of origin for intestinal inflammation. Nature 2013;503(7475):272–6.

100. Buchta Rosean C, Bostic RR, Ferey JCM, et al. Preexisting Commensal Dysbiosis Is a Host-Intrinsic Regulator of Tissue Inflammation and Tumor Cell Dissemination in Hormone Receptor-Positive Breast Cancer. Cancer Res 2019;79(14): 3662–75.

101. Plottel CS, Blaser MJ. Microbiome and malignancy. Cell Host Microbe 2011; 10(4):324–35.

102. Parida S, Sharma D. The Microbiome-Estrogen Connection and Breast Cancer Risk. Cells 2019;8(12):1642.

103. Donovan SM. Introduction to the special focus issue on the impact of diet on gut microbiota composition and function and future opportunities for nutritional modulation of the gut microbiome to improve human health. Gut Microbes 2017;8(2):75–81.

104. Martinez Steele E, Baraldi LG, Louzada ML, et al. Ultra-processed foods and added sugars in the US diet: evidence from a nationally representative cross-sectional study. BMJ Open 2016;6(3):e009892.
105. World Cancer Research Fund/American Institute for Cancer Research. Diet, Nutrition, Physical Activity and Cancer: A Global Perspective. Continuous Update Project Expert Report. 2018;50.
106. Buckland G, Ros MM, Roswall N, et al. Adherence to the Mediterranean diet and risk of bladder cancer in the EPIC cohort study. Int J Cancer 2014;134(10): 2504–11.
107. Cade JE, Taylor EF, Burley VJ, et al. Does the Mediterranean dietary pattern or the Healthy Diet Index influence the risk of breast cancer in a large British cohort of women? Eur J Clin Nutr 2011;65(8):920–8.
108. Zhu Y, Kawaguchi K, Kiyama R. Differential and directional estrogenic signaling pathways induced by enterolignans and their precursors. PLoS One 2017;12(2): e0171390.
109. Iglesias-Vazquez L, Van Ginkel Riba G, Arija V, et al. Composition of gut microbiota in children with autism spectrum disorder: a systematic review and meta-analysis. Nutrients 2020;12(3):792.
110. Golofast B, Vales K. The connection between microbiome and schizophrenia. Neurosci Biobehav Rev 2020;108:712–31.
111. Coretti L, Paparo L, Riccio MP, et al. Gut microbiota features in young children with autism spectrum disorders. Front Microbiol 2018;9:3146.
112. Strati F, Cavalieri D, Albanese D, et al. New evidences on the altered gut microbiota in autism spectrum disorders. Microbiome 2017;5(1):24.
113. MacFabe DF. Enteric short-chain fatty acids: microbial messengers of metabolism, mitochondria, and mind: implications in autism spectrum disorders. Microb Ecol Health Dis 2015;26:28177.
114. Shimmura C, Suda S, Tsuchiya KJ, et al. Alteration of plasma glutamate and glutamine levels in children with high-functioning autism. PLoS One 2011; 6(10):e25340.
115. Israelyan N, Margolis KG. Serotonin as a link between the gut-brain-microbiome axis in autism spectrum disorders. Pharmacol Res 2018;132:1–6.
116. Lange KW, Hauser J, Reissmann A. Gluten-free and casein-free diets in the therapy of autism. Curr Opin Clin Nutr Metab Care 2015;18(6):572–5.
117. Newell C, Bomhof MR, Reimer RA, et al. Ketogenic diet modifies the gut microbiota in a murine model of autism spectrum disorder. Mol Autism 2016;7(1):37.
118. Suskind DL, Wahbeh G, Gregory N, et al. Nutritional therapy in pediatric Crohn disease: the specific carbohydrate diet. J Pediatr Gastroenterol Nutr 2014; 58(1):87–91.
119. Biesalski HK. Nutrition meets the microbiome: micronutrients and the microbiota. Ann N Y Acad Sci 2016;1372(1):53–64.
120. Selma-Royo M, Tarrazo M, Garcia-Mantrana I, et al. Shaping Microbiota During the First 1000 Days of Life. Adv Exp Med Biol 2019;1125:3–24.
121. Sun J. Dietary vitamin D, vitamin D receptor, and microbiome. Curr Opin Clin Nutr Metab Care 2018;21(6):471–4.
122. Bakke D, Sun J. Ancient nuclear receptor VDR with new functions: microbiome and inflammation. Inflamm Bowel Dis 2018;24(6):1149–54.
123. Wu S, Zhang YG, Lu R, et al. Intestinal epithelial vitamin D receptor deletion leads to defective autophagy in colitis. Gut 2015;64(7):1082–94.

124. Kabbani TA, Koutroubakis IE, Schoen RE, et al. Association of vitamin D level with clinical status in inflammatory bowel disease: a 5-year longitudinal study. Am J Gastroenterol 2016;111(5):712–9.

125. Ananthakrishnan AN, Khalili H, Higuchi LM, et al. Higher predicted vitamin D status is associated with reduced risk of Crohn's disease. Gastroenterology 2012;142(3):482–9.

126. Lv Z, Wang Y, Yang T, et al. Vitamin A deficiency impacts the structural segregation of gut microbiota in children with persistent diarrhea. J Clin Biochem Nutr 2016;59(2):113–21.

127. Liu J, Liu X, Xiong XQ, et al. Effect of vitamin A supplementation on gut microbiota in children with autism spectrum disorders - a pilot study. BMC Microbiol 2017;17(1):204.

128. Pierre JF, Hinterleitner R, Bouziat R, et al. Dietary antioxidant micronutrients alter mucosal inflammatory risk in a murine model of genetic and microbial susceptibility. J Nutr Biochem 2018;54:95–104.

129. Xu J, Xu C, Chen X, et al. Regulation of an antioxidant blend on intestinal redox status and major microbiota in early weaned piglets. Nutrition 2014;30(5):584–9.

130. Yang Q, Liang Q, Balakrishnan B, et al. Role of dietary nutrients in the modulation of gut microbiota: a narrative review. Nutrients 2020;12(2):381.

131. Fergus C, Barnes D, Alqasem MA, et al. The queuine micronutrient: charting a course from microbe to man. Nutrients 2015;7(4):2897–929.

132. Kozlovski I, Agami R. Queuing up the ribosome: nutrition and the microbiome control protein synthesis. EMBO J 2018;37(18):e100405.

133. Okada N, Shindo-Okada N, Sato S, et al. Detection of unique tRNA species in tumor tissues by Escherichia coli guanine insertion enzyme. Proc Natl Acad Sci U S A 1978;75(9):4247–51.

134. Aytac U, Gündüz U. Q-modification of tRNAs in human brain tumors. Cancer Biochem Biophys 1994;14(2):93–8.

135. Baranowski W, Dirheimer G, Jakowicki JA, et al. Deficiency of queuine, a highly modified purine base, in transfer RNAs from primary and metastatic ovarian malignant tumors in women. Cancer Res 1994;54(16):4468–71.

136. Emmerich B, Zubrod E, Weber H, et al. Relationship of queuine-lacking transfer RNAs to the grade of malignancy in human leukemias and lymphomas. Cancer Res 1985;45(9):4308–14.

137. Huang B-S, Wu R-T, Chien K-Y. Relationship of the queuine content of transfer ribonucleic acids to histopathological grading and survival in human lung cancer. Cancer Res 1992;52(17):4696–700.

138. Singhal RP, Vakharia VN. The role of queuine in the aminoacylation of mammalian aspartate transfer RNAs. Nucleic Acids Res 1983;11(12):4257–72.

139. Gündüz U, Elliott MS, Seubert PH, et al. Absence of tRNA-guanine transglycosylase in a human colon adenocarcinoma cell line. Biochim Biophys Acta 1992;1139(3):229–38.

140. Zackular JP, Moore JL, Jordan AT, et al. Dietary zinc alters the microbiota and decreases resistance to Clostridium difficile infection. Nat Med 2016;22(11):1330–4.

141. Shao Y, Lei Z, Yuan J, et al. Effect of zinc on growth performance, gut morphometry, and cecal microbial community in broilers challenged with Salmonella enterica serovar typhimurium. J Microbiol 2014;52(12):1002–11.

142. Berglund S, Domellof M. Meeting iron needs for infants and children. Curr Opin Clin Nutr Metab Care 2014;17(3):267–72.

143. Ellermann M, Gharaibeh RZ, Maharshak N, et al. Dietary iron variably modulates assembly of the intestinal microbiota in colitis-resistant and colitis-susceptible mice. Gut Microbes 2020;11(1):32–50.

144. Nairz M, Schroll A, Sonnweber T, et al. The struggle for iron - a metal at the host-pathogen interface. Cell Microbiol 2010;12(12):1691–702.

145. Constante M, Fragoso G, Lupien-Meilleur J, et al. Iron Supplements Modulate Colon Microbiota Composition and Potentiate the Protective Effects of Probiotics in Dextran Sodium Sulfate-induced Colitis. Inflamm Bowel Dis 2017;23(5): 753–66.

146. Gibson GR, Roberfroid MB. Dietary modulation of the human colonic microbiota: introducing the concept of prebiotics. J Nutr 1995;125(6):1401–12.

147. Depeint F, Tzortzis G, Vulevic J, et al. Prebiotic evaluation of a novel galactoo-ligosaccharide mixture produced by the enzymatic activity of Bifidobacterium bifidum NCIMB 41171, in healthy humans: a randomized, double-blind, cross-over, placebo-controlled intervention study. Am J Clin Nutr 2008;87(3):785–91.

148. He Y, Lawlor NT, Newburg DS. Human Milk Components Modulate Toll-Like Re-ceptor-Mediated Inflammation. Adv Nutr 2016;7(1):102–11.

149. Kulinich A, Liu L. Human milk oligosaccharides: the role in the fine-tuning of innate immune responses. Carbohydr Res 2016;432:62–70.

150. Wijnands MV, Schoterman HC, Bruijntjes JB, et al. Effect of dietary galacto-oligosaccharides on azoxymethane-induced aberrant crypt foci and colorectal cancer in Fischer 344 rats. Carcinogenesis 2001;22(1):127–32.

151. Gibson GR, Hutkins R, Sanders ME, et al. Expert consensus document: the In-ternational Scientific Association for Probiotics and Prebiotics (ISAPP) consensus statement on the definition and scope of prebiotics. Nat Rev Gastro-enterol Hepatol 2017;14(8):491–502.

152. de Vrese M, Schrezenmeir J. Probiotics, prebiotics, and synbiotics. Adv Bio-chem Eng Biotechnol 2008;111:1–66.

153. De Vadder F, Kovatcheva-Datchary P, Goncalves D, et al. Microbiota-generated metabolites promote metabolic benefits via gut-brain neural circuits. Cell 2014; 156(1–2):84–96.

154. Blekhman R, Goodrich JK, Huang K, et al. Host genetic variation impacts micro-biome composition across human body sites. Genome Biol 2015;16:191.

155. Turpin W, Espin-Garcia O, Xu W, et al. Association of host genome with intestinal microbial composition in a large healthy cohort. Nat Genet 2016;48(11):1413–7.

156. Wang J, Thingholm LB, Skieceviciene J, et al. Genome-wide association anal-ysis identifies variation in vitamin D receptor and other host factors influencing the gut microbiota. Nat Genet 2016;48(11):1396–406.

157. Bonder MJ, Kurilshikov A, Tigchelaar EF, et al. The effect of host genetics on the gut microbiome. Nat Genet 2016;48(11):1407–12.

158. Chatterjee I, Lu R, Zhang Y, et al. Vitamin D receptor promotes healthy microbial metabolites and microbiome. Sci Rep 2020;10:7340.

159. Zhang YG, Lu R, Wu S, et al. Vitamin D Receptor Protects Against Dysbiosis and Tumorigenesis via the JAK/STAT Pathway in Intestine. Cell Mol Gastroenterol Hepatol 2020.

160. Ogbu D, Xia E, Sun J. Gut instincts: vitamin D/vitamin D receptor and micro-biome in neurodevelopment disorders. Open Biol 2020;10:200063.

Colorectal Cancer and Diet
Risk Versus Prevention, Is Diet an Intervention?

Elinor Zhou, MD[a],*, Samara Rifkin, MD, ScM[b]

KEYWORDS

- Colorectal cancer • Diet • Fiber • Red meat • Processed meat
- n-3 polyunsaturated fatty acids (PUFAs) • Vitamin D • Calcium

KEY POINTS

- This article reviews prior studies involving certain food items and their relation to colorectal cancer (CRC), as dietary modification may have the potential to decrease CRC incidence.
- There is biological plausibility regarding the beneficial potential of fiber on CRC, but the human data are inconclusive.
- There is convincing evidence regarding the harmful effect of red meat and especially processed meat on the risk of CRC.
- There is strong evidence that consuming dairy products and dietary calcium decreases the risk of CRC. The evidence for vitamin D is limited.
- Further studies are needed to conclude with certainty the relationships between diet and CRC risk.

INTRODUCTION

Colorectal cancer (CRC) is the third most common cause of cancer in men and women in the United States and the world.[1,2] CRC varies globally and increasing rates have followed in the footsteps of Westernization.[3] Epidemiologic studies and migrant studies have provided evidence that rising CRC rates are associated with increased alcohol use; smoking; physical inactivity; high intake of fat, red and processed meat, and processed foods; and low intake of fiber, including whole grains and leafy vegetables.[4–6] Rates of CRC have stabilized in Western countries in part because of colon cancer screening. Still, CRC rates have been rising in younger age groups and continue to increase in westernizing low-income countries.[4,7] Given ongoing CRC despite recommended colon cancer screening and increased rates in individuals

[a] Division of Gastroenterology and Hepatology, Johns Hopkins University School of Medicine, 1830 East Monument Street, Suite 431, Baltimore, MD, USA; [b] Department of Medicine, Division of Gastroenterology and Hepatology, University of Michigan School of Medicine, 1150 West Medical Center Drive, 6520 MSRB1, Ann Arbor, MI, USA
* Corresponding author.
E-mail address: zhou.elinor@gmail.com
Twitter: @ElinorZhouMD (E.Z.)

Gastroenterol Clin N Am 50 (2021) 101–111
https://doi.org/10.1016/j.gtc.2020.10.012
0889-8553/21/© 2020 Elsevier Inc. All rights reserved.

before screening age, future progress in CRC prevention should leverage prevention efforts by reducing modifiable risk factors, including tobacco cessation, weight loss, and diet modification.

Epidemiologic research approximates that more than one-half of colon cancer risk is preventable by modifiable risk factors, including diet.[8,9] Data suggest a potential role for intestinal microbiota in mediating the association between diet and colorectal neoplasia.[10]

Based on prior studies, including observational data, a protective diet against CRC has been defined to include avoidance of processed and charred red meat, the inclusion of vegetables (especially cruciferous) and fiber. This article reviews prior studies involving certain food items and their relation to CRC, as dietary modification may have the potential to decrease CRC incidence.

FIBER

Fiber protects against colorectal carcinogenesis in part by limiting the exposure of epithelial mucosa to fecal carcinogens by bulking fecal stream, binding fecal carcinogens (ie, secondary bile acids), increasing motility, and decreasing stool transit time and building biomass of beneficial colonizers.[11] Fermentation of fiber by colonic anaerobic bacteria creates an acidic milieu limiting toxin production, and leads to the production of short-chain fatty acids with a myriad of beneficial effects, including butyrate, propionate, and acetate.[11–13] Butyrate, the preferred energy source of colonic epithelial cells, stabilizes gut barrier function, improves peripheral insulin sensitivity, and protects against colorectal carcinogenesis.[14] Butyrate accumulates in colon cancer cell cytoplasm, where it acts as a histone deacetylase inhibitor suppressing proliferation and leading to apoptosis.[11,15] In fiber-deficient settings, researchers have demonstrated how *Akkermansia muciniphila,* a mucus-degrading bacteria, uses mucus glycoproteins as a nutrition source, thinning the mucus barrier and permitting access to the epithelium.[11,16] Conversely, supplementation with fiber and *Bifidobacterium* strengthened gut barrier function and reduced inflammation.[17]

The human data regarding protective effects against CRC is compelling but inconclusive. Numerous case-controls and prospective cohort studies have found inverse associations,[18–20] but many have found null associations.[21–24] The World Cancer Research Fund aggregated 43 cohort studies and randomized control trials and found that 10 g fiber per day was inversely associated with a 10% reduction in CRC.[25] Several studies, including a large meta-analysis combining 25 prospective studies, have noted an association with cereal fiber and whole grains rather than fruits and vegetables.[18,26–30] Studies with significant findings are marked by study populations with a higher upper level of fiber intake and higher amount of fiber from cereal and whole grains, including those in European countries described in the EPIC (European Investigation into Cancer and Nutrition) study.[19] Higher fiber intake after the diagnosis of nonmetastatic CRC has also been associated with lower CRC-specific and overall mortality.[31]

Notably, 7 randomized controlled trials evaluating the use of fiber to prevent secondary colorectal adenomas and carcinomas have failed to demonstrate a protective association.[32–39] The Polyp Prevention Study randomized patients to a high-fiber low-fat diet, and found no association between increased fiber intake and reduced risk of colorectal neoplasia. Notably, a subgroup analysis found a significant inverse association among patients who consumed the highest quartile of dry bean consumption and reduced risk of adenomas.[40] Other fiber interventions with intermediate outcomes present convincing evidence of preventing early procarcinogenic changes to the colonic epithelium. In the Dietary Switch study, African American individuals at high risk of colon cancer were given 50 g of fiber per day. After only 2 weeks, suggestive changes were observed in microbiota and short-chain fatty acids, and colonic mucosa cancer biomarkers were improved.[41]

RED AND PROCESSED MEAT

The International Agency for Research on Cancer issued a review that classified red meat as "probably carcinogenic to humans" (group 2A) and processed meat as Class I, "carcinogenic to humans."[42] The systemic review and meta-analysis performed by the World Cancer Research Fund's Continuous Update Project included 19 case-controls and 7 prospective observational studies and found a relative risk of 12% and 16% increased fold of CRC for every 100 g of red meat and processed meat consumed, respectively.[43] Several studies have also described stronger associations with distal colon cancer compared with proximal.[44,45]

Several compounds within meat likely contribute to carcinogenesis, including N-nitroso compounds (NOCs), heme, heterocyclic amines (HCAs), and polycyclic aromatic hydrocarbons (PAHs) created during the process of cooking red meat at high temperature.[42] NOCs are alkylating agents formed from nitrites or nitrates added as preservatives to processed meat.[46,47] In the colon, NOCs are transformed into DNA adducts by bacteria and go on to cause mutations during DNA replication.[47] Heme contained in myoglobin can lead to oxidative stress and endogenous NOC formation. Observational studies have found a significant association between dietary HCAs and PAHs and CRC incidence, even after adjusting for red meat consumption.[48–52] Genetic variation in certain enzymes that activate or deactivate HCAs and PAHs have been shown to strengthen or weaken the relationship between meat exposure and CRC.[50,53–55] A large US prospective study on meat type and cooking methods demonstrated an increased risk of CRC associated with red meat intake and processed meat intake and also detected association between heme iron, nitrates from processed meat, and heterocyclic amine intake.[52,56,57]

Related to meat consumption is the high sulfur content contained in animal tissue, which has also been associated with CRC. Processed meat is rich in sulfur amino acids. Fermentation of meat by sulfate-reducing bacteria produces hydrogen sulfide (H_2S). H_2S breaks down the disulfide bonds that hold the mucus layer together, permitting epithelial access and colitis, and in addition, causes DNA damage and alters intraepithelial immune cell populations.[58–60] Elevated levels of sulfate-reducing bacteria and fecal H_2S content have been described in men with distal CRC.[61] A large US cohort study found an association between elevated sulfur microbial dietary score and distal colon and rectal cancer risk in men.[61] Another case-control study discovered that sulfidogenic bacteria were observed more frequently in African American patients with CRC when compared with controls.[62]

HIGH-FAT DIET

In 1973, Drasar and Irving[63] first described that colon cancer was highly correlated with fat intake. Reddy[64] reaffirmed this linkage by reporting an ecologic correlation between per-capita consumption of animal fat and national rates of CRC. Based on animal studies, high-fat diets are proposed to increase the intestinal excretion of bile acids, which can be metabolized by gut bacteria to deoxycholic acid, damage colonic mucosa, and promote CRC development.[65] High-fat diets are also proposed to induce changes in the intestinal microbiome composition, causing alterations in intestinal immune and inflammatory factors involved in gut tumorigenesis.[66]

In human studies, the correlation between fat intake and CRC remains controversial. Previous studies have shown that high-fat-intake groups have a higher CRC risk than low-fat-intake groups. For example, in 1990, the Nurses' Health Study, a prospective cohort study, found that the highest quintile of animal fat intake compared with the lowest was associated with an increased colon cancer risk, with a relative risk (RR) of 1.89 (95% CI 1.13–3.15, $P = .01$).[67] A study evaluating different fat intake types found that both saturated fat and cholesterol were significantly associated with the risk of developing CRC (OR 5.23, 95% CI 2.33–11.76; and OR 2.48, 95% CI 1.18–5.21, respectively)[68]; however, many studies have failed to find associations between total fat or fatty acids with the risk of CRC.[32,69]

A 2011 meta-analysis of 13 prospective cohort studies with 459,910 participants showed that the combined RR of CRC was 0.99 (95% CI 0.89–1.09) when the highest level of total dietary fat was compared with the lowest level.[70] A 2018 meta-analysis of 18 studies found that the pooled RRs for the risk of CRC were 1.00 (95% CI 0.90–1.12), 0.97 (95% CI 0.86–1.10), 1.08 (95% CI 0.92–1.26), and 0.99 (95% CI 0.93–1.04) for total fat, saturated fatty acid, monounsaturated fatty acid, and polyunsaturated fatty acid, respectively.[71] The meta-analyses suggest that dietary fats and fatty acids have no effects on the risk of CRC.

In animal studies, n-3 polyunsaturated fatty acids (PUFAs) appear to have anti-inflammatory properties and may protect against CRC, whereas n-6 PUFAs have inflammatory potential and may lead to colorectal tumorigenesis.[72] n-3 PUFAs compete with n-6 PUFAs, blocking cyclooxygenase-mediated production of inflammatory eicosanoids, prostaglandin E_2 (PGE$_2$), associated with colorectal adenomas and cancers, through competitive inhibition of n-6 PUFAs.[73–78] n-3 PUFAs also may act through anti-inflammatory eicosanoids, which reduce cell proliferation, enhance cell apoptosis, and promote cell differentiation.[79,80]

Human studies are equivocal regarding antitumorigenic roles of n-3 PUFAs. A meta-analysis of 20 prospective observational studies found that the highest category of n-3 PUFA serum levels were inversely associated with CRC, whereas the association by n-3 PUFA intake calculated by food frequency questionnaire (FFQ) was null.[81] Studies using FFQs to measure n-3 PUFA more frequently find null associations as they introduce considerable variability in terms of self-reported intake of fish as well as bioavailability of nutrients as PUFA amounts vary by food source, fishing season, and cooking methods.[59,82] Also, the biosynthesis of long-chain PUFAs is minimal and varies from person to person.[83]

Randomized controlled trials evaluating the effect of n-3 PUFA intervention on colorectal neoplasia have produced mixed results. Treatment with 2 g of eicosapentaenoic acid (EPA) in subjects with familial adenomatous polyposis for 6 months was associated with a mean reduction in polyp number and polyp size.[84] The seAFOod RCT treated high-risk patients with EPA 200 mg, aspirin (ASA) 300 mg, both EPA and ASA, or placebo, and failed to detect a difference in adenoma detection rate for EPA, ASA or the combined arm compared with placebo. Although the trial did not find an association with the primary outcome, they demonstrated some evidence of chemoprevention, as EPA reduced mean left-sided adenomas and conventional adenomas.[85,86]

There have been few studies evaluating n-3 PUFA as chemotherapy. A prospective study found that patients with stage III colon cancer who consumed higher intake of marine omega-3 fatty acid derived from FFQs had improved 3-year disease-free survival for KRAS wild-type tumors and deficient mismatch repair.[87]

FRUITS AND NONSTARCHY VEGETABLES

Fruits and vegetables may protect against CRC because of their high levels of several potential anticarcinogenic and antimutagenic compounds, including fiber, carotenoids, flavonoids, folate, other B vitamins, vitamins C and E, minerals, and antioxidants.[88,89] Many of these compounds have potent antioxidative properties, which could inhibit cell damage and exposure to reactive oxygen species, and thus potentially protect against CRC. The suggested mechanisms for prevention of cancer include induction of detoxifying phase II enzymes, antioxidant activity, protection against DNA damage, modulation of DNA methylation, and promotion of apoptosis.[89]

Prior epidemiologic studies of fruits and vegetables have been inconsistent and inconclusive. This is probably due to a large amount of unaccounted variation, including the amount of consumption, nutrient content, and varied cooking and preparation and storage.[59] A 2013 meta-analysis of 9 studies on fruit and 8 studies on vegetables found that low intakes of these foods were significant risk factors for CRC.[90] A 2007 pooled analysis of 14 cohort studies reported that fruit and vegetable intake was not strongly associated with colon cancer overall, but may be associated with a lower risk of distal colon cancer (when comparing total fruit and vegetable intakes of 800 g/d or more vs <200 g/d, multivariate RR was 0.74; 95% CI 0.57–0.95; P = .02).[91] A 2016 prospective study found that total fruit and vegetable intake was not associated with reduced incident or recurrent colon adenoma risk overall, but a significant inverse association was observed for multiple adenomas (OR third tertile vs first tertile = 0.61, 95% CI 0.38–1.00).[92]

With regard to fruits, the World Cancer Research Fund's 2018 update reviewed 21 studies (24 publications) and concluded that there is limited evidence suggesting that low consumption of fruit increases the risk of CRC. With regard to nonstarchy vegetables, they identified 23 studies (32 publications) reviewing the evidence for nonstarchy plants and the development of CRC. They concluded that there is limited evidence suggesting that low consumption of nonstarchy vegetables increases the risk of CRC.[93]

DAIRY, CALCIUM, VITAMIN D

Dairy products are hypothesized to be protective against CRC because of high calcium content, vitamin D content, conjugated linoleic acid, butyric acid, and fermented dairy products.[94] Ionized calcium can form insoluble soaps with tumor-promoting free fatty acids and bile acids in the colonic lumen. This led to the hypothesis that calcium was antitumorigenic and protective against CRC.[95] In addition, extracellular dietary calcium activates calcium-sensing receptors in intestinal epithelial cells, which are capable of activating diverse intracellular signaling pathways involved in proliferation, differentiation, and the control of apoptosis, suggesting that dietary calcium plays an essential role in the prevention of colonic cancer through its pleiotropic effects on normal and preneoplastic colonic epithelial cells.[96] Laboratory studies have demonstrated that vitamin D may be involved in a wide spectrum of anticancer activities: antiproliferation, apoptosis, anti-inflammation, prevention of invasion and metastasis, and suppression of angiogenesis.[97]

With regard to dairy products, the World Cancer Research Fund's 2018 update identified 14 studies (16 publications) reviewing the evidence for dairy products and CRC. Their dose-response meta-analysis (14,859 cases) showed a 13% decreased risk per 400 g of dairy per day (RR 0.87, 95% CI 0.83–0.90).[93] They concluded that the consumption of dairy products likely protects against CRC, and is supported with good quality of evidence. A 2011 meta-analysis (19 cohort studies) looked at the dose-response relationship between different dairy products and CRC risk and found that milk and total dairy products, but not cheese or other dairy products, were associated with a reduction in CRC risk.[98]

For dietary calcium, the World Cancer Research Fund's 2018 update identified 20 studies (26 publications) reviewing the evidence for dietary calcium and CRC. A pooled analysis of 10 studies reported a significant inverse association.[93] Thirteen studies were included in a dose-response meta-analysis (11,519 cases) that showed a 6% decreased risk per 200 mg of dietary calcium per day (RR 0.94 [95% CI 0.93–0.96]). The evidence consistently demonstrated an inverse association between dietary calcium and CRC risk.

With regard to foods containing vitamin D, the World Cancer Research Fund's 2018 update identified 15 studies reviewing the evidence on foods containing vitamin D and CRC. They noted a significant 5% decreased risk per 100 IU of Vitamin D per day (RR 0.95; 95% CI 0.93–0.98; I^2 = 11%, n = 5171, 10 studies). They concluded that the evidence for vitamin D was limited but generally consistent.[93]

SUMMARY

This article reviews prior studies involving certain food items and their relation to CRC. The data are conflicting, with most protective foods lacking convincing randomized control trials; however, some observational studies and laboratory studies provide compelling evidence that diet may have the potential to modify CRC incidence, as in the case of fiber, dairy and calcium, and red meat and processed meat. Recent research suggests that the intestinal microbiome, which is heavily influenced and shaped by dietary intake, may play a role in modifying the risk of colorectal carcinogenesis. Further studies are needed to definitively investigate the relationships between diet and CRC risk and map out the interactions between food and microbiome.

DISCLOSURE

The authors have nothing to disclose.

REFERENCES

1. Cancer Stat Facts: Colorectal Cancer. National Cancer Institute Surveillance, Epidemoiology, and End Results Program Web site. 2019. Available at: https://seer.cancer.gov/statfacts/html/colorect.html. Accessed March 1, 2020.
2. Ferlay J, Soerjomataram I, Dikshit R, et al. Cancer incidence and mortality worldwide: sources, methods and major patterns in GLOBOCAN 2012. Int J Cancer 2015;136(5):E359–86.
3. Keum N, Giovannucci E. Global burden of colorectal cancer: emerging trends, risk factors and prevention strategies. Nat Rev Gastroenterol Hepatol 2019; 16(12):713–32.
4. Murphy N, Moreno V, Hughes DJ, et al. Lifestyle and dietary environmental factors in colorectal cancer susceptibility. Mol Aspects Med 2019;69:2–9.
5. Hughes LAE, Simons CCJM, Brandt PAvd, et al. Lifestyle, diet, and colorectal cancer risk according to (epi)genetic instability: current evidence and future directions of molecular pathological epidemiology. Curr Colorectal Cancer Rep 2017;13(6):455–69.
6. Thomas DB, Karagas MR. Cancer in first and second generation Americans. Cancer Res 1987;47(21):5771–6.

7. Stoffel EM, Murphy CC. Epidemiology and mechanisms of the increasing incidence of colon and rectal cancers in young adults. Gastroenterology 2020; 158(2):341–53.
8. Platz EA, Willett WC, Colditz GA, et al. Proportion of colon cancer risk that might be preventable in a cohort of middle-aged US men. Cancer Causes Control 2000; 11(7):579–88.
9. Erdrich J, Zhang X, Giovannucci E, et al. Proportion of colon cancer attributable to lifestyle in a cohort of US women. Cancer Causes Control 2015;26(9):1271–9.
10. Mehta RS, Nishihara R, Cao Y, et al. Association of dietary patterns with risk of colorectal cancer subtypes classified by fusobacterium nucleatum in tumor tissue. JAMA Oncol 2017;3(7):921–7.
11. Ocvirk S, Wilson AS, Appolonia CN, et al. Fiber, fat, and colorectal cancer: new insight into modifiable dietary risk factors. Curr Gastroenterol Rep 2019; 21(11):62.
12. Zeng H, Lazarova DL, Bordonaro M. Mechanisms linking dietary fiber, gut microbiota and colon cancer prevention. World J Gastrointest Oncol 2014;6(2):41–51.
13. Smith EA, Macfarlane GT. Enumeration of human colonic bacteria producing phenolic and indolic compounds: effects of pH, carbohydrate availability and retention time on dissimilatory aromatic amino acid metabolism. J Appl Bacteriol 1996;81(3):288–302.
14. McNabney SM, Henagan TM. Short chain fatty acids in the colon and peripheral tissues: a focus on butyrate, colon cancer, obesity and insulin resistance. Nutrients 2017;9(12):1348.
15. Donohoe DR, Holley D, Collins LB, et al. A gnotobiotic mouse model demonstrates that dietary fiber protects against colorectal tumorigenesis in a microbiota- and butyrate-dependent manner. Cancer Discov 2014;4(12):1387–97.
16. Desai MS, Seekatz AM, Koropatkin NM, et al. A dietary fiber-deprived gut microbiota degrades the colonic mucus barrier and enhances pathogen susceptibility. Cell 2016;167(5):1339–53.e1.
17. Schroeder BO, Birchenough GMH, Ståhlman M, et al. Bifidobacteria or fiber protects against diet-induced microbiota-mediated colonic mucus deterioration. Cell Host Microbe 2018;23(1):27–40.e27.
18. Aune D, Chan DSM, Lau R, et al. Dietary fibre, whole grains, and risk of colorectal cancer: systematic review and dose-response meta-analysis of prospective studies. BMJ 2011;343:d6617.
19. Bingham SA, Day NE, Luben R, et al. Dietary fibre in food and protection against colorectal cancer in the European Prospective Investigation into Cancer and Nutrition (EPIC): an observational study. Lancet 2003;361(9368):1496–501.
20. Dahm CC, Keogh RH, Spencer EA, et al. Dietary fiber and colorectal cancer risk: a nested case-control study using food diaries. J Natl Cancer Inst 2010;102(9):614–26.
21. Fuchs CS, Giovannucci EL, Colditz GA, et al. Dietary fiber and the risk of colorectal cancer and adenoma in women. N Engl J Med 1999;340(3):169–76.
22. Park Y, Hunter DJ, Spiegelman D, et al. Dietary fiber intake and risk of colorectal cancer: a pooled analysis of prospective cohort studies. JAMA 2005;294(22):2849–57.
23. Terry P, Giovannucci E, Michels KB, et al. Fruit, vegetables, dietary fiber, and risk of colorectal cancer. J Natl Cancer Inst 2001;93(7):525–33.
24. Pietinen P, Malila N, Virtanen M, et al. Diet and risk of colorectal cancer in a cohort of Finnish men. Cancer Causes Control 1999;10(5):387–96.

25. Norat T, Aune D, Chan D, et al. Fruits and vegetables: updating the epidemiologic evidence for the WCRF/AICR lifestyle recommendations for cancer prevention. Cancer Treat Res 2014;159:35–50.
26. Kunzmann AT, Coleman HG, Huang W-Y, et al. Dietary fiber intake and risk of colorectal cancer and incident and recurrent adenoma in the Prostate, Lung, Colorectal, and Ovarian Cancer Screening Trial. Am J Clin Nutr 2015;102(4): 881–90.
27. He X, Wu K, Zhang X, et al. Dietary intake of fiber, whole grains and risk of colorectal cancer: an updated analysis according to food sources, tumor location and molecular subtypes in two large US cohorts. Int J Cancer 2019;145(11):3040–51.
28. Schatzkin A, Mouw T, Park Y, et al. Dietary fiber and whole-grain consumption in relation to colorectal cancer in the NIH-AARP Diet and Health Study. Am J Clin Nutr 2007;85(5):1353–60.
29. Ben Q, Sun Y, Chai R, et al. Dietary fiber intake reduces risk for colorectal adenoma: a meta-analysis. Gastroenterology 2014;146(3):689–99.e6.
30. Hansen L, Skeie G, Landberg R, et al. Intake of dietary fiber, especially from cereal foods, is associated with lower incidence of colon cancer in the HELGA cohort. Int J Cancer 2012;131(2):469–78.
31. Song M, Wu K, Meyerhardt JA, et al. Fiber intake and survival after colorectal cancer diagnosis. JAMA Oncol 2018;4(1):71–9.
32. Beresford SAA, Johnson KC, Ritenbaugh C, et al. Low-fat dietary pattern and risk of colorectal cancer: the Women's Health Initiative Randomized Controlled Dietary Modification Trial. JAMA 2006;295(6):643–54.
33. MacLennan R, Macrae F, Bain C, et al. Randomized trial of intake of fat, fiber, and beta carotene to prevent colorectal adenomas. J Natl Cancer Inst 1995;87(23): 1760–6.
34. Schatzkin A, Lanza E, Corle D, et al. Lack of effect of a low-fat, high-fiber diet on the recurrence of colorectal adenomas. Polyp Prevention Trial Study Group. N Engl J Med 2000;342(16):1149–55.
35. Alberts DS, Martínez ME, Roe DJ, et al. Lack of effect of a high-fiber cereal supplement on the recurrence of colorectal adenomas. N Engl J Med 2000;342(16): 1156–62.
36. Mathers JC, Movahedi M, Macrae F, et al. Long-term effect of resistant starch on cancer risk in carriers of hereditary colorectal cancer: an analysis from the CAPP2 randomised controlled trial. Lancet Oncol 2012;13(12):1242–9.
37. Burn J, Bishop DT, Mecklin J-P, et al. Effect of aspirin or resistant starch on colorectal neoplasia in the Lynch syndrome. N Engl J Med 2008;359(24):2567–78.
38. Yao Y, Suo T, Andersson R, et al. Dietary fibre for the prevention of recurrent colorectal adenomas and carcinomas. Cochrane Database Syst Rev 2017;2017(1): CD003430.
39. Bonithon-Kopp C, Kronborg O, Giacosa A, et al. Calcium and fibre supplementation in prevention of colorectal adenoma recurrence: a randomised intervention trial. European Cancer Prevention Organisation Study Group. Lancet 2000; 356(9238):1300–6.
40. Lanza E, Hartman TJ, Albert PS, et al. High dry bean intake and reduced risk of advanced colorectal adenoma recurrence among participants in the polyp prevention trial. J Nutr 2006;136(7):1896–903.
41. O'Keefe SJ, Li JV, Lahti L, et al. Fat, fibre and cancer risk in African Americans and rural Africans. Nat Commun 2015;6:6342.
42. Bouvard V, Loomis D, Guyton KZ, et al. Carcinogenicity of consumption of red and processed meat. Lancet Oncol 2015;16(16):1599–600.

43. Vieira AR, Abar L, Chan DSM, et al. Foods and beverages and colorectal cancer risk: a systematic review and meta-analysis of cohort studies, an update of the evidence of the WCRF-AICR Continuous Update Project. Ann Oncol 2017; 28(8):1788–802.

44. Etemadi A, Abnet CC, Graubard BI, et al. Anatomical subsite can modify the association between meat and meat compounds and risk of colorectal adenocarcinoma: findings from three large US cohorts. Int J Cancer 2018;143(9):2261–70.

45. Ferrucci LM, Sinha R, Huang W-Y, et al. Meat consumption and the risk of incident distal colon and rectal adenoma. Br J Cancer 2012;106(3):608–16.

46. Aykan NF. Red meat and colorectal cancer. Oncol Rev 2015;9(1):38–44.

47. Alisson-Silva F, Kawanishi K, Varki A. Human risk of diseases associated with red meat intake: analysis of current theories and proposed role for metabolic incorporation of a non-human sialic acid. Mol Aspects Med 2016;51:16–30.

48. Demeyer D, Mertens B, De Smet S, et al. Mechanisms linking colorectal cancer to the consumption of (processed) red meat: a review. Crit Rev Food Sci Nutr 2016; 56(16):2747–66.

49. Rohrmann S, Hermann S, Linseisen J. Heterocyclic aromatic amine intake increases colorectal adenoma risk: findings from a prospective European cohort study. Am J Clin Nutr 2009;89(5):1418–24.

50. Fu Z, Shrubsole MJ, Smalley WE, et al. Associations between dietary fiber and colorectal polyp risk differ by polyp type and smoking status. J Nutr 2014; 144(5):592–8.

51. Sinha R, Cross AJ, Graubard BI, et al. Meat intake and mortality: a prospective study of over half a million people. Arch Intern Med 2009;169(6):562–71.

52. Cross AJ, Ferrucci LM, Risch A, et al. A large prospective study of meat consumption and colorectal cancer risk: an investigation of potential mechanisms underlying this association. Cancer Res 2010;70(6):2406–14.

53. Murtaugh MA, Sweeney C, Ma K-n, et al. The CYP1A1 genotype may alter the association of meat consumption patterns and preparation with the risk of colorectal cancer in men and women. J Nutr 2005;135(2):179–86.

54. Ferrucci LM, Cross AJ, Gunter MJ, et al. Xenobiotic metabolizing genes, meat-related exposures, and risk of advanced colorectal adenoma. World Rev Nutr Diet 2010;101:34–45.

55. Gilsing AMJ, Berndt SI, Ruder EH, et al. Meat-related mutagen exposure, xenobiotic metabolizing gene polymorphisms and the risk of advanced colorectal adenoma and cancer. Carcinogenesis 2012;33(7):1332–9.

56. Martínez Góngora V, Matthes KL, Castaño PR, et al. Dietary heterocyclic amine intake and colorectal adenoma risk: a systematic review and meta-analysis. Cancer Epidemiol Biomarkers Prev 2019;28(1):99–109.

57. Chiavarini M, Bertarelli G, Minelli L, et al. Dietary intake of meat cooking-related mutagens (HCAs) and risk of colorectal adenoma and cancer: a systematic review and meta-analysis. Nutrients 2017;9(5):514.

58. Ijssennagger N, Belzer C, Hooiveld GJ, et al. Gut microbiota facilitates dietary heme-induced epithelial hyperproliferation by opening the mucus barrier in colon. Proc Natl Acad Sci U S A 2015;112(32):10038–43.

59. Song M, Garrett WS, Chan AT. Nutrients, foods, and colorectal cancer prevention. Gastroenterology 2015;148(6):1244–60.e6.

60. Attene-Ramos MS, Nava GM, Muellner MG, et al. DNA damage and toxicogenomic analyses of hydrogen sulfide in human intestinal epithelial FHs 74 Int cells. Environ Mol Mutagen 2010;51(4):304–14.

61. Nguyen LH, Ma W, Wang DD, et al. Association between sulfur-metabolizing bacterial communities in stool and risk of distal colorectal cancer in men. Gastroenterology 2020;158(5):1313–25.
62. Yazici C, Wolf PG, Kim H, et al. Race-dependent association of sulfidogenic bacteria with colorectal cancer. Gut 2017;66(11):1983–94.
63. Drasar BS, Irving D. Environmental factors and cancer of the colon and breast. Br J Cancer 1973;27:167–72.
64. Reddy BS. Types and amount of dietary fat and colon cancer risk: prevention by omega-3 fatty acid-rich diets. Environ Health Prev Med 2002;7:95–102.
65. Nauss KM, Locniskar M, Newberne PM. Effect of alterations in the quality and quantity of dietary fat on 1,2-dimethylhydrazine-induced colon tumorigenesis in rats. Cancer Res 1983;43(9):4083–90.
66. Schulz M, Atay Ç, Heringer J, et al. High-fat-diet-mediated dysbiosis promotes intestinal carcinogenesis independently of obesity. Nature 2014;514:508–12.
67. Willett WC, Stampfer MJ, Colditz GA, et al. Relation of meat, fat, and fiber intake to the risk of colon cancer in a prospective study among women. N Engl J Med 1990;323(24):1664–72.
68. Tayyem RFB, Bawadi HA, Shehadah IN, et al. Macro- and micronutrients consumption and the risk for colorectal cancer among Jordanians. Nutrients 2015;(7):1769–86.
69. Lin JZ SM, Cook NR, Lee IM, et al. Dietary fat and fatty acids and risk of colorectal cancer in women. Am J Epidemiol 2004;160:1011–22.
70. Liu LZW, Wang RQ, Mukherjee R, et al. Is dietary fat associated with the risk of colorectal cancer? A meta-analysis of 13 prospective cohort studies. Eur J Nutr 2011;50:173–84.
71. Kim MPK. Dietary fat intake and risk of colorectal cancer: a systematic review and meta-analysis of prospective studies. Nutrients 2018;10(12) [pii:E1963].
72. Reddy BS. Omega-3 fatty acids in colorectal cancer prevention. Int J Cancer 2004;112(1):1–7.
73. Giardiello FM, Yang VW, Hylind LM, et al. Primary chemoprevention of familial adenomatous polyposis with sulindac. N Engl J Med 2002;346(14):1054–9.
74. Hansen-Petrik MB, McEntee MF, Jull B, et al. Prostaglandin E(2) protects intestinal tumors from nonsteroidal anti-inflammatory drug-induced regression in Apc(-Min/+) mice. Cancer Res 2002;62(2):403–8.
75. Cai Q, Gao Y-T, Chow W-H, et al. Prospective study of urinary prostaglandin E2 metabolite and colorectal cancer risk. J Clin Oncol 2006;24(31):5010–6.
76. Wang D, DuBois RN. Urinary PGE-M: a promising cancer biomarker. Cancer Prev Res 2013;6(6):507–10.
77. Murff HJ, Shrubsole MJ, Cai Q, et al. Dietary intake of PUFAs and colorectal polyp risk. Am J Clin Nutr 2012;95(3):703–12.
78. Shrubsole MJ, Cai Q, Wen W, et al. Urinary prostaglandin E2 metabolite and risk for colorectal adenoma. Cancer Prev Res 2012;5(2):336–42.
79. Rose DP, Connolly JM. Omega-3 fatty acids as cancer chemopreventive agents. Pharmacol Ther 1999;83(3):217–44.
80. Cheng J, Ogawa K, Kuriki K, et al. Increased intake of n-3 polyunsaturated fatty acids elevates the level of apoptosis in the normal sigmoid colon of patients polypectomized for adenomas/tumors. Cancer Lett 2003;193(1):17–24.
81. Kim Y, Kim J. Intake or blood levels of n-3 polyunsaturated fatty acids and risk of colorectal cancer: a systematic review and meta-analysis of prospective studies. Cancer Epidemiol Biomarkers Prev 2020;29(2):288–99.

82. Rifkin SB, Shrubsole MJ, Cai Q, et al. PUFA levels in erythrocyte membrane phospholipids are differentially associated with colorectal adenoma risk. Br J Nutr 2017;117(11):1615–22.
83. Cottet V, Collin M, Gross A-S, et al. Erythrocyte membrane phospholipid fatty acid concentrations and risk of colorectal adenomas: a case-control nested in the French E3N-EPIC cohort study. Cancer Epidemiol Biomarkers Prev 2013;22(8):1417–27.
84. West NJ, Clark SK, Phillips RKS, et al. Eicosapentaenoic acid reduces rectal polyp number and size in familial adenomatous polyposis. Gut 2010;59(7):918–25.
85. Hull MA, Sprange K, Hepburn T, et al. Eicosapentaenoic acid and aspirin, alone and in combination, for the prevention of colorectal adenomas (seAFOod Polyp Prevention trial): a multicentre, randomised, double-blind, placebo-controlled, 2 × 2 factorial trial. Lancet 2018;392(10164):2583–94.
86. Hull MA, Sprange K, Hepburn T, et al. Eicosapentaenoic acid and/or aspirin for preventing colorectal adenomas during colonoscopic surveillance in the NHS Bowel Cancer Screening Programme: the seAFOod RCT. Southampton (UK): NIHR Journals Library; 2019.
87. Song M, Chan AT, Fuchs CS, et al. Dietary intake of fish, ω-3 and ω-6 fatty acids and risk of colorectal cancer: a prospective study in U.S. men and women. Int J Cancer 2014;135(10):2413–23.
88. Steinmetz KA, Potter JD. Vegetables, fruit, and cancer. II. Mechanisms. Cancer Causes Control 1991;2(6):427–42.
89. Zhang SJZ, Yan Z, Yang J. Consumption of fruits and vegetables and risk of renal cell carcinoma: a meta-analysis of observational studies. Oncotarget 2017;8(17):27892–903.
90. Johnson CM, Wei C, Ensor JE, et al. Meta-analyses of colorectal cancer risk factors. Cancer Causes Control 2013;24(6):1207–22.
91. Koushik AHD, Spiegelman D, Beeson WL, et al. Fruits, vegetables, and colon cancer risk in a pooled analysis of 14 cohort studies. J Natl Cancer Inst 2007;99:1471–83.
92. Kunzmann ATCH, Huang WY2 Cantwell MM, Kitahara CM, et al. Fruit and vegetable intakes and risk of colorectal cancer and incident and recurrent adenomas in the PLCO cancer screening trial. Int J Cancer 2016;138(8):1851–61.
93. Research WCRFAIfC. Diet, nutrition, physical activity and colorectal cancer. Revised 2018.
94. Norat T, Riboli E. Dairy products and colorectal cancer. A review of possible mechanisms and epidemiological evidence. Eur J Clin Nutr 2003;57(1):1–17.
95. Newmark HL, Wargovich MJ, Bruce WR. Colon cancer and dietary fat, phosphate, and calcium: a hypothesis. J Natl Cancer Inst 1984;72(6):1323–5.
96. Lamprecht SA, Lipkin M. Cellular mechanisms of calcium and vitamin D in the inhibition of colorectal carcinogenesis. Ann N Y Acad Sci 2001;952:73–87.
97. Feldman D, Krishnan AV, Swami S1, et al. The role of vitamin D in reducing cancer risk and progression. Nat Rev Cancer 2014;14(5):342–57.
98. Aune D, Lau R, Chan DS, et al. Dairy products and colorectal cancer risk: a systematic review and meta-analysis of cohort studies. Ann Oncol 2012;23(1):37–45.

Treatment of Obesity
Beyond the Diet

Sina Gallo, PhD, MSc, RD[a],*, Lawrence J. Cheskin, MD, FACP, FTOS[b]

KEYWORDS

- Adult obesity • Treatment • Nutrition • Dietary • Lifestyle • Comprehensive

KEY POINTS

- In order for weight loss to lead to clinically meaningful results, weight loss must be maintained.
- Energy restriction is effective for immediate weight loss, but approaches tailored to the patient's lifestyle that target changes in nutrition and physical activity are most effective for long-term weight maintenance.
- Monitoring of health-related outcomes is necessary to show intervention effectiveness, and monitoring of behavioral changes (ie, nutrition and physical activity related) also increases effectiveness.

INTRODUCTION

Although treatment of obesity has always proved challenging, the adverse health impact of obesity has long been recognized. As Flemyng pointed out 260 years ago, "*Corpulency, when in extraordinary degree, may be reckoned a disease, as it in some measure obstructs the free exercise of the animal functions; and hath a tendency to shorten life, by paving the way to dangerous distempers.*"[1]

In the present day, data show that 42% of US adults suffer from obesity and 9% suffer from severe obesity.[2] Obesity is often accompanied by metabolic diseases, notably coronary heart disease and type 2 diabetes, which also carry their own morbidity and mortality risks. Disparities in obesity are apparent by race and ethnicity, as Hispanic men and women had a 1.2-fold increased risk of obesity and non-Hispanic black women had a 1.4-fold increased risk compared with their white counterparts. The prevalence also varies by age, urbanization, and education level.[3]

Among adults who are overweight or obese, there is strong evidence to suggest that a reduction of body weight of 2% to 5% leads to improvements in cardiovascular health outcomes.[4] However, to sustain these improvements, weight loss needs to be maintained. Intensive lifestyle interventions have been found to reduce

a Foods and Nutrition, University of Georgia, Dawson Hall room 209, 305 Sanford Drive, Athens, GA 30602, USA; b Nutrition and Food Studies, George Mason University, Johns Hopkins School of Medicine, Peterson Hall, 4114, 1F7, 4400 University Drive, Fairfax, VA 22030, USA
* Corresponding author.
E-mail address: sina.gallo@uga.edu

Gastroenterol Clin N Am 50 (2021) 113–125
https://doi.org/10.1016/j.gtc.2020.10.003
0889-8553/21/© 2020 Elsevier Inc. All rights reserved.

weight and prevent or treat obesity-associated comorbidities. The *Look AHEAD* (Action for Health in Diabetes) study provided intensive lifestyle intervention over 8 years to more than 5000 adults with type 2 diabetes. It found that 39% of participants who lost 10% of their initial body weight by year 1 maintained it at year 8, and another 26% maintained between 5% and 10% loss at year 8.[5] Among the morbidly obese, however, weight loss maintenance is a greater challenge, as less than 5% succeed in losing a significant amount of weight and maintaining the weight loss.[6]

To sustain weight loss changes over time, interventions are necessary that target lifestyle behaviors to decrease energy intake along with improvements in diet quality, combined with increases in energy expenditure. These interventions should be combined with supportive behavioral therapy for best outcomes. The objective of this article is to provide a review of the treatment of adult obesity, primarily focused on dietary interventions, using primarily evidence from randomized clinical trials (RCTs), systematic and meta-analyses, and guidelines on the topic.

DIETARY INTERVENTIONS
Food-Based Changes

The concept of small changes in nutrition and physical activity behaviors is worth highlighting. Although patients often seek aggressive, rapid change, and this does result in greater initial weight loss in some, large regain of weight is a frequent occurrence. Small changes that result in an energy deficit between 100 and 200 kcal per day may be more feasible and sustainable to support weight management and prevent gradual weight gain.[7] Two family-based interventions have tested the "small-changes" approach among those with a child who was overweight/obese.[8,9] The first found a significant difference in the mean change in both percentage body mass index (BMI), for age (−1.1%, P<.05) and percentage body fat (−1.4%, P<.01) between target children in the intervention versus control groups.[8] The latter identified significantly more children maintaining or decreasing their BMI-for-age in the intervention versus control group (67% vs 53%, P<.05).[9] In these interventions, families were asked to make small changes to daily routines, such as consuming cereal for breakfast, replacing dietary sugar with a noncaloric sweetener, or increasing physical activity by an additional 2000 steps per day.

Among adults participating in the Aspiring for Lifelong Health (ASPIRE) program, the small changes group resulted in a clinically significant 5% body weight loss after the 16-week intervention.[10] Unfortunately, the intervention was insufficient to sustain weight loss through the second year among veterans who suffered from overweight/obesity and participated in ASPIRE-VA.[11] The investigators propose that much of the weight regain seen in the second year may have been due to participants with diabetes, as these participants lost weight initially but started regaining weight as sessions became increasingly less frequent.[11] Hence, this suggests that veterans with diabetes may need longer-term and more intensive treatment. Approaches that focus solely on consumption of fruits and vegetables, however, do not appear to promote significant weight loss.[12,13] Among adults who were overweight/obese, replacing caloric with noncaloric beverages (either water or diet beverages) had a greater benefit, an average of 2% to 2.5% body weight loss over 6 months,[14] and additional weight loss was observed among women participating in a 12-month follow-up that replaced diet beverages with water.[15] Of note, the magnitude of weight loss found for these small, food-based changes is less than those thought to result in improvement in cardiometabolic heath.[4]

Restricted-Energy Diets

Although energy-restricted diets vary greatly in level and source of daily caloric restriction, as well as in the level of structure required, both the low-calorie diet (LCD) and the very-low-calorie diet (VLCD) have been mainstays of treatment of obesity since the 1970s. LCDs typically range from 1200 to 1600 kcal/d and impose structure through use of meal plans that specify food choices and portion sizes. Meal replacements (ie, bars, shakes) may be used to help with improving adherence, as these have a pre-specified caloric intake and limit food choices. A partial meal replacement diet was found to be more effective for short-term weight loss than an LCD with conventional foods,[16] and 2 daily meal replacements were more effective than 1 daily among obese/overweight individuals with type 2 diabetes.[17]

A medically supervised VLCD is fewer than 800 calories per day and appropriate for individuals who are severely obese (generally BMI $\geq$40) and/or those with serious medical conditions related to their obesity and a BMI $\geq$30. They are also increasingly being used among patients before undergoing bariatric surgery to reduce risks associated with surgery.[18] A VLCD may consist of whole foods, commercially available meal replacements/liquids, or a combination of the two. It is recommended that patients being considered for VLCDs undergo a comprehensive medical evaluation. Absolute contraindications include the presence of untreated or severe cardiac, hepatic, renal, or thromboembolic disease; type 1 diabetes; current cancer; and severe eating disorders. Regular visits for medical supervision are recommended while on the VLCD. With full adherence, weight loss averages 1.1 to 1.8 kg per week, depending on initial body mass (more rapid weight loss typically with more severe obesity) and physical activity level. The high-protein fraction of most VLCDs (typically 70–100 g/ d or 0.8–1.5 g protein/kg body weight) may minimize muscle wasting as rapid weight loss occurs. The more rapid weight loss phase is followed by progressive refeeding. Multidisciplinary treatment, which includes education on nutrition, exercise, and behavior modification, will help the patient maintain his or her weight loss during and beyond the refeeding phase. A meta-analysis reported that among adults with class III obesity, VLCDs administered mostly via liquid meal replacement products, and used for 6 weeks or greater, resulted in a clinically relevant weight loss (which ranged from 10.2% to 28.0% of initial body weight).[19]

Intermittent fasting or caloric restriction regimens allow for fasting and nonfasting cycles over a given period and were designed to improve adherence compared with other energy-restricted diets. Alternate-day fasting (ADF) is 1 such method that has emerged recently and involves a partial fasting day, similar to a VLCD, followed by a normal feeding day when foods and beverages are consumed ad libitum. ADF has been found to be associated with better compliance, greater reduction of fat mass, and preservation of lean body mass as compared with VLCDs.[20] However, VLCDs do not appear to result in greater long-term weight losses than LCDs.[18]

Macronutrient-Focused Diets

Macronutrient-based dietary changes focus on 1 target macronutrient (usually carbohydrates or protein); however, changes in 1 macronutrient will result in changes in other macronutrients in the diet. The Institute of Medicine established the acceptable macronutrient distribution ranges for macronutrients based on percentage of total caloric intake (protein: 10%–35%, fat: 20%–35%, carbohydrate: 45%–65%) by considering the epidemiologic evidence that suggests consumption within these ranges is associated with a reduction in the risk of chronic diseases.[21] However, macronutrient-focused diets are often outside of this range.

Many RCTs have been conducted to determine the optimal macronutrient distribution of the diet and recently have focused on the low-carbohydrate, high-protein diet. The low-carbohydrate, high-protein diet is most common among participants in the National Weight Loss Registry, a database of greater than 4000 adults who have been successful at long-term weight loss and maintenance. The National Weight Loss Registry is reporting following a low-calorie, low-fat diet to achieve weight control,[22] yet low-fat diets' popularity has declined more recently.

Low-carbohydrate dieting was popularized by Atkins and is usually defined as less than 20 g of total carbohydrate per day, without restriction of energy or other macronutrients. Once a desired weight loss is achieved, carbohydrate intake is somewhat liberalized to 50 g per day. A meta-analysis of 5 RCTs compared low-carbohydrate versus low-fat diets and found that although low-carbohydrate diets were more effective for weight loss at 6 months, the benefit disappeared by 12 months. In addition, the low-fat diet was found to lead to a greater decrease in total and low-density lipoprotein (LDL)-cholesterol compared with the low-carbohydrate diet, whereas the low-carbohydrate diets reduced blood triglycerides and increased high-density lipoprotein-cholesterol levels more than the low-fat LCD.[23]

An increasingly popular diet that results in a more extreme restriction in carbohydrates to induce serum and urinary ketones has been the "ketogenic" diet. Results from meta-analyses, which compared RCTs of the ketogenic versus low-fat diet, found significant improvements in weight with the ketogenic for diet up to 24 months. However, a significant increase in LDL-cholesterol was observed, although the clinical significance of this increase has been questioned.[24,25] It is noted that dropout rates for ketogenic diets ranged from 13% to 84% across studies.[24] Ketogenic diets and a modified form of this diet may play a promising role in epilepsy treatment.[26]

The positive weight outcomes associated with low-carbohydrate diets have been suggested to be due in part by the high-protein content. A high-protein diet is defined as consuming at least 20% of energy from protein, with no restriction on fat or carbohydrates.[27] A meta-analysis that included 24 RCTs comparing isocaloric high versus low-protein diets found that the high-protein diets resulted not only in weight loss but also in greater fat mass loss. Weight loss may be enhanced by the increased satiety and resting energy expenditure that accompany high-protein intake.[28] However, these diets, like ketogenic diets, suffer from reduced adherence and eventual weight regain. Many high-protein diets are actualized through use of portion-controlled liquid and solid meal replacements. Among participants with obesity and the metabolic syndrome, those consuming 2 high-protein meal replacements daily, compared with a conventional protein diet, lost more body weight and more fat mass.[29] This finding aligns with prior work that found that meal replacements may be more effective for weight loss irrespective of the macronutrient composition of the diet,[16] possibly because of the additional control of intake levels inherent in replacing regular meals with a strict formula of calorie-controlled feedings. A very recent meta-analysis also found that among patients with type 2 diabetes, low-calorie, low-carbohydrate meal replacements or diets combined with education appear the most promising interventions to achieve the largest weight and BMI reductions.[30] One concern with high-protein intake is that greater renal decline may occur, as demonstrated in women with impaired renal function.[31] More recently, long-term low carbohydrate diets comprising animal-derived foods have been found to be associated with increased overall mortality.[32]

Pattern-Based Diets

Long-term weight loss and attendant metabolic and cardiovascular disease (CVD) control may require more permanent alterations in diet and lifestyle than what short-term diets provide. Dietary pattern-based changes focus on the overall diet by providing recommendations on the types of foods to consume as compared with the amount of energy or macronutrients. The Dietary Guidelines for Americans (DGA) provide recommendations on a high nutrient-density eating pattern, which is associated with weight maintenance and a reduction in chronic disease risk.[33] The DGA are a resource for health professionals and policymakers, particularly those working on the design and implementation of food assistance programs, but can also be used by the public to make healthier food choices for those 2 years and older. Five overarching guidelines are specified, and key recommendations (**Fig. 1**) provide further guidance on how individuals can follow the 5 guidelines.

The *Dietary Approaches to Stop Hypertension* (DASH) diet was developed through research funded by the National Institutes of Health to reduce hypertension among those with moderate to higher blood pressure.[34,35] The DASH dietary pattern is high in fruits, vegetables, fat-free/low-fat dairy products, whole grains, lean meats, nuts, legumes, and seeds and contains few sweets, added sugars, and red meat. The consumption of dietary sodium is reduced to 2300 mg/d (standard DASH) or 1500 mg/d (low-sodium DASH), the latter in line with the American Heart Association recommendation.[36] The original DASH diet does not stipulate daily energy restrictions; however, the addition of exercise and weight loss to the DASH diet results in even larger reductions in blood pressure compared with DASH alone.[37] However, compliance to

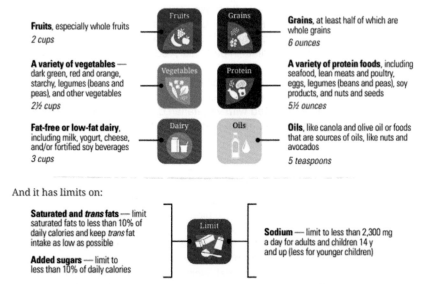

What's in a Healthy Eating Pattern?

The *2015–2020 Dietary Guidelines* has recommendations for a healthy eating pattern.

For someone who needs 2,000 calories a day, a healthy eating pattern includes:

Fruits, especially whole fruits
2 cups

Grains, at least half of which are whole grains
6 ounces

A variety of vegetables — dark green, red and orange, starchy, legumes (beans and peas), and other vegetables
2½ cups

A variety of protein foods, including seafood, lean meats and poultry, eggs, legumes (beans and peas), soy products, and nuts and seeds
5½ ounces

Fat-free or low-fat dairy, including milk, yogurt, cheese, and/or fortified soy beverages
3 cups

Oils, like canola and olive oil or foods that are sources of oils, like nuts and avocados
5 teaspoons

And it has limits on:

Saturated and *trans* fats — limit saturated fats to less than 10% of daily calories and keep *trans* fat intake as low as possible

Added sugars — limit to less than 10% of daily calories

Sodium — limit to less than 2,300 mg a day for adults and children 14 y and up (less for younger children)

Fig. 1. How to build a healthy eating pattern. DGA, 2015 to 2020. (*From* U.S. Department of Health and Human Services, U.S. Department of Agriculture. 2015-2020 Dietary Guidelines for Americans.; 2015. http://health.gov/dietaryguidelines/2015/guidelines/.)

the DASH diet was found to be lower among African Americans compared with whites, suggesting culturally adapted dietary strategies may be needed for minority populations.[38]

The traditional *Mediterranean diet* is generally based on the diet pattern observed in Mediterranean regions (particularly Greece and Italy) during the 1960s. It focused on plant-based foods, including fruits, vegetables, grains, nuts and seeds, minimally processed foods, olive oil as the main fat source, dairy, fish, and poultry, consumed moderately, with very limited red meat and the frequent, but moderate intake of wine.[39] Early studies found the Mediterranean diet resulted in similar caloric deficits, yet more favorable effects on glycemic markers (glucose, insulin) compared with a low-fat diet, with a high adherence rate (85% at 2 years[40]). More recently, the Prevención con Dieta Mediterránea (PREDIMED) multicenter, randomized, nutritional trial was conducted among those at high risk for CVD in Spain to test 2 modified versions of the Mediterranean diet, with extravirgin olive oil (EVOO) or supplemented with nuts, versus advice on adhering to a low-fat diet. PREDIMED further demonstrated that the Mediterranean diet supplemented with either EVOO or nuts, in addition to improvements in other cardiovascular end points, also led to decreases in diastolic blood pressure, and more so than on a low-fat diet.[41] These improvements are frequently the same magnitude as effects observed with statin therapy, although further work is needed in this area.[42] Many of the benefits associated with the Mediterranean diet are thought to be due to the high unsaturated fat and antioxidant intake of the diet.

Overall, vegetable-based dietary patterns, which recommended replacing plant-based protein foods with animal proteins, have become increasing popular and widespread. Both the Academy of Nutrition and Dietetics and DGA highlight the benefits of plant-based diet patterns, while acknowledging the need for appropriate planning to ensure vegetarian and vegan diets are nutritionally adequate.[33,43] Such foods include legumes, nuts, and grains, and in lacto-ovo-vegetarian diets, dairy products and eggs. However, in vegan diets, all animal-derived products are avoided, limiting some of these options.

In observational studies, compared with those consuming animal sources, vegetarians generally have lower body weight, lower blood pressure, less diabetes and other health issues, as well as less weight gain.[44,45] Evidence from clinical trials supports that vegetarians diets, and vegan diets in particular, reduce body weight.[46] However, the long-term effects of vegetarian diets or the effects on weight maintenance remain unclear, as most studies reviewed have been less than 1 year in duration.[47] Furthermore, similar to other diets that target either energy, macronutrients, or other patterns, the positive health results associated with vegetarian diets may be due to the energy restriction and resulting weight loss, more than an effect independent of weight loss.

Timing of Food Intake

Dietary interventions have also focused on the factors that influence timing of the diet, although this literature is limited. It has been shown that consuming more energy earlier in the day is conducive to weight loss.[48] Overweight and obese women randomized to a high-calorie breakfast versus a high-calorie dinner for 12 weeks showed a 2.5-fold greater weight loss (-8.7 ± 1.4 vs -3.6 ± 1.5 kg, respectively, $P<.01$) and reduction in waist circumference (8.5 ± 1.9 vs -3.9 ± 1.4 cm, respectively, $P<.01$).[49]

Irregular feeding patterns, however, may induce desynchronization of the circadian rhythm system via decoupling of peripheral oscillators from the suprachiasmatic nucleus.[48] This finding is consistent with epidemiologic evidence suggesting that those who reported having regular breakfast consumption habits (whether eating breakfast every day or never eating breakfast) were less likely to be obese compared with those with irregular patterns (eating breakfast 3 or 4 times per week).[50] Although this was a cross-sectional study, differences in diet quality or total caloric intake related to breakfast consumption did not appear to explain these results, as these variables were included in multivariable modeling. Hence, these results suggest the distribution of calories throughout the day may be more effective for weight loss and maintenance than large swings in consumption. More recently, diets based on time-restriction, which limits caloric consumption to a 10-hour window, a form of intermittent fasting as described earlier, resulted in weight loss and significant improvements in blood parameters among a group of adults with metabolic syndrome.[51]

ACTIVITY INTERVENTION

Physical activity will help induce weight loss to the extent it leads to negative energy balance because of increases in energy expenditure. The current physical activity guidelines for Americans recommend at least 150 minutes of moderate to vigorous physical activity (MVPA) per week for weight control.[52] Still longer durations of physical activity may be necessary for weight loss and maintenance, and up to 300 minutes of MVPA weekly are recommended as necessary for improvements in health outcomes. A reduction of sedentary activity defined as sitting or reclining activities with very-low-energy expenditure is also associated with improvements in weight and cardiometabolic heath.[53] The health benefits observed may be either due to a reallocation of sedentary time to light activity, which increases energy expenditure, or through a reduction of food activities often associated with sedentary time, such as TV watching. Although interventions have been successfully implemented to decrease sedentary time, particularly using sit-stand workstations, the effects on weight managements are not clear.[54] It is clear that combined behavioral weight management programs, which include both diet and exercise interventions, result in greater long-term weight loss (between 12 and 18 months) compared with exercise-only programs, with a mean difference of −6.29 kg; 95% confidence interval −7.33 to −5.25.[55] It seems that addition of physical activity to diet may not be beneficial for initial weight loss, yet more so for maintenance of weight loss possibly through a reduction in energy intake.

CULTURAL ADAPTATIONS

Health promotion interventions, which incorporate the target populations' sociocultural values, norms, and stressors, may better influence behavior change and lead to improved program effectiveness. Considering the large disparities that exist in obesity rates among US ethnic minority populations compared with whites,[3] culturally tailored interventions may be needed to close this gap. These techniques have been successfully applied in the psychology field to adapt treatments, yet are increasingly used across other health fields.[56] Trials such as the ORBIT (*Obesity Reduction Black Intervention Trial*) and TRIMM (*Tailored Rapid Interactive Mobile Messaging*) among African Americans have found evidence that greater weight loss can be achieved with a culturally adapted weight-loss program compared with a more general health program.[57,58] In addition, trials that are both culturally and gender-adapted are currently ongoing.[59] Most studies, however, continue to rely on surface-level structural adaptations, which include visual and auditory cues for messaging (ie, ethnic foods, pictures, and music). Deep structure adaptations, which involve gathering information from target community members on cultural norms, beliefs, and structures, may improve outcomes, however, are more complicated and more difficult to attain.[60] Thus, culturally adapted weight management programs are needed, which include deep structure adaptations. These strategies need to be adequately documented, so that they can be replicated and enable comparisons of effectiveness among interventions.

Multidisciplinary Team Approach

Most comprehensive lifestyle intervention programs combine caloric restriction of at least 500 kcal/d with a physical activity prescription of at least 150 minutes of MVPA per week and structured behavior change strategies. A multidisciplinary team should include a primary physician or nurse practitioner with expertise in medical complications of obesity and obesity pharmacotherapy, a dietitian, an exercise specialist, and a counselor for behavior change. This team can best provide a comprehensive, in-depth, personalized weight loss program by combining the most effective interventions from each discipline. This personalized weight loss program can be complemented by a pharmacist, case manager, and specialty physicians, including bariatric surgeon, psychiatrist, and gastroenterologist, or others if specific comorbidities are present (eg, a podiatrist, cardiologist, or nephrologist). Patients should, however, be the center of the team's focus. Weight management programs, such as the *Look AHEAD* and *Diabetes Prevention Program*, are examples of comprehensive intervention with proven success.[5,61] These programs used cognitive behavioral therapy (CBT) to assist with changing eating and activity behaviors. The most common CBT strategies include self-monitoring, goal setting, problem-solving and preplanning, stimulus control, and relapse prevention. Intensive lifestyle interventions are based in part on the Chronic Care Model of health care delivery,[62,63] the core principles of which include a multidisciplinary team, long-term commitment, patient-centered care, and evidence-based and protocol-driven treatment choices.[64] Jensen and colleagues[4] provides a treatment algorithm to guide primary care practitioners in weight management decision making, which encompasses evaluation, prevention, and management. There is a need to have well-informed providers to effectively manage a chronic condition like obesity.

INTENSITY AND DELIVERY OF INTERVENTIONS

It is clear that the intensity and frequency of treatment visits for weight control are important predictors of outcome success. Guidelines suggest that 1 to 2 treatment sessions per month (6–12/6 months), which are face to face and on site, produce 2- to 4-kg weight loss in 6 to 12 months, and high intensity (>14 sessions/6 months) yields greater weight loss compared with low to moderate intensity intervention.[4] There is probably some limit to the benefit of increasing intensity of interventions, however, as "diet fatigue" may occur with very prolonged or very taxing intervention schemes. A break from intensive interventions of modest duration may be useful in resetting engagement with interventions.

Interventions can be delivered with the use of technology to decrease costs, reach, and possibly attrition yet produce less weight loss compared with face-to-face interventions.[65] Smartphone-based delivery may have additional benefits compared with computer-based delivery, as can be more frequent/ever-present, can be interactive, and can more readily incorporate tailored messaging. Efficacy compared with other methods is not yet clear, however.

COMMERCIAL PROGRAMS AND SUPPLEMENTS

Commercial programs are widespread in the developed world and have no inherent reason that they should be less effective than freely available programs.

Commercial programs are less likely to be subjected to controlled trials than other programs, but some notable exceptions exist, including studies of Weight Watchers. One study of the popular weight control program, "Lose It," found that users who exhibited more consistent patterns of consumption, particularly not eating more on weekends, tended to lose more weight than those who did not.[66] Also of note in the context of dietary interventions, provision of foods in the form of low-calorie meal replacements has been shown in a meta-analysis to yield greater at least initial weight loss than interventions that do not use meal replacement.[67] Weight loss is likely due to portion control being more automatic and convenient when providing meal replacement than when relying on consistent adherence to advice to alter diet.

SUMMARY

The high prevalence of adult obesity in the United States necessitates both a public health approach and a health care system approach to its treatment. Medical team care coordination is required, which may include partnerships between registered dietitians, nurses, pharmacists, psychologists, physical therapists, social workers, and so forth, with use of auxiliary support from weight loss medications, devices, and surgeries when more invasive therapy is medically required. However, modification of factors at the community, organizational, and government level is also required to help mitigate this problem. Reimbursement for obesity treatment for all members of the medical team is 1 example of a government initiative, which is essential for treatment. A weight loss and maintenance in the range of 5% can produce clinically important changes in health, with greater increases resulting in greater health improvements. Successful maintenance of weight loss, which is the ultimate goal, requires adapting lifestyle behaviors that influence both energy intake and energy expenditure sides of the energy balance equation. This review focused primarily on dietary interventions, whether these be macronutrient focused or pattern based; interventions that can be best tailored to the patient's current lifestyle will have the chance of weight loss success and long-term weight maintenance.

CLINICS CARE POINTS

- Counsel patients who are overweight and obese that lifestyle changes which produce 5% weight loss can result in clinical health benefits.
- Diets should be prescribed in consultation with a nutrition professional such as an registered dietitian and as part of a comprehensive lifestyle intervention which aims to reduce caloric intake in the range of 500-750 kcal per day.
- Evidence based dietary approaches should be used to reduce food intake and very low calorie diets (<800 kcal/day) should be limited to when medically necessary and be provided in a medical setting which has the ability to support potential health complications.

DISCLOSURE

The authors have nothing to disclose.

REFERENCES

1. Flemyng M. A discourse on the nature causes and cure of corpulency. Illustrated by a Remarkable Case, Read before the Royal Society, November 1757. and

Now First Published, by Malcolm Flemyng, M.D. (Paperback). London, England: L Davis and C Reymers; 1760.

2. Hales C, Carroll M, Fryar C, et al. Prevalence of obesity and severe obesity among adults: United States, 2017–2018. Hyattsville, MD: National Center for Health Statistics.; 2020.

3. Hales CM, Fryar CD, Carroll MD, et al. Differences in obesity prevalence by demographic characteristics and urbanization level among adults in the United States, 2013-2016. JAMA 2018;319(23):2419.

4. Jensen MD, Ryan DH, Apovian CM, et al. 2013 AHA/ACC/TOS guideline for the management of overweight and obesity in adults: a report of the American College of Cardiology/American Heart Association Task Force on Practice Guidelines and The Obesity Society. J Am Coll Cardiol 2014;63(25 Pt B):2985–3023.

5. Look AHEAD Research Group. Eight-year weight losses with an intensive lifestyle intervention: the look AHEAD study. Obesity (Silver Spring) 2014;22(1):5–13.

6. Fildes A, Charlton J, Rudisill C, et al. Probability of an obese person attaining normal body weight: cohort study using electronic health records. Am J Public Health 2015;105(9):e54–9.

7. Hills AP, Byrne NM, Lindstrom R, et al. "Small changes" to diet and physical activity behaviors for weight management. Obes Facts 2013;6(3):228–38.

8. Rodearmel SJ, Wyatt HR, Barry MJ, et al. A family-based approach to preventing excessive weight gain. Obesity (Silver Spring) 2006;14(8):1392–401.

9. Rodearmel SJ, Wyatt HR, Stroebele N, et al. Small changes in dietary sugar and physical activity as an approach to preventing excessive weight gain: the America on the Move family study. Pediatrics 2007;120(4):e869–79.

10. Lutes LD, Winett RA, Barger SD, et al. Small changes in nutrition and physical activity promote weight loss and maintenance: 3-month evidence from the ASPIRE randomized trial. Ann Behav Med 2008;35(3):351–7.

11. Lutes LD, Damschroder LJ, Masheb R, et al. Behavioral treatment for veterans with obesity: 24-month weight outcomes from the ASPIRE-VA Small Changes Randomized Trial. J Gen Intern Med 2017;32(Suppl 1):40–7.

12. Kaiser KA, Brown AW, Bohan Brown MM, et al. Increased fruit and vegetable intake has no discernible effect on weight loss: a systematic review and meta-analysis. Am J Clin Nutr 2014;100(2):567–76.

13. Mytton OT, Nnoaham K, Eyles H, et al. Systematic review and meta-analysis of the effect of increased vegetable and fruit consumption on body weight and energy intake. BMC Public Health 2014;14:886.

14. Tate DF, Turner-McGrievy G, Lyons E, et al. Replacing caloric beverages with water or diet beverages for weight loss in adults: main results of the Choose Healthy Options Consciously Everyday (CHOICE) randomized clinical trial. Am J Clin Nutr 2012;95(3):555–63.

15. Madjd A, Taylor MA, Delavari A, et al. Effects of replacing diet beverages with water on weight loss and weight maintenance: 18-month follow-up, randomized clinical trial. Int J Obes 2018;42(4):835–40.

16. Heymsfield SB, van Mierlo CAJ, van der Knaap HCM, et al. Weight management using a meal replacement strategy: meta and pooling analysis from six studies. Int J Obes Relat Metab Disord 2003;27(5):537–49.

17. Leader NJ, Ryan L, Molyneaux L, et al. How best to use partial meal replacement in managing overweight or obese patients with poorly controlled type 2 diabetes. Obesity (Silver Spring) 2013;21(2):251–3.

18. Tsai AG, Wadden TA. The evolution of very-low-calorie diets: an update and meta-analysis. Obesity (Silver Spring) 2006;14(8):1283–93.

19. Maston G, Gibson AA, Kahlaee HR, et al. Effectiveness and characterization of severely energy-restricted diets in people with class III obesity: systematic review and meta-analysis. Behav Sci (Basel) 2019;9(12):144.

20. Alhamdan BA, Garcia-Alvarez A, Alzahrnai AH, et al. Alternate-day versus daily energy restriction diets: which is more effective for weight loss? A systematic review and meta-analysis. Obes Sci Pract 2016;2(3):293–302.

21. Institute of Medicine. Dietary reference intakes for energy, carbohydrate. Fiber, fat, fatty acids, cholesterol, protein, and amino acids. Washington, DC: The National Academies Press; 2005. https://doi.org/10.17226/10490.

22. Wing RR, Phelan S. Long-term weight loss maintenance. Am J Clin Nutr 2005; 82(1 Suppl):222S–5S.

23. Nordmann AJ, Nordmann A, Briel M, et al. Effects of low-carbohydrate vs low-fat diets on weight loss and cardiovascular risk factors: a meta-analysis of randomized controlled trials. Arch Intern Med 2006;166(3):285–93.

24. Bueno NB, de Melo ISV, de Oliveira SL, et al. Very-low-carbohydrate ketogenic diet v. low-fat diet for long-term weight loss: a meta-analysis of randomised controlled trials. Br J Nutr 2013;110(7):1178–87.

25. Mansoor N, Vinknes KJ, Veierød MB, et al. Effects of low-carbohydrate diets v. low-fat diets on body weight and cardiovascular risk factors: a meta-analysis of randomised controlled trials. Br J Nutr 2016;115(3):466–79.

26. Martin K, Jackson CF, Levy RG, et al. Ketogenic diet and other dietary treatments for epilepsy. Cochrane Database Syst Rev 2016;(2):CD001903.

27. Westerterp-Plantenga MS, Lemmens SG, Westerterp KR. Dietary protein - its role in satiety, energetics, weight loss and health. Br J Nutr 2012;108(Suppl 2): S105–12.

28. Wycherley TP, Moran LJ, Clifton PM, et al. Effects of energy-restricted high-protein, low-fat compared with standard-protein, low-fat diets: a meta-analysis of randomized controlled trials. Am J Clin Nutr 2012;96(6):1281–98.

29. Flechtner-Mors M, Boehm BO, Wittmann R, et al. Enhanced weight loss with protein-enriched meal replacements in subjects with the metabolic syndrome. Diabetes Metab Res Rev 2010;26(5):393–405.

30. Maula A, Kai J, Woolley AK, et al. Educational weight loss interventions in obese and overweight adults with type 2 diabetes: a systematic review and meta-analysis of randomized controlled trials. Diabet Med 2020;37(4):623–35.

31. Knight EL, Stampfer MJ, Hankinson SE, et al. The impact of protein intake on renal function decline in women with normal renal function or mild renal insufficiency. Ann Intern Med 2003;138(6):460–7.

32. Seidelmann SB, Claggett B, Cheng S, et al. Dietary carbohydrate intake and mortality: a prospective cohort study and meta-analysis. Lancet Public Health 2018; 3(9):e419–28.

33. U.S. Department of Health and Human Services, U.S. Department of Agriculture. 2015-2020 Dietary guidelines for Americans. 2015. Available at: http://health.gov/dietaryguidelines/2015/guidelines/. Accessed August 29th, 2020.

34. Appel LJ, Moore TJ, Obarzanek E, et al. A clinical trial of the effects of dietary patterns on blood pressure. DASH Collaborative Research Group. N Engl J Med 1997;336(16):1117–24.

35. Sacks FM, Obarzanek E, Windhauser MM, et al. Rationale and design of the Dietary Approaches to Stop Hypertension trial (DASH). A multicenter controlled-feeding study of dietary patterns to lower blood pressure. Ann Epidemiol 1995; 5(2):108–18.

36. Arnett DK, Blumenthal RS, Albert MA, et al. 2019 ACC/AHA guideline on the primary prevention of cardiovascular disease: executive summary: a report of the American College of Cardiology/American Heart Association Task Force on Clinical Practice Guidelines. J Am Coll Cardiol 2019;74(10):1376–414.

37. Blumenthal JA, Babyak MA, Hinderliter A, et al. Effects of the DASH diet alone and in combination with exercise and weight loss on blood pressure and cardiovascular biomarkers in men and women with high blood pressure: the ENCORE study. Arch Intern Med 2010;170(2):126–35.

38. Epstein DE, Sherwood A, Smith PJ, et al. Determinants and consequences of adherence to the dietary approaches to stop hypertension diet in African-American and white adults with high blood pressure: results from the ENCORE trial. J Acad Nutr Diet 2012;112(11):1763–73.

39. Willett WC, Sacks F, Trichopoulou A, et al. Mediterranean diet pyramid: a cultural model for healthy eating. Am J Clin Nutr 1995;61(6 Suppl):1402S–6S.

40. Shai I, Schwarzfuchs D, Henkin Y, et al. Weight loss with a low-carbohydrate, Mediterranean, or low-fat diet. N Engl J Med 2008;359(3):229–41.

41. Toledo E, Hu FB, Estruch R, et al. Effect of the Mediterranean diet on blood pressure in the PREDIMED trial: results from a randomized controlled trial. BMC Med 2013;11:207.

42. Ros E, Martínez-González MA, Estruch R, et al. Mediterranean diet and cardiovascular health: teachings of the PREDIMED study. Adv Nutr 2014;5(3):330S–6S.

43. Melina V, Craig W, Levin S. Position of the Academy of Nutrition and Dietetics: vegetarian diets. J Acad Nutr Diet 2016;116(12):1970–80.

44. Orlich MJ, Fraser GE. Vegetarian diets in the Adventist Health Study 2: a review of initial published findings. Am J Clin Nutr 2014;100(Suppl 1):353S–8S.

45. Rosell M, Appleby P, Spencer E, et al. Weight gain over 5 years in 21,966 meat-eating, fish-eating, vegetarian, and vegan men and women in EPIC-Oxford. Int J Obes 2006;30(9):1389–96.

46. Barnard ND, Levin SM, Yokoyama Y. A systematic review and meta-analysis of changes in body weight in clinical trials of vegetarian diets. J Acad Nutr Diet 2015;115(6):954–69.

47. Huang R-Y, Huang C-C, Hu FB, et al. Vegetarian diets and weight reduction: a meta-analysis of randomized controlled trials. J Gen Intern Med 2016;31(1): 109–16.

48. Garaulet M, Gómez-Abellán P, Alburquerque-Béjar JJ, et al. Timing of food intake predicts weight loss effectiveness. Int J Obes 2013;37(4):604–11.

49. Jakubowicz D, Barnea M, Wainstein J, et al. High caloric intake at breakfast vs. dinner differentially influences weight loss of overweight and obese women. Obesity (Silver Spring) 2013;21(12):2504–12.

50. Guinter MA, Park Y-M, Steck SE, et al. Day-to-day regularity in breakfast consumption is associated with weight status in a prospective cohort of women. Int J Obes 2020;44(1):186–94.

51. Wilkinson MJ, Manoogian ENC, Zadourian A, et al. Ten-hour time-restricted eating reduces weight, blood pressure, and atherogenic lipids in patients with metabolic syndrome. Cell Metab 2020;31(1):92–104.e5.

52. US Department of Health and Human Services. Physical activity guidelines for Americans. Available at: https://www.hhs.gov/fitness/be-active/physical-activity-guidelines-for-americans/index.html. Accessed March 15, 2020.

53. Dunstan DW, Howard B, Healy GN, et al. Too much sitting–a health hazard. Diabetes Res Clin Pract 2012;97(3):368–76.

54. Chau JY, Daley M, Dunn S, et al. The effectiveness of sit-stand workstations for changing office workers' sitting time: results from the Stand@Work randomized controlled trial pilot. Int J Behav Nutr Phys Act 2014;11:127.
55. Johns DJ, Hartmann-Boyce J, Jebb SA, et al. Behavioural Weight Management Review Group. Diet or exercise interventions vs combined behavioral weight management programs: a systematic review and meta-analysis of direct comparisons. J Acad Nutr Diet 2014;114(10):1557–68.
56. Bernal G, Domenech Rodríguez MM. Cultural adaptations: tools for evidence-based practice with diverse populations. Washington, DC: American Psychological Association; 2012.
57. Lin M, Mahmooth Z, Dedhia N, et al. Tailored, interactive text messages for enhancing weight loss among African American adults: the TRIMM randomized controlled trial. Am J Med 2015;128(8):896–904.
58. Fitzgibbon ML, Stolley MR, Schiffer L, et al. Obesity reduction black intervention trial (ORBIT): 18-month results. Obesity (Silver Spring) 2010;18(12):2317–25.
59. Garcia DO, Valdez LA, Bell ML, et al. A gender- and culturally-sensitive weight loss intervention for Hispanic males: the ANIMO randomized controlled trial pilot study protocol and recruitment methods. Contemp Clin Trials Commun 2018;9: 151–63.
60. Resnicow K, Baranowski T, Ahluwalia JS, et al. Cultural sensitivity in public health: defined and demystified. Ethn Dis 1999;9(1):10–21.
61. Knowler WC, Barrett-Connor E, Fowler SE, et al. Reduction in the incidence of type 2 diabetes with lifestyle intervention or metformin. N Engl J Med 2002; 346(6):393–403.
62. Coleman K, Austin BT, Brach C, et al. Evidence on the Chronic Care Model in the new millennium. Health Aff 2009;28(1):75–85.
63. Wagner EH, Austin BT, Von Korff M. Organizing care for patients with chronic illness. Milbank Q 1996;74(4):511–44.
64. Foster D, Sanchez-Collins S, Cheskin LJ. Multidisciplinary team-based obesity treatment in patients with diabetes: current practices and the state of the science. Diabetes Spectr 2017;30(4):244–9.
65. Wieland LS, Falzon L, Sciamanna CN, et al. Interactive computer-based interventions for weight loss or weight maintenance in overweight or obese people. Cochrane Database Syst Rev 2012;(8):CD007675.
66. Hill C, Weir BW, Fuentes LW, et al. Relationship between weekly patterns of caloric intake and reported weight loss outcomes: retrospective cohort study. JMIR MHealth UHealth 2018;6(4):e83.
67. Astbury NM, Piernas C, Hartmann-Boyce J, et al. A systematic review and meta-analysis of the effectiveness of meal replacements for weight loss. Obes Rev 2019;20(4):569–87.

Precision Medicine and Obesity

Maria Daniela Hurtado A, MD, PhD[a,b], Andres Acosta, MD, PhD[c],*

KEYWORDS

- Obesity • Precision medicine • Phenotype • Personalized nutrition • Nutrigenomics

KEY POINTS

- Obesity has reached epidemic proportions. Weight loss outcomes with current available therapeutic options are not only modest but also variable among patients. Precision medicine is an emerging arena that offers new opportunities to dealing with this condition.
- High-resolution biotechnologies have provided evidence that there are numerous intermediary processes that contribute to obesity.
- These processes have led to partially understand some of the pathophysiologic processes involved in obesity and its clinical consequences, and have been targeted to individualize obesity therapy with some success.
- As clinicians continue to gather information, it is anticipated that the prediction, prevention and treatment of obesity will be substantially improved.

INTRODUCTION

In the last decades, the prevalence of obesity has increased globally, reaching epidemic proportions.[1] Its worldwide prevalence has almost tripled between 1980 and 2016.[2] In the United States, in 2013 to 2014, the prevalence of obesity among Americans was 39%.[1,3] Obesity has been attributed to about $480 billion in increased medical spending.[4]

The cause, clinical presentation, and complications of obesity differ significantly from patient to patient, making it difficult to prevent and treat this disease. Within the current health care system, the treatment of obesity follows an algorithm that starts with lifestyle modification and later progresses to the use of pharmacologic agents,

[a] Division of Endocrinology, Diabetes, Metabolism and Nutrition, Department of Medicine, Mayo Clinic Health System, 700 West Ave South, La Crosse, WI 54601, USA; [b] Division of Endocrinology, Diabetes, Metabolism and Nutrition, Department of Medicine, Mayo Clinic, 200 1st Street Southwest, Rochester, MN 55905, USA; [c] Division of Gastroenterology and Hepatology, Department of Medicine, Mayo Clinic, 200 1st Street Southwest, Rochester, MN 55905, USA
* Corresponding author.
E-mail address: Acosta.andres@mayo.edu
Twitter: MDanielaHurtado (M.D.H.A.); dr_aac (A.A.)

Gastroenterol Clin N Am 50 (2021) 127–139
https://doi.org/10.1016/j.gtc.2020.10.005
0889-8553/21/© 2020 Elsevier Inc. All rights reserved.

endoscopic devices, and/or bariatric surgery based on the patient's response. Lifestyle modification is not always successful, and even when combined with behavioral therapy and pharmacologic agents, weight loss outcomes are not only modest but also vary among patients.

The rising prevalence of obesity and the lack of established and validated treatment options warrant the exploration of alternative therapeutic strategies that can complement current paradigms. Preferably, novel strategies would be personalized to the individual for enhanced effectiveness and tolerability in the form of precision medicine. Although there are many ongoing initiatives with this goal, much needs to be resolved before precision obesity medicine becomes common practice.

WHAT IS PRECISION MEDICINE?

Precision medicine is constructed on the premise that most current therapeutic and prevention approaches for a certain disease are based on the average patient and do not take into consideration interpersonal variability. This approach is successful for some people but not for others. Contrary to this one-size-fits-all tactic, precision medicine takes into consideration individual variability in genetics, metabolites, intestinal microbiome, and environmental factors that can affect all these, with the objective of predicting which disease treatment and/or prevention strategy will work better in which group of people.[5]

The human genome sequencing and subsequent development of population genetics are the foundation of precision medicine. These tools have been used to help identify hundreds of gene variants associated with obesity and its related traits through genome-wide association studies (GWAS). The recent advances in high-resolution characterization of a variety of biologic variants, such as transcripts, proteins, metabolites, microbiota, and epigenetic markers, among others, has expanded the capability to understand the conduits that link a person's biologic idiosyncrasies to disease susceptibility.

Although precision medicine could potentially improve the prevention and treatment of common multifactorial diseases, its application for obesity has been limited to date. Currently, obesity is classified based on the degree of excess weight, fat distribution, and its complications. Approaches centered on data mining of high-resolution biotechnologies have the potential to identify subgroups without bias to generate new pathophysiologic hypotheses. Identifying specific subgroups may lead to gene-oriented treatments, more novel therapeutic strategies, and drug discovery and development.

CURRENT OBESITY CLASSIFICATIONS

Traditionally, obesity classification is based on body mass index (BMI). Although all individuals with obesity have excess body fat, there are important heterogenic differences among this population. Anthropometric classification of obesity therefore has limitations when it comes to guiding clinical decisions in patients. Research over the past decades has provided new knowledge that has led to identifying different subtypes among patients with obesity. These classifications have provided important information on underlying pathophysiologic mechanisms driving obesity and its complications, and have helped pave the way toward precision obesity medicine.

- *BMI:* Obesity has been traditionally diagnosed by calculating the BMI (ratio of body weight in kilograms and height squared in meters). BMI allows classification of individuals by grade, from overweight to morbid obesity (**Table 1**).[6] BMI

Table 1 Body mass index classification	
Weight Status	BMI (kg/m^2)
Underweight	<18.5
Normal range	18.5–24.9
Overweight	25.0–29.9
Obesity class I	30.0–34.9
Obesity class II	35.0–39.9
Obesity class III	$\geq$40

correlates well with percentage of body fat, with the exception of people who have increased lean weight (eg, body builders). However, because of obesity's remarkable heterogeneity, this index does not always discriminate the risk of metabolic abnormalities and complications that are frequently associated with obesity. For instance, although patients with obesity are as a group at a higher risk of comorbidities compared with normal-weight individuals, some patients with obesity may show no metabolic complications (ie, the metabolically healthy individuals with obesity).[7]

- *Distribution of fat/body shape:* Various studies have shown that the common complications of obesity, such as cardiovascular disease, metabolic syndrome, dyslipidemia, and type 2 diabetes mellitus, are more closely associated to the body fat distribution than to the absolute fat percentage. Central obesity, characterized by proportionally greater amount of fat in the trunk compared with the hips and lower extremities, has been associated with increased risk for the aforementioned obesity complications. However, lower-body adiposity is less associated with those complications.[8,9] This classification has led to some understanding of obesity pathophysiology, but its use in precision medicine has been limited to date.

- *The Edmonton Obesity Staging system:* This five-stage system classifies obesity considering physical, metabolic and psychological parameters with the goal to determine the optimal treatment (**Table 2**).[10] It was developed to assist in identifying and prioritizing individuals who would benefit the most from resource-intensive and aggressive management, allowing a more individualized approach. This system has been suggested to be a better mortality predictor compared with BMI.[11]

- *Genetics:* Obesity is classified into polygenic or monogenic disorders. Most obesity cases are multifactorial or polygenic, that is, attributed to the interaction between multiple loci. Research has shown that there are many genetic factors that play a permissive role and when interacting with environmental factors result in obesity.[12] On the contrary, monogenic disorders are the result of a single mutated gene and account for the minority of cases of obesity (less than 1%). Clinically, monogenic disorders are associated or not with a syndrome. In nonsyndromic monogenic obesity, there are well characterized genes that play a role in energy homeostasis regulation by the leptin-melanocortin pathway.[13] In syndromic monogenic disorders, obesity presents in association with other features, such as dysmorphic features, cognitive delay and other abnormalities.[14] Understanding the genetics

Table 2
The Edmonton Obesity Staging System

Stage	Description	Management
0	No apparent obesity-related risk factors, no physical symptoms, no psychopathology, no functional limitations, and/or impairment of well-being.	Identification of factors contributing to increased body weight. Counseling to prevent further weight gain through lifestyle measures including healthy eating and increased physical activity.
1	Presence of obesity-related subclinical risk factors (eg, borderline hypertension, impaired fasting glucose, elevated liver enzymes), mild physical symptoms (eg, dyspnea on moderate exertion, occasional aches and pains, fatigue), mild psychopathology, mild functional limitations, and/or mild impairment of well-being.	Investigation for other (nonweight-related) contributors to risk factors. More intense lifestyle interventions, including diet and exercise, to prevent further weight gain. Monitoring of risk factors and health status.
2	Presence of established obesity-related chronic disease, moderate limitations in activities of daily living and/or well-being.	Initiation of obesity treatments including considerations of all behavioral, pharmacologic, and surgical treatment options. Close monitoring and management of comorbidities as indicated.
3	Established end-organ damage, such as myocardial infarction, heart failure, diabetic complications, incapacitating osteoarthritis, significant psychopathology, significant functional limitations, and/or impairment of well-being.	More intensive obesity treatment including consideration of all behavioral, pharmacologic, and surgical treatment options. Aggressive management of comorbidities as indicated.
4	Severe (potentially end-stage) disabilities from obesity-related chronic diseases, severe disabling psychopathology, severe functional limitations, and/or severe impairment of well-being.	Aggressive obesity management as deemed feasible. Palliative measures including pain management, occupational therapy, and psychosocial support.

From Sharma AM, Kushner RF. A proposed clinical staging system for obesity. *International Journal of Obesity.* 2009;33(3):289-295.

of a disease can potentially lead to developing genetics-based treatments, particularly for monogenic disorders.

OVERVIEW OF MAJOR OBESITY PRECISION MEDICINE INITIATIVES

Through complex mechanisms, genetic and environmental factors impact the two processes that are key drivers of obesity: caloric intake and physical activity levels. Although genetic studies have helped untangle this complex landscape, genetic polymorphisms alone do not explain the obesity epidemic. Nowadays, high-resolution biotechnologies have helped characterize other biologic variants, such as transcripts, proteins, metabolites, microbiota, and epigenetic markers among others, that could potentially provide a detailed fingerprint of a person's phenotype and how they might respond to different antiobesity treatments. This knowledge can substantially improve the prediction, prevention, and treatment of obesity. Here we summarize how these biologic variants may be targeted to individualize obesity treatment.

Genetics

The heritability of BMI is between 40% and 70%.[15,16] GWAS for adiposity traits (waist-to-hip ratio, BMI, visceral adiposity, and total body fat among others) have so far identified greater than 300 single nucleotide polymorphisms (SNPs). **Table 3** lists the better characterized SNPs and their associated phenotype. Individually, these SNPs have a

Table 3
Common SNPs, epigenetically modified genes, SNP-diet interactions, and metabolic pathways associated with obesity and obesity traits

SNPs[12]		
Gene	**Phenotype**	
FTO	BMI, waist circumference, fat percentage, extreme obesity	
MC4R	BMI, waist circumference, extreme obesity	
MC3R, SLC6A14	Obesity	
BDNF, TMEM18	BMI, extreme obesity	
POMC, NEGR1, PCSK1, GNPDA2, MAP2K5, SEC16 B	BMI	
Epigenetically Modified Genes[26]		
Gene	**Phenotype**	
POMC, NPY, SLC6A4, MCHR1	Overall obesity	
FTO, LPL, IRS 1, TMEM18	Fat distribution	
PPARG	Percentage body fat	
LEP	Overall obesity, fat distribution, BMI	
SNP-Diet Interactions[63]		
Gene	**Diet Interaction**	**Putative Disease Risk**
FTO	High fat and high carbohydrate	Obesity
LCT	Dairy products	
PPARG, G1PR	High fat	
TXN	Low vitamin E	Abdominal obesity
MC4R	Western dietary pattern and high saturated fatty acids	Metabolic syndrome
APOB	High fat	
TCF7L2	High saturated fatty acids	
APOC3, APOA1	Western dietary pattern	
Deregulated Metabolic Signatures[64]		
Metabolic Pathway	**Phenotype**	
Branched-chain amino acid metabolism	Obesity and insulin resistance	
Androgen synthesis	Childhood obesity	

Data from Refs.[12,26,63,64]

modest effect on the risk of obesity and simulation studies have shown that currently known SNPs do not account for more than 20% of variance in BMI.[17,18] The discovery of SNPs may potentially lead to the development of new preventative and therapeutic options to treat obesity. However, such developments will take time because they require a deep understanding of how a SNP influences the expression of target genes, and how these affect phenotype. At the moment, this information is largely unavailable for most SNPs.

The potential of genetics-directed therapy is exemplified with monogenic obesity disorders, such as in the case of leptin and proopiomelanocortin (POMC) deficiency. Recombinant leptin and setmelanotide (a melanocortin-4 receptor agonist, receptor through which POMC signals) used, respectively, in patients with leptin and POMC deficiency have resulted in significant weight loss.[19,20] Both treatments have been used in common obesity with variable results, suggesting that some SNPs may have a common mechanistic gene of action.[20,21] If these SNPs are identified, it could potentially recognize a subset of patients with common obesity that may benefit from these treatments.

Gene by Environment Interactions

Studies have suggested that when individuals have a genetic predisposition to obesity, they are more prone to gain weight when they are exposed to hostile environments. Because SNPs have modest effect size on obesity traits, researchers have aggregated several risk-increasing SNP variants into genetic risk scores. Genetic risk scores have a superior power compared with individual SNPs to detect the interaction between genes and environment.[22] Data suggest that the following factors amplify the association of genetic risk scores with BMI: low socioeconomic status, chronic psychosocial stress, decreased sleep duration, gender, increased consumption of sugar-containing beverages, increased fried food intake, and decreased physical activity.[12]

The clinical application of this knowledge is still limited. Data from genes by environment interaction studies have provided ground to commercially available GWAS-based genetic profiling. GWAS-based genetic profiling is now easily accessible for individuals to learn their risk of obesity or difficulties with weight loss. Although this has potential for precision-medicine, data suggest that genetic risk-based knowledge does not change behavior.[23] Specifically, for obesity, although genetic risk-based counseling increased the participant's motivation to make lifestyle changes, this did not translate necessarily into weight loss.[24]

Epigenetics

The rapid emergence of the obesity epidemic is not fully explained by genetics, which could not have changed dramatically over such a short period of time. Unlike genetics, many key environmental factors have changed over this timeframe, most notably diet and physical activity. Environmental factors interact with our genes through epigenetic modifications of the genome that can alter gene activity.[25] Epigenetic changes are dynamic and removing the inducing factors can often reverse these changes.

There are many studies providing evidence for a strong correlation between epigenetic modifications with obesity traits. For instance, researchers have analyzed methylation patterns of genes that may participate in obesity pathophysiology, such as eating behavior, glucose metabolism, lipid metabolism, adipogenesis, circadian rhythm, and inflammation, among others. Data show that methylation of these genes correlates with obesity, obesity traits, and its complications.[26] Emphasizing the importance of epigenetic modifications in obesity, interventional studies have demonstrated that physical activity and bariatric surgery alter epigenetic modification patterns that are sometimes tissue-specific and may consequentially result in beneficial metabolic changes.[27,28]

There are currently inexpensive microarrays permitting high-throughput epigenetic change profiling. Although these changes may be highly relevant in the pathophysiology of obesity, their net effect in human populations has yet to be quantified. This information taken together suggests that epigenetic markers by themselves may not be enough to come up with precision obesity therapies. However, the effect size of the correlation with obesity traits could potentially be informative as a prognostic and diagnostic tool. **Table 3** lists the better characterized epigenetic modifications and their associated phenotype.

Metabolomics

Metabolites are elemental units of cellular function. Disruption in their regulation results in changes that can have clinical ramifications. Consequently, the metabolome contains information that can provide insights into the mechanisms of a specific disease. Metabolomics is a tool aimed at detecting and measuring changes in metabolite profiles in response to physiologic or pathologic conditions. Researchers have identified profound disruption of the metabolome in obesity and metabolic signatures of this condition that are strongly correlated with BMI, other obesity traits, and metabolic comorbidities.[29] **Table 3** lists the better characterized metabolic pathways disruptions and their associated phenotype. Within patients with obesity, studies in this field have been able to identify different metabolomic patterns between healthy individuals with obesity and individuals with obesity and metabolic complications, such as cardiovascular disease, dyslipidemia, metabolic syndrome, and diabetes. Furthermore, studies show that in healthy obese and even healthy lean individuals, an abnormal metabolome is associated with increased cardiovascular events compared with control subjects matched for BMI and with opposite metabolomes.[30]

In this era of precision medicine, researchers have investigated the potential of weight loss interventions based on metabolome signatures. Published data suggest that weight loss variation among individuals following a low-calorie diet can be predicted by their baseline metabolic profile.[31,32] Although this field is actively evolving, metabolomics can identify clinically meaningful heterogeneity in obesity that could potentially lead to the identification of a metabolic fingerprint that cannot only help phenotype a patient but can also help select certain patients for certain specific therapies.

Microbiome

Gut microbiome genes have unique functions that complement the genetic catalog of humans.[33] Growing evidence reveals that the gut microbiome is sensitive to dietary, environmental, and host factors. These factors can alter microbiome precisely, resulting in metabolic changes that can consequently cause a disease. Despite the mounting evidence establishing a robust association between alterations of the gut microbiome and obesity, the exact underlying mechanisms have yet to be characterized.

In animal studies, the gut microbiome was observed to regulate the host's ability to harvest energy from food.[34] Further work has provided direct evidence of a transmissible obesity microbiota[35] where opportunistic pathogens could participate in the development of obesity by altering host gene expression and by inducing insulin resistance mediated by metabolic endotoxemia[36] or by altering the brain-gut-axis.[37] On the contrary, certain bacteria clusters have been associated with reduced risk of cardiometabolic disease by having genomes with higher capability for methane production and mucin degradation, for instance.[38]

Most human data come from studies that have compared the gut microbiome of exceedingly different populations: individuals from westernized and industrialized countries versus individuals from hunter-gatherer societies. The main difference is in the diversity of the gut microbiome, with the former having decreased diversity compared with the latter.[39,40] Weight loss intervention clinical studies have shown shifts in the gut microbiome that have been implicated in the resulting reduction in weight and improved metabolic function.[41,42] Specific microbiome changes associated with obesity or the risk of developing obesity include higher *Bifidobacterial* and lower *Staphylococcus aureus* concentrations, and an increased in the ratio of *Firmicutes/Bacteroidetes*, with the latter increasing abundantly with weight loss.[43,44]

Microbiome manipulation could lead to prevention and/or treatment of obesity. Approaches could potentially include designer probiotics and fecal matter transplant. Currently, there is little information available on the efficacy and safety of probiotic formulations.[45] In terms of fecal matter transplant, few human studies have shown that this treatment is efficacious for metabolic disorders; results have been variable and therefore utility is limited.[46] Currently, any potential ability to foster the growth of "healthy" bacteria through diet changes could be highly valuable in optimizing the use of nutrition to combat disease. Achieving this intermediate objective could provide a practical alternative, while serving as a stepping stone as the physiologic (or pathophysiologic) roles of singular microbes continue to be investigated.

Pharmacogenomics

Pharmacogenomics studies how genetics affect an individual's response to particular pharmaceutical compounds. This field integrates pharmacology and genomics to develop effective, safe medications and dosages that are tailored to variations in an individual's genes. Pharmacogenomics could play an important role in obesity management. First, there are several medications that result in weight gain as an adverse effect,[47] and researchers have demonstrated the impact of genetic variants and the risk of metabolic adverse events associated with weight gain–promoting medications.[48–52] Second, the effect of antiobesity medications on weight loss is highly variable among patients[53] and studies have shown that gene variants may partially explain the variability in response to treatment. For instance, genetic variants in the insulin receptor gene and the GLP-1 receptor gene have been associated with differential weight loss in those treated with topiramate and liraglutide, respectively.[54,55] No genetic variants associated with differential weight loss have been identified for the other currently Food and Drug Administration–approved antiobesity medications.

Personalized pharmacotherapy for obesity has been slowly adopted by clinical practice; however, emerging evidence has shown its substantial potential. Incorporating genetic variants that may affect the susceptibility of an individual to drug-induced weight gain and/or the susceptibility for antiobesity drug weight loss into obesity medicine is useful in drug selection and/or dose optimization, positively affecting the efficacy and safety of pharmacologic agents for a determined individual.

Nutrigenetics and Nutrigenomics

Diet is an important environmental factor that interacts with genes. Furthermore, nutrients do not affect individuals in the same way. With the information currently available, there has been a growing necessity to improve personalized nutrition to treat obesity and its associated medical conditions taking into consideration the interaction between diet and the genome. From this interest, the fields of nutrigenetics and nutrigenomics have evolved. Nutrigenetics is the science of the effect of genetic variation on dietary response. However, nutrigenomics is defined as the role of nutrients and bioactive food components in gene expression.[56] Exploitation of this information is essential to understanding how nutrient-gene interactions are affected by the genotype, with the ultimate goal of developing targeted and clinically useful dietary and lifestyle recommendations for optimal health and disease prevention. **Table 3** lists the better characterized SNPs-diet interactions and their putative disease risk.

Studies have demonstrated the importance of these fields in individualizing the obesity patient's care. For instance, researchers have developed personalized weight reduction programs based on calorie-controlled diets using gene variants that are involved in metabolism. In one study, participants receiving dietary advice to optimize nutrient intake tailored to their genotype lost more weight during the weight loss period, and also had better weight loss retention over time.[57] Although these results are promising, larger studies have failed to demonstrate the interaction between genetic variants, dietary recommendations and weight loss.[58]

Clinical Quantitative Traits

Improving phenotyping in large numbers of patients with obesity is crucial to elucidating the factors that account for variability in response to the different treatments for obesity. In this respect, researchers have identified the following quantitative traits in food intake regulation that may be specifically targeted by current available therapies: satiety and satiation, gastric motility, behavioral influences, and gastric sensorimotor factors.[59] In a proof of concept clinical trial, these quantitative traits predicted response to antiobesity pharmacotherapy.[60–62] These data suggest that phenotypic subgroups identified based on pathophysiologic mechanisms offers the opportunity to select patients for antiobesity drugs based on the mechanisms of action of the medication. This approach could potentially enhance drug efficacy.

CHALLENGES

Precision medicine implementation in clinical practice poses various challenges. First, precision medicine practice contrasts with the practice of evidence-based medicine that has modeled the one-size-fits-all approach. This traditional approach has provided inadequate solutions for outliers that can potentially be better served by precision medicine. Responsible data sharing permits bridging of both approaches.

Second, health practitioners may be skeptical about ordering specialized testing that may allow a better characterization of a condition. Furthermore, in health professions' curricula, topics on this individualized approach are scarce. The achievability of obesity precision medicine will depend on the cooperation of all actors involved.

Third, although there exists a vast amount of information that will help pave the way to obesity precision medicine, there is a knowledge gap between the association of biologic markers and obesity, and the mechanisms behind these associations. This gap needs to be filled to be able to develop specific interventions that facilitate individualized medicine for obesity.

Finally, precision medicine research depends deeply on large and interconnected cohorts and biobanks. These data are highly sensitive and could be broadly disseminated to address research questions that cannot yet be conceived. Emphasis should be placed on protecting privacy, while facilitating the responsible and safe storage, transmission, and use of data.

SUMMARY

Current obesity therapies are still based on the assumption that one treatment fits all. This treatment strategy varies in its effectiveness from individual to individual and suggests that specific patient characteristics dictate risk factor susceptibility and treatment response. Precision medicine has offered a new ground that theoretically provides the basis that will allow individualized treatments based on data obtained from bio samples, digital images, wearable devices, and conventional data from medical records.

Although there have been major advances in this field, much needs to be resolved before obesity precision medicine becomes a prevailing practice. Current available information gathered from genetic, epigenetic, metabolic, pharmacologic, microbiologic and clinical studies has revealed that there are numerous intermediary processes that contribute to obesity. These intermediary processes have provided an outline to partially understand the pathophysiologic mechanisms behind the heterogeneity of obesity and its clinical consequences. Some of these processes have or are currently being targeted to individualize obesity therapy with some success.

Although the evolving arena of precision medicine grants new opportunities for fighting obesity, it also presents with new challenges related to integration of data, health literacy, and data privacy. As clinicians continue to gather information, new disease classifications, which can be coupled with more effective, cheaper, and with fewer side effects, will be defined.

DISCLOSURE

M.D. Hurtado A has nothing to disclose. A. Acosta is a stockholder in Gila Therapeutics and Phenomix Sciences; and serves as a consultant for Rhythm Pharmaceuticals and General Mills.

FUNDING SOURCE

Dr. A. Acosta is supported by NIH grant: NIDDK K23DK114460.

REFERENCES

1. Collaborators TGO. Health effects of overweight and obesity in 195 countries over 25 years. N Engl J Med 2017;377(1):13–27.
2. World Health Organization. Noncommunicable diseases country profiles 2018. Available at: https://www.who.int/nmh/publications/ncd-profiles-2018/en/. Accessed April 10, 2020.
3. Flegal KM, Kruszon-Moran D, Carroll MD, et al. Trends in obesity among adults in the United States, 2005 to 2014. JAMA 2016;315(21):2284–91.
4. Waters H, Graf M. America's obesity crisis: the health and economic costs of excess weight. The Milken Institute; 2018. Available at: https://milkeninstitute.org/sites/default/files/reports-pdf/Mi-Americas-Obesity-Crisis-WEB.pdf. Accessed April 5, 2020.
5. Collins FS, Varmus H. A new initiative on precision medicine. N Engl J Med 2015; 372(9):793–5.
6. Clinical guidelines on the identification, evaluation, and treatment of overweight and obesity in adults: the evidence report. National Institutes of Health. Obes Res 1998;6(Suppl 2):51s–209s.
7. Blüher M. The distinction of metabolically 'healthy' from 'unhealthy' obese individuals. Curr Opin Lipidol 2010;21(1):38–43.
8. Larsson B, Svärdsudd K, Welin L, et al. Abdominal adipose tissue distribution, obesity, and risk of cardiovascular disease and death: 13 year follow up of

participants in the study of men born in 1913. Br Med J (Clin Res ed) 1984; 288(6428):1401–4.

9. Pischon T, Boeing H, Hoffmann K, et al. General and abdominal adiposity and risk of death in Europe. N Engl J Med 2008;359(20):2105–20.

10. Sharma AM, Kushner RF. A proposed clinical staging system for obesity. Int J Obes 2009;33(3):289–95.

11. Kuk JL, Ardern CI, Church TS, et al. Edmonton Obesity Staging System: association with weight history and mortality risk. Appl Physiol Nutr Metab 2011;36(4): 570–6.

12. Goodarzi MO. Genetics of obesity: what genetic association studies have taught us about the biology of obesity and its complications. Lancet Diabetes Endocrinol 2018;6(3):223–36.

13. Saeed S, Arslan M, Froguel P. Genetics of obesity in consanguineous populations: toward precision medicine and the discovery of novel obesity genes. Obesity (Silver Spring) 2018;26(3):474–84.

14. Kaur Y, de Souza RJ, Gibson WT, et al. A systematic review of genetic syndromes with obesity. Obes Rev 2017;18(6):603–34.

15. Schousboe K, Visscher PM, Erbas B, et al. Twin study of genetic and environmental influences on adult body size, shape, and composition. Int J Obes Relat Metab Disord 2004;28(1):39–48.

16. Stunkard AJ, Harris JR, Pedersen NL, et al. The body-mass index of twins who have been reared apart. N Engl J Med 1990;322(21):1483–7.

17. Yang J, Bakshi A, Zhu Z, et al. Genetic variance estimation with imputed variants finds negligible missing heritability for human height and body mass index. Nat Genet 2015;47(10):1114–20.

18. Locke AE, Kahali B, Berndt SI, et al. Genetic studies of body mass index yield new insights for obesity biology. Nature 2015;518(7538):197–206.

19. Farooqi IS, Matarese G, Lord GM, et al. Beneficial effects of leptin on obesity, T cell hyporesponsiveness, and neuroendocrine/metabolic dysfunction of human congenital leptin deficiency. J Clin Invest 2002;110(8):1093–103.

20. Collet TH, Dubern B, Mokrosinski J, et al. Evaluation of a melanocortin-4 receptor (MC4R) agonist (Setmelanotide) in MC4R deficiency. Mol Metab 2017;6(10): 1321–9.

21. Roth JD, Roland BL, Cole RL, et al. Leptin responsiveness restored by amylin agonism in diet-induced obesity: evidence from nonclinical and clinical studies. Proc Natl Acad Sci U S A 2008;105(20):7257–62.

22. Marigorta UM, Gibson G. A simulation study of gene-by-environment interactions in GWAS implies ample hidden effects. Front Genet 2014;5:225.

23. Hollands GJ, French DP, Griffin SJ, et al. The impact of communicating genetic risks of disease on risk-reducing health behaviour: systematic review with meta-analysis. BMJ 2016;352:i1102.

24. Meisel SF, Beeken RJ, van Jaarsveld CHM, et al. Genetic susceptibility testing and readiness to control weight: results from a randomized controlled trial. Obesity (Silver Spring) 2015;23(2):305–12.

25. Jaenisch R, Bird A. Epigenetic regulation of gene expression: how the genome integrates intrinsic and environmental signals. Nat Genet 2003;33(Suppl):245–54.

26. Rohde K, Keller M, la Cour Poulsen L, et al. Genetics and epigenetics in obesity. Metabolism 2019;92:37–50.

27. Fabre O, Ingerslev LR, Garde C, et al. Exercise training alters the genomic response to acute exercise in human adipose tissue. Epigenomics 2018;10(8): 1033–50.

28. Kirchner H, Nylen C, Laber S, et al. Altered promoter methylation of PDK4, IL1 B, IL6, and TNF after Roux-en Y gastric bypass. Surg Obes Relat Dis 2014;10(4): 671–8.

29. Rangel-Huerta OD, Pastor-Villaescusa B, Gil A. Are we close to defining a metabolomic signature of human obesity? A systematic review of metabolomics studies. Metabolomics 2019;15(6):93.

30. Cirulli ET, Guo L, Leon Swisher C, et al. Profound perturbation of the metabolome in obesity is associated with health risk. Cell Metab 2019;29(2):488–500.e482.

31. Stroeve JH, Saccenti E, Bouwman J, et al. Weight loss predictability by plasma metabolic signatures in adults with obesity and morbid obesity of the DiOGenes study. Obesity (Silver Spring) 2016;24(2):379–88.

32. Geidenstam N, Magnusson M, Danielsson APH, et al. Amino acid signatures to evaluate the beneficial effects of weight loss. Int J Endocrinol 2017;2017: 6490473.

33. Ley RE, Peterson DA, Gordon JI. Ecological and evolutionary forces shaping microbial diversity in the human intestine. Cell 2006;124(4):837–48.

34. Backhed F, Ding H, Wang T, et al. The gut microbiota as an environmental factor that regulates fat storage. Proc Natl Acad Sci U S A 2004;101(44):15718–23.

35. Ridaura VK, Faith JJ, Rey FE, et al. Gut microbiota from twins discordant for obesity modulate metabolism in mice. Science 2013;341(6150):1241214.

36. Cani PD, Amar J, Iglesias MA, et al. Metabolic endotoxemia initiates obesity and insulin resistance. Diabetes 2007;56(7):1761–72.

37. Bauer PV, Hamr SC, Duca FA. Regulation of energy balance by a gut–brain axis and involvement of the gut microbiota. Cell Mol Life Sci 2016;73(4):737–55.

38. Dao MC, Everard A, Aron-Wisnewsky J, et al. *Akkermansia muciniphila* and improved metabolic health during a dietary intervention in obesity: relationship with gut microbiome richness and ecology. Gut 2016;65(3):426–36.

39. Yatsunenko T, Rey FE, Manary MJ, et al. Human gut microbiome viewed across age and geography. Nature 2012;486(7402):222–7.

40. Schnorr SL, Candela M, Rampelli S, et al. Gut microbiome of the Hadza hunter-gatherers. Nat Commun 2014;5:3654.

41. Palleja A, Kashani A, Allin KH, et al. Roux-en-Y gastric bypass surgery of morbidly obese patients induces swift and persistent changes of the individual gut microbiota. Genome Med 2016;8(1):67.

42. Ryan KK, Tremaroli V, Clemmensen C, et al. FXR is a molecular target for the effects of vertical sleeve gastrectomy. Nature 2014;509(7499):183–8.

43. Duncan SH, Lobley GE, Holtrop G, et al. Human colonic microbiota associated with diet, obesity and weight loss. Int J Obes (Lond) 2008;32(11):1720–4.

44. Kalliomäki M, Collado MC, Salminen S, et al. Early differences in fecal microbiota composition in children may predict overweight. Am J Clin Nutr 2008;87(3): 534–8.

45. Sivamaruthi BS, Kesika P, Suganthy N, et al. A review on role of microbiome in obesity and antiobesity properties of probiotic supplements. Biomed Res Int 2019;2019:3291367.

46. Hartstra AV, Bouter KEC, Bäckhed F, et al. Insights into the role of the microbiome in obesity and type 2 diabetes. Diabetes Care 2015;38(1):159–65.

47. Verhaegen AA, Van Gaal LF. Drug-induced obesity and its metabolic consequences: a review with a focus on mechanisms and possible therapeutic options. J Endocrinol Invest 2017;40(11):1165–74.

48. Zhang JP, Lencz T, Zhang RX, et al. Pharmacogenetic associations of antipsychotic drug-related weight gain: a systematic review and meta-analysis. Schizophr Bull 2016;42(6):1418–37.
49. Secher A, Bukh J, Bock C, et al. Antidepressive-drug-induced bodyweight gain is associated with polymorphisms in genes coding for COMT and TPH1. Int Clin Psychopharmacol 2009;24(4):199–203.
50. Bai X, Xu C, Wen D, et al. Polymorphisms of peroxisome proliferator-activated receptor gamma (PPARgamma) and cluster of differentiation 36 (CD36) associated with valproate-induced obesity in epileptic patients. Psychopharmacology (Berl) 2018;235(9):2665–73.
51. Molnar A, Kovesdi A, Szucs N, et al. Polymorphisms of the GR and HSD11B1 genes influence body mass index and weight gain during hormone replacement treatment in patients with Addison's disease. Clin Endocrinol (Oxf) 2016;85(2): 180–8.
52. Kang ES, Cha BS, Kim HJ, et al. The 11482G >A polymorphism in the perilipin gene is associated with weight gain with rosiglitazone treatment in type 2 diabetes. Diabetes Care 2006;29(6):1320–4.
53. Heymsfield SB, Wadden TA. Mechanisms, pathophysiology, and management of obesity. N Engl J Med 2017;376(3):254–66.
54. Li QS, Lenhard JM, Zhan Y, et al. A candidate-gene association study of topiramate-induced weight loss in obese patients with and without type 2 diabetes mellitus. Pharmacogenet Genomics 2016;26(2):53–65.
55. Jensterle M, Pirs B, Goricar K, et al. Genetic variability in GLP-1 receptor is associated with inter-individual differences in weight lowering potential of liraglutide in obese women with PCOS: a pilot study. Eur J Clin Pharmacol 2015;71(7):817–24.
56. Fenech M, El-Sohemy A, Cahill L, et al. Nutrigenetics and nutrigenomics: viewpoints on the current status and applications in nutrition research and practice. J Nutrigenet Nutrigenomics 2011;4(2):69–89.
57. Arkadianos I, Valdes AM, Marinos E, et al. Improved weight management using genetic information to personalize a calorie controlled diet. Nutr J 2007;6:29.
58. Gardner CD, Trepanowski JF, Del Gobbo LC, et al. Effect of low-fat vs low-carbohydrate diet on 12-month weight loss in overweight adults and the association with genotype pattern or insulin secretion: the DIETFITS randomized clinical trial. JAMA 2018;319(7):667–79.
59. Camilleri M, Acosta A. Gastrointestinal traits: individualizing therapy for obesity with drugs and devices. Gastrointest Endosc 2016;83(1):48–56.
60. Acosta A, Camilleri M, Shin A, et al. Quantitative gastrointestinal and psychological traits associated with obesity and response to weight-loss therapy. Gastroenterology 2015;148(3):537–46.e534.
61. Acosta A, Camilleri M, Burton D. Exenatide in obesity with accelerated gastric emptying: a randomized, pharmacodynamics study. Phys Rep 2015;3(11): e12610.
62. Halawi H, Khemani D, Eckert D, et al. Effects of liraglutide on weight, satiation, and gastric functions in obesity: a randomised, placebo-controlled pilot trial. Lancet Gastroenterol Hepatol 2017;2(12):890–9.
63. Ramos-Lopez O, Milagro FI, Allayee H, et al. Guide for current nutrigenetic, nutrigenomic, and nutriepigenetic approaches for precision nutrition involving the prevention and management of chronic diseases associated with obesity. Lifestyle Genom 2017;10(1–2):43–62.
64. Newgard CB. Metabolomics and metabolic diseases: where do we stand? Cell Metab 2017;25(1):43–56.

Nutritional Management of Acute Pancreatitis

Kavin A. Kanthasamy, MD[a],*, Venkata S. Akshintala, MD[b], Vikesh K. Singh, MD, MSc[c]

KEYWORDS

- Acute pancreatitis • Nutrition • Enteral nutrition

KEY POINTS

- Acute pancreatitis (AP) remains among the most common gastrointestinal disorders requiring hospital admission.
- EN further preserves gut function by reducing gut dysmotility and ileus promoted by pancreatic and systemic inflammation.
- However, poor tolerance of EN and the spectrum of disease severity in patients with AP present unique challenges for clinicians in determining the appropriate type, timing, route, and composition of nutritional support, which results in significant variation in management across centers.

INTRODUCTION

Acute pancreatitis (AP) remains among the most common gastrointestinal disorders requiring hospital admission. The burden and cost of AP on the health care system continues to rise accounting for nearly 280,000 hospitalizations and more than $2.6 billion dollars spent annually in the United States.[1] The management of AP is largely supportive and focuses on intravenous fluid therapy, analgesics, and nutritional support. Enteral nutrition (EN) is one of the few interventions that has been shown to reduce mortality in AP[2] and plays a key role in limiting disease progression and accelerating patient recovery.

The pathogenesis of AP across all etiologies involves a complex cascade of intra-acinar pancreatic zymogen activation, most notably trypsinogen, resulting in acinar injury and upregulation of proinflammatory mediators and cytokines that contribute to a profound local and systemic inflammatory response syndrome (SIRS).[2] Nutritional support plays a key role in mitigating the sequelae of the SIRS response with specific attention to hypoperfusion of the gut barrier mediated by inflammatory and microcirculatory damage.[3] EN is thought to promote the integrity of the damaged gut barrier by

[a] Division of Gastroenterology, Johns Hopkins Medical Institutions, 1800 Orleans Street, Baltimore, MD 21287, USA; [b] 1800 Orleans Street, Sheikh Zayed Tower, Baltimore, MD 21287, USA; [c] 1830 East Monument Street, Room 428, Baltimore, MD 21205, USA
* Corresponding author.
E-mail address: kkantha1@jhmi.edu

Gastroenterol Clin N Am 50 (2021) 141–150
https://doi.org/10.1016/j.gtc.2020.10.014
0889-8553/21/

preventing luminal mucosal atrophy, hence reducing gut permeability and the resulting translocation of gut microbiota that potentiates AP-associated SIRS, multiorgan failure, and infection (**Fig. 1**).[4,5] EN further preserves gut function by reducing gut dysmotility and ileus promoted by pancreatic and systemic inflammation. Ileus has been associated with infected pancreatic necrosis in patients with necrotizing AP, likely a reflection of the paradigm of bacterial translocation.[6] The inflammatory response also induces a highly catabolic state that increases metabolic demand causing a negative nitrogen balance of up to 20 to 40 g per day that promotes malnutrition.[7,8]

For these reasons, optimizing nutritional support and maintaining gut function is instrumental in the recovery of patients with AP. However, poor tolerance of EN and the spectrum of disease severity in patients with AP present unique challenges for clinicians in determining the appropriate type, timing, route, and composition of nutritional support, which results in significant variation in management across centers.[9] This review summarizes the current evidence with regard to these questions and provides recommendations in line with current consensus opinions to guide the clinical management of AP from the perspective of nutritional support.

ORAL NUTRITION AND TIMING

Historically, the initial management of AP prioritized bowel rest with *nil per os* (NPO) status with the rationale that avoiding EN would minimize pancreatic stimulation and any exacerbation of ongoing inflammation. In normal patients, oral/duodenal feeding leads to greater stimulation of pancreatic exocrine function compared with fasting and intravenous nutrition as measured by rates of duodenal trypsin secretion (**Table 1**).[10,11] Middistal jejunal feeding, however, does not seem to stimulate pancreas exocrine secretion.[9] AP has been shown to diminish pancreatic exocrine function and the effect seems proportional to morphologic disease severity with the lowest rates of trypsin secretion seen in necrotizing pancreatitis (see **Table 1**).[12] This suggests that pancreatic exocrine function may be "stunned" in AP and EN, regardless of the route, especially in necrotizing AP, may not produce appreciable pancreatic stimulation to contribute to worsening disease severity. Furthermore, EN has been shown to promote gut integrity and function, introducing the concept of

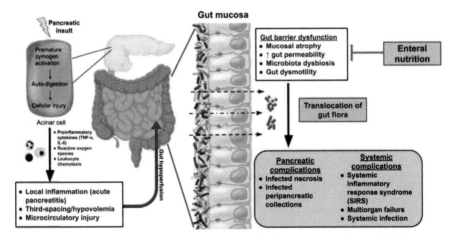

Fig. 1. Pathophysiology of acute pancreatitis and mitigation of associated gut barrier dysfunction by enteral nutrition. IL, interleukin; TNF, tumor necrosis factor.

Table 1	
Pancreatic enzyme secretory response to various forms of diet	
Mode of Feeding	**Trypsin (u/h)**
Normal patients	
Fasting (n = 7)	134 (22)
Intravenous (n = 5)	171 (33)
Duodenal total (n = 13)	408 (51)
Polymeric (n = 6)	471 (73)
Elemental (n = 7)	335 (65)
Middistal jejunal (n = 11)	119 (16)
Disease Severity	**Trypsin (u/h)**
AP	
Control, no AP (n = 8)	514 ± 86
Mild/moderate (n = 8)	214 ± 83
Necrotizing (n = 4)	32 ± 7

Duodenal trypsin secretion rates in normal patients given various modes of feeding and in patients with AP given duodenal feeding. Values are listed as group means with standard error.

Data from Kaushik N, Pietraszewski M, Holst JJ, O'keefe SJ. Enteral feeding without pancreatic stimulation. Pancreas. 2005;31(4):353-9; and O'keefe SJ, Lee RB, Anderson FP, et al. Physiological effects of enteral and parenteral feeding on pancreaticobiliary secretion in humans. Am J Physiol Gastrointest Liver Physiol. 2003;284(1):G27-36.

"gut rousing, but not resting."[13,14] In line with this, contemporary evidence supports early enteral feeding, ideally *per os* in AP.

A recent systematic review of 11 randomized control trials (RCTs) by Vege and colleagues[15] compared the role of early feeding (within 48 hours of admission) with delayed feeding across all severities of AP and found no difference in outcomes including mortality, rates of multiorgan failure, and complications related to pancreatic necrosis. Prior systematic reviews have also shown decreased length of stay (LOS)[16] and potentially lower infectious complications[17,18] with early feeding within 48 hours of admission. The American Gastroenterological Association (AGA) guidelines for AP currently strongly recommend early (within 24 hours) oral feeding as tolerated rather than keeping patients NPO based on this moderate quality body of evidence.[19] Multiple RCTs suggest initiation of oral feeding upfront with a soft low-fat, low-residue diet because it provides more calories without worsening of symptoms or difference in LOS when compared with an initial diet of clear liquids.[20–22]

It is important to acknowledge that oral refeeding is sometimes not feasible in patients with significant symptoms, gastrointestinal dysmotility, and in severe AP (SAP)/necrotizing disease. For these patients, timely initiation of EN via a nasogastric tube (NGT) or nasojejunal tube (NJT) becomes appropriate. However, the administration of prompt EN via NGT/NJT as a substitute for oral intake in patients with predicted SAP is not associated with improved outcomes. The PYTHON trial, a multicenter RCT from the Netherlands, that randomized patients with predicted SAP (defined as Acute Physiology and Chronic Health Evaluation II score of ≥8, an Imrie or modified Glasgow score of ≥3, or a serum C-reactive protein level of >150 mg/L) to either early EN via NGT within 24 hours of admission or to "on-demand" oral feeding within 72 hours, found no differences in the composite end points of major infection and death or in secondary end points of rates of pancreatic necrosis or need for intensive care unit level care.[23] Of note nearly 70% of patients in the on-demand group were able to tolerate oral feeding in the early stages of disease and had shorter time to tolerance of full oral feeding (6 days for oral group vs 9 days for EN group). Additional studies have demonstrated no difference in inflammatory profiles/cytokine production in oral versus EN in SAP.[24] Although more research is needed to clarify the optimal timing and administration of EN in severe and acute necrotizing pancreatitis, early oral feeding in this subgroup may be trialed cautiously and directed by patient symptoms.

TYPE OF NUTRITION (ENTERAL NUTRITION VS PARENTERAL NUTRITION)

The previously held dogma of gut and pancreatic rest in AP established parenteral nutrition (PN) as the primary means of providing nutrition while patients were kept NPO. Current evidence, however, has clearly shown worse outcomes with PN relative to EN. In a technical review of 12 RCTs that compared EN with PN across all severities of pancreatitis, there was more than a two-fold reduction in the rate of multiorgan failure (odds ratio, 0.41; 95% confidence interval, 0.27–063) and nearly a four-fold reduction in infected peripancreatic necrosis (odds ratio, 0.28; 95% confidence interval, 0.15–0.51) with the use of EN.[15] Other meta-analyses have also shown increased cost, infectious complications, and LOS with the use of PN.[25,26] These findings were similarly shown in a Cochrane review by Al-Omran and colleagues of eight RCTs that also demonstrated increased mortality in the subset of patients with SAP receiving PN.[27] These findings are likely reflective of known complications inherent to PN, such as to catheter-related bloodstream infections and sepsis, metabolic derangements,[11] and compromise of gut barrier function and microbiota dysbiosis that has been demonstrated with the withdrawal of EN in critically ill patients.[28,29]

In patients unable to tolerate oral feeding within the first 48 to 72 hours because of symptoms, ileus, or SAP, EN via NGT or NJT should be prioritized over PN in line with the current strong recommendation from the AGA that was based on moderate-quality evidence.[30] Given the relative harm associated with PN, it should be reserved only for patients unable to tolerate EN over a prolonged period, when an NGT/NJT cannot be placed, or when minimal caloric needs cannot be met with EN alone.

ROUTE OF ENTERAL NUTRITION (NASOGASTRIC VS NASOJEJUNAL)

Despite clear evidence supporting the use of EN in patients intolerant of oral feeding, there is less compelling evidence for a preferred route: NGT versus NJT. A meta-analysis of three RCTs that compared NGT with NJT feeding in SAP demonstrated no difference in mortality, infectious complications, or LOS.[31] The distal delivery of EN via NJT offers a theoretic reduction in aspiration risk and middistal jejunal nutrition has been shown to minimize pancreatic stimulation. However, RCTs and meta-analyses have shown no difference in tracheal aspiration,[30] exacerbation of pain, or energy balance between the two routes.[32] These studies had several limitations including large heterogeneity, high risk of bias because of a lack of blinding, small sample sizes, and poorly specified outcomes. A large multicenter trial comparing NGT with NJT feeding in AP was unfortunately terminated because of lack of adequate patient recruitment (ClinicalTrials.gov NCT00580749). The lack of clear evidence suggesting a superior route of EN in SAP may reflect stunning of pancreatic exocrine function observed in necrotizing disease.

Although available evidence is not robust, NGT represents a more pragmatic option for EN in AP given the relative ease of bedside placement compared with endoscopic placement of NJT. There are new bedside transnasal systems that have been developed for the placement of NGT and NJT. Additional research is required to more definitively establish the optimal and safest route of EN in SAP; however, results of the PYTHON trial demonstrating equal tolerance of oral feeding compared with tube feeding in SAP may make the comparison less relevant for clinical management.

COMPOSITION OF ENTERAL NUTRITION AND IMMUNONUTRITION

There is a wide range of EN formulations with varying purported benefits in AP and, for simplicity, is divided into three categories: (1) oligomeric feeds, (2) polymeric feeds, and (3) "immunonutrition." Oligomeric, also known as semielemental, formulations contain small peptides, medium-chain fatty acids, and simple polysaccharides that do not require digestion by pancreatic enzymes and theoretically offer greater pancreatic rest than more complex polymeric formulations that contain full proteins, complex lipids, and carbohydrates.[33,34] Two meta-analyses, however, comparing oligomeric with polymeric formulations found no difference in terms of feeding intolerance, mortality, or LOS between the two formulations.[35] There is no apparent clinical advantage to the use of oligomeric formulations and more inexpensive polymeric formulations should be readily used.

Immunonutrition broadly refers to specialized formulations containing immunomodulatory supplements that are thought to offer benefit by modifying the immune response associated with AP. The most well studied of these include formulations supplemented with one of either glutamine, arginine, omega-3 fatty acids, nucleotides, and fiber enrichment. Trials in other clinical settings involving critically ill patients given immunonutrition-supplemented EN, specifically with glutamine and arginine, have described trends toward lower infectious complications and mortality compared with standard EN.[36–38] The benefit of immunonutrition-supplemented EN in AP is less established and based on low-quality studies. A Cochrane systematic review by Poropat and colleagues[39] of 15 trials investigating EN formulations specifically containing immunonutrition components given to patients with AP found no difference in all-cause mortality or occurrence of SIRS when compared with other EN formulations. Nearly all the trials in this review were noted to be of low quality with a high risk for bias. A separate meta-analysis by Petrov and colleagues[40] similarly did not demonstrate a clinical benefit with immunonutrition formulations in regard to LOS or infectious complications.

There are trials, largely from China, showing clinical benefit of PN supplemented with glutamine or glutamine administered intravenously in SAP with regards to lower infectious complications, LOS, and resolution of inflammatory markers.[41–44] Glutamine is postulated to exert an immunomodulatory effect via increasing lymphocyte mitogenic function, whereas decreasing production of proinflammatory cytokines, such as interleukin-6 and tumor necrosis factor-α and antioxidant properties. Glutamine also supports the growth of other rapidly dividing cells, such as enterocytes.[45] These benefits have not been demonstrated in trials with glutamine-supplemented EN,[43,46] currently limiting the clinical relevance of glutamine in AP until further investigation with high-quality trials can be performed.

Patients with AP are known to have gut dysbiosis or unfavorable imbalance of gut microbiota that may contribute to associated inflammation.[3,47] The use of probiotics, substances containing live microorganisms of healthy gut flora, however, has been shown to be detrimental in AP. The PROPATRIA trial, a multicenter, double-blind, placebo-controlled RCT of nearly 300 patients with predicted SAP conducted in the Netherlands aimed to reduce infectious complications in patients with SAP through the use of enteral probiotic preparations. The study compared the use a multispecies mixture of two different *Bifidobacterium* species, three different *Lactobacillus* species, and one *Lactococcus* species with placebo. Findings from the trial demonstrated no significant difference in the primary end point of infectious complications and a two- to three-fold increase in mortality in patients who received probiotics.[48] Until more studies can establish an acceptable safety margin and consistent dosing for probiotic administration, their use should be avoided in AP.

The benefit of immunonutrition in AP is currently unclear and, as recommended by the AGA, warrants further investigation with high-quality RCTs to support routine use. Current evidence is lacking in supporting the use of immunonutrition-supplemented EN but there may be some benefit of glutamine-supplemented PN in patients with SAP requiring PN. A Cochrane systematic review and network meta-analysis by DiMartino and colleagues[49] is ongoing to further clarify the benefit of immunonutrition supplementation in EN and PN in AP.

SUMMARY AND RECOMMENDATIONS

In addition to supportive care, nutritional support is a cornerstone of the management of AP across all disease severities. EN serves to preserve the gut barrier as a means to mitigate immune dysregulation and systemic inflammation inherent to the clinical syndrome of AP. Based on the current body of evidence, oral feeding trials should be initiated generally within 24 hours with a soft, low-residue diet as tolerated rather than routinely keeping patients NPO. Polymeric EN should be given via tube feeding for patients unable to tolerate an oral feeding challenge within 48 to 72 hours. NGT may be the preferred route of feeding in patients without gastric outlet obstruction, ileus, or of high aspiration risk because of its relative convenience and lack of evidence supporting the superiority of NJT (**Fig. 2**). It is important to actively reassess patients reported symptoms to attempt oral feeding trials as feasible. PN should be avoided because of worse clinical outcomes relative to EN and is reserved only for select situations where EN cannot be administered. Immunonutrition formulations cannot be routinely

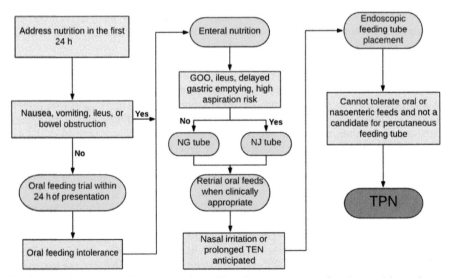

Fig. 2. Flow diagram on the suggested nutritional management of patients with moderate to severe acute pancreatitis (pancreatic necrosis). GOO, gastric outlet obstruction; NG, nasogastric; NJ, nasojejunal; TEN, total enteral nutrition; TPN, total parenteral nutrition.

recommended based on current evidence and additional investigation is required to clarify its benefit in AP. Probiotic use should be avoid in AP.

CLINICS CARE POINTS

- Oral and enteral nutrition (EN) significantly reduces the risk of mortality, infection, and organ failure in patients with acute pancreatitis and should be prioritized along with fluid therapy and analgesia.

- Oral feeding using a soft low-fat and low-residue diet should be attempted within 24 hours of presentation as tolerated by symptoms rather than keeping patients *nil per os* (NPO). Early oral feeding is safe and has been shown to decrease hospital length of stay.

- Patients unable to tolerate oral feeding trials over 48 to 72 hours should receive EN through a feeding tube. There is no difference between nasogastric or nasojejunal tubes and the choice of which to use is left to the discretion of the clinician and available resources.

- Parenteral nutrition should be avoided in acute pancreatitis because of increased rates of infection and mortality relative to EN. Its use is reserved for only select circumstances where EN is not tolerated.

- The benefit of "immunonutrition" and other nutritional supplements in acute pancreatitis requires further investigation. Probiotic use should be avoided.

DISCLOSURE

All included authors disclose no commercial or financial conflicts of interest.

REFERENCES

1. Peery AF, Crockett SD, Murphy CC, et al. Burden and cost of gastrointestinal, liver, and pancreatic diseases in the United States: update 2018. Gastroenterology 2019;156(1):254–72.e11.
2. Lee PJ, Papachristou GI. New insights into acute pancreatitis. Nat Rev Gastroenterol Hepatol 2019;16(8):479–96.
3. Akshintala VS, Talukdar R, Singh VK, et al. The gut microbiome in pancreatic disease. Clin Gastroenterol Hepatol 2019;17(2):290–5.
4. Tenner S, Baillie J, DeWitt J, et al. American College of Gastroenterology guideline: management of acute pancreatitis. Am J Gastroenterol 2013;108(9): 1400–15, 1416.
5. Wu LM, Sankaran SJ, Plank LD, et al. Meta-analysis of gut barrier dysfunction in patients with acute pancreatitis. Br J Surg 2014;100:1644–56.
6. Moran RA, Jalaly NY, Kamal A, et al. Ileus is a predictor of local infection in patients with acute necrotizing pancreatitis. Pancreatology 2016;16(6):966–72.
7. Gianotti L, Meier R, Lobo DN, et al. ESPEN guidelines on parenteral nutrition: pancreas. Clin Nutr 2009;28(4):428–35.
8. Meir RF, Sobotka L. Basics in clinical nutrition: nutritional support in acute and chronic pancreatitis. Clinical Nutriton and Metabolism 2010;5:e58–62.
9. Dua MM, Worhunsky DJ, Tran TB, et al. Severe acute pancreatitis in the community: confusion reigns. J Surg Res 2015;199(1):44-50.
10. Kaushik N, Pietraszewski M, Holst JJ, et al. Enteral feeding without pancreatic stimulation. Pancreas 2005;31(4):353–9.

11. O'keefe SJ, Lee RB, Anderson FP, et al. Physiological effects of enteral and parenteral feeding on pancreaticobiliary secretion in humans. Am J Physiol Gastrointest Liver Physiol 2003;284(1):G27–36.

12. O'keefe SJ, Lee RB, Li J, et al. Trypsin secretion and turnover in patients with acute pancreatitis. Am J Physiol Gastrointest Liver Physiol 2005;289(2):G181–7.

13. Petrov MS. Moving beyond the 'pancreatic rest' in severe and critical acute pancreatitis. Crit Care 2013;17(4):161.

14. Petrov MS, Windsor JA. Nutritional management of acute pancreatitis: the concept of 'gut rousing'. Curr Opin Clin Nutr Metab Care 2013;16:557–63.

15. Vege SS, Dimagno MJ, Forsmark CE, et al. Initial medical treatment of acute pancreatitis: American Gastroenterological Association Institute Technical Review. Gastroenterology 2018;154(4):1103–39.

16. Horibe M, Nishizawa T, Suzuki H, et al. Timing of oral refeeding in acute pancreatitis: a systematic review and meta-analysis. United European Gastroenterol J 2016;4(6):725–32.

17. Vaughn VM, Shuster D, Rogers MAM, et al. Early versus delayed feeding in patients with acute pancreatitis: a systematic review. Ann Intern Med 2017;166(12):883–92.

18. Bakker OJ, van Brunschot S, Farre A, et al. Timing of enteral nutrition in acute pancreatitis: meta-analysis of individuals using a single-arm of randomised trials. Pancreatology 2014;14:340–6.

19. Crockett SD, Wani S, Gardner TB, et al. American Gastroenterological Association Institute Guideline on initial management of acute pancreatitis. Gastroenterology 2018;154(4):1096–101.

20. Jacobson BC, Vander vliet MB, Hughes MD, et al. A prospective, randomized trial of clear liquids versus low-fat solid diet as the initial meal in mild acute pancreatitis. Clin Gastroenterol Hepatol 2007;5(8):946–51.

21. Moraes JM, Felga GE, Chebli LA, et al. A full solid diet as the initial meal in mild acute pancreatitis is safe and result in a shorter length of hospitalization: results from a prospective, randomized, controlled, double-blind clinical trial. J Clin Gastroenterol 2010;44(7):517–22.

22. Zhao XL, Zhu SF, Xue GJ, et al. Early oral refeeding based on hunger in moderate and severe acute pancreatitis: a prospective controlled, randomized clinical trial. Nutrition 2015;31(1):171–5.

23. Bakker OJ, van Brunschot S, van Santvoort HC, et al. Early versus on-demand nasoenteric tube feeding in acute pancreatitis. N Engl J Med 2014;371(21):1983–93.

24. Powell JJ, Murchison JT, Fearon KC, et al. Randomized controlled trial of the effect of early enteral nutrition on markers of the inflammatory response in predicted severe acute pancreatitis. Br J Surg 2000;87(10):1375–81.

25. Yi F, Ge L, Zhao J, et al. Meta-analysis: total parenteral nutrition versus total enteral nutrition in predicted severe acute pancreatitis. Intern Med 2012;51:523–30.

26. Mutch KL, Heidal KB, Gross KH, et al. Cost-analysis of nutrition support in patients with severe acute pancreatitis. Int J Health Care Qual Assur 2011;24(7):540–7.

27. Al-omran M, Albalawi ZH, Tashkandi MF, et al. Enteral versus parenteral nutrition for acute pancreatitis. Cochrane Database Syst Rev 2010;(1):CD002837.

28. Ralls MW, Demehri FR, Feng Y, et al. Enteral nutrient deprivation in patients leads to a loss of intestinal epithelial barrier function. Surgery 2015;157(4):732–42.

29. Ralls MW, Miyasaka E, Teitelbaum DH. Intestinal microbial diversity and perioperative complications. JPEN J Parenter Enteral Nutr 2014;38(3):392–9.
30. Petrov MS, Correia MI, Windsor JA. Nasogastric tube feeding in predicted severe acute pancreatitis: a systematic review of the literature to determine safety and tolerance. JOP 2008;9:440–8.
31. Zhu Y, Yin H, Zhang R, et al. Nasogastric nutrition versus nasojejunal nutrition in patients with severe acute pancreatitis: a meta-analysis of randomized controlled trials. Gastroenterol Res Pract 2016;2016:6430632.
32. Chang Y, Fu H, Xiao Y, et al. Nasogastric or nasojejunal feeding in predicted severe acute pancreatitis: a meta-analysis. Crit Care 2013;17:R118.
33. Makola D, Krenitsky J, Parrish C, et al. Efficacy of enteral nutrition for the treatment of pancreatitis using standard enteral formula. Am J Gastroenterol 2006; 101(10):2347–55.
34. Tiengou LE, Gloro R, Pouzoulet J, et al. Semi-elemental formula or polymeric formula: is there a better choice for enteral nutrition in acute pancreatitis? Randomized comparative study. JPEN J Parenter Enteral Nutr 2006;30(1):1–5.
35. Petrov MS, Loveday BP, Pylypchuk RD, et al. Systematic review and meta-analysis of enteral nutrition formulations in acute pancreatitis. Br J Surg 2009; 96:1243–52.
36. Beale RJ, Bryg DJ, Bihari DJ. Immunonutrition in the critically ill: a systematic review of clinical outcome. Crit Care Med 1999;27:2799–805.
37. Heys SD, Walker LG, Smith I, et al. Enteral nutritional supplementation with key nutrients in patients with critical illness and cancer: a meta-analysis of randomized controlled clinical trials. Ann Surg 1999;229:467–77.
38. Heyland DK, Novak F, Drover JW, et al. Should immunonutrition become routine in critically ill patients: a systematic review of the evidence. JAMA 2001;286:944–53.
39. Poropat G, Giljaca V, Hauser G, et al. Enteral nutrition formulations for acute pancreatitis. Cochrane Database Syst Rev 2015;(3):CD010605.
40. Petrov MS, Atduev VA, Zagainov VE. Advanced enteral therapy in acute pancreatitis: is there a room for immunonutrition? A meta-analysis. Int J Surg 2008;6: 119–24.
41. Hajdú N, Belágyi T, Issekutz A, et al. [Intravenous glutamine and early nasojejunal nutrition in severe acute pancreatitis: a prospective randomized clinical study]. Magy Seb 2012;65(2):44–51.
42. Xue P, Deng LH, Xia Q, et al. Impact of alanyl-glutamine dipeptide on severe acute pancreatitis in early stage. World J Gastroenterol 2008;14(3):474–8.
43. Yong L, Lu QP, Liu SH, et al. Efficacy of glutamine-enriched nutrition support for patients with severe acute pancreatitis: a meta-analysis. JPEN J Parenter Enteral Nutr 2016;40(1):83–94.
44. Liu X, Sun XF, Ge QX. The role of glutamine supplemented total parenteral nutrition (TPN) in severe acute pancreatitis. Eur Rev Med Pharmacol Sci 2016;20(19): 4176–80.
45. Barash M, Jayshil JP. Gut luminal and clinical benefits of early enteral nutrition in shock. Curr Surg Rep 2019;7(10):21.
46. Petrov MS, Whelan K. Comparison of complications attributable to enteral and parenteral nutrition in predicted severe acute pancreatitis: a systematic review and meta-analysis. Br J Nutr 2010;103(9):1287–95.
47. Tan C, Ling Z, Huang Y, et al. Dysbiosis of intestinal microbiota associated with inflammation involved in the progression of acute pancreatitis. Pancreas 2015; 44(6):868–75.

48. Besselink MG, Van santvoort HC, Buskens E, et al. Probiotic prophylaxis in predicted severe acute pancreatitis: a randomised, double-blind, placebo-controlled trial. Lancet 2008;371(9613):651–9.

49. Di Martino M, Madden AM, Gurusamy KS. Nutritional supplementation in enteral and parenteral nutrition for people with acute pancreatitis. Cochrane Database Syst Rev 2019;(1):CD013250.

Nutrition in the Management of Inflammatory Bowel Diseases

Alexa N. Sasson, MD, FRCPC[a], Richard J.M. Ingram, MRCP, PhD[b],
Maitreyi Raman, MD, MSc, FRCPC[c],
Ashwin N. Ananthakrishnan, MD, MPH[d],*

KEYWORDS

- Nutrition • Diet • Crohn's disease • Ulcerative colitis • Micronutrient deficiency
- Screening

KEY POINTS

- Inflammatory bowel disease is a complex, multifactorial immune-mediated disease in which an understanding of patient nutritional status should be a cornerstone of clinical care.
- Malnutrition is common in inflammatory bowel disease and cumulative evidence suggests that micronutrient deficiency and supplementation play an essential role in disease process and management.
- Dietary intake is modifiable and there is growing literature on the potential benefit of therapeutic dietary interventions and nutritional support for individuals with inflammatory bowel disease.

INTRODUCTION

Inflammatory bowel diseases (IBD), comprising Crohn's disease (CD) and ulcerative colitis (UC), are complex immune-mediated diseases arising out of an interaction between genetic, immunologic, microbial, and environmental factors. Although treatment of these diseases has traditionally focused on immunosuppression to modulate the dysregulated gastrointestinal and systemic immune response, diet and nutrition are increasingly recognized as key components of comprehensive IBD management and among the topics most frequently inquired about by patients.

[a] Division of Gastroenterology, University of Toronto, 27 King's College Circle, Toronto, Ontario M5S 2E4, Canada; [b] Division of Gastroenterology, University of Calgary, 6D27 TRW Building, 3280 Hospital Drive Northwest, Calgary, Alberta T2N 4Z6, Canada; [c] Division of Gastroenterology, University of Calgary, 6D33 TRW Building, 3280 Hospital Drive Northwest, Calgary, Alberta T2N 4Z6, Canada; [d] Division of Gastroenterology, Massachusetts General Hospital and Harvard Medical School, 165 Cambridge Street, 9th Floor, Boston, MA 02114, USA
* Corresponding author.
E-mail address: aananthakrishnan@mgh.harvard.edu

Gastroenterol Clin N Am 50 (2021) 151–167
https://doi.org/10.1016/j.gtc.2020.10.001
0889-8553/21/© 2020 Elsevier Inc. All rights reserved.

General malnutrition is prevalent among individuals with IBD. The identification of individuals at risk through systematic nutritional assessment may allow early effective interventions.[1] Individual micronutrient deficiencies are also present in more than one-half of patients with IBD.[2] The identification, treatment, and monitoring of these factors play an important role in disease management. Finally, dietary factors have been implicated in disease pathogenesis, arising both as a consequence and potential cause of persistent inflammation, and are amenable to modification. On this background, we review the existing literature for screening and assessment of malnutrition and overnutrition; micronutrient deficiency identification, monitoring, and supplementation; and enteral and parenteral nutrition (PN) support, in intestinal failure and perioperatively. We have recently reviewed the role of diet and its role as primary therapy in IBD[3]; therefore, this topic will only be mentioned in brief in this article.

UNDERNUTRITION IN INFLAMMATORY BOWEL DISEASE: CLINICAL IMPACT AND ASSESSMENT

Undernutrition among individuals with IBD is common with a prevalence of 18% to 62% in UC and 65% to 75% in CD.[4,5] The spectrum of involvement includes macronutrient and micronutrient deficiencies, and sarcopenia.[6] There are several factors contributing to malnutrition in IBD.[1] These include decreased oral intake owing to disease-associated symptoms or prolonged inpatient nil per os orders; maldigestion and malabsorption, including through small bowel inflammation; bacterial overgrowth and rapid transit; loss of intestinal function and area, particularly following surgical resection(s) including short bowel syndrome; and increased intestinal losses, including high-output stomas, increased catabolic drive and side-effects of medications. These factors can co-occur and compound through the disease course.

Undernutrition in people with IBD is associated with increased mortality, postoperative complications, length of stay, and cost.[7,8] Undernourished children with IBD are at risk for growth impairment and metabolic bone disease.[9] Sarcopenia, defined as depletion in lean muscle mass with decreased muscle strength, arises from multifactorial etiologies, including chronic inflammation, decreased mobility, and malnutrition, all of which have relevance to IBD.[10] Sarcopenia is associated with undesirable surgical outcomes, including major postoperative complications.[11] Tools have been developed to assess nutritional status and screen for malnutrition in clinical practice.

ASSESSING NUTRITIONAL STATUS

Although the European Society for Clinical Nutrition and Metabolism guidelines on clinical nutrition in IBD recommend routine screening for malnutrition using a validated tool,[8] nutrition screening is frequently not performed in ambulatory clinics.[12] Several screening and assessment tools exist, as reviewed by Li and colleagues[13] and summarized in **Table 1**. Few instruments have been specifically validated for clinical outcomes in IBD. For screening, 4 tools hold particular promise (the Malnutrition Universal Screening Tool, Nutrition Risk Screening tool, Malnutrition Screening Tool, Malnutrition Inflammatory Risk Tool, and the Saskatchewan IBD Nutrition Risk Tool),[13] in addition to patient-administered self-screening.[14] For example, the Nutrition Risk Screening tool comprises a 7-point scale based on age of 70 years or greater, the impact of current disease severity on nutritional requirements, and nutritional impairment (determined by percentage weight loss in the past 1–3 months, low or low to normal body mass index [BMI], and decreased dietary intake in the preceding week against normal requirement).[15] However, the Nutrition Risk Screening tool has only been successfully validated for inpatients. Other screening tools assess similar

Table 1
Nutrition assessment and screening tools

Evaluation Criteria	Subjective Global Assessment	Nutrition Risk Screening	Malnutrition Inflammatory Risk Tool	Malnutrition Universal Screening Tool	Canadian Nutrition Screening Tool	Nutrition Risk Index	Malnutrition Screening Tool	Saskatchewan IBD Nutrition Risk Tool
Body mass index	X	X	X	X				
Weight loss	X	X	X	X	X	X	X	X
Decreased appetite	X	X			X		X	X
Active symptoms	X	X		X				X
Food restriction								X
Laboratory markers			X			X		
Physical examination	X							

components of dietary restriction, BMI, and weight loss, together with C-reactive protein (in the Malnutrition Inflammatory Risk Tool) and recent gastrointestinal symptoms (in the Saskatchewan IBD Nutrition Risk Tool). The Nutritional Risk Index predicted clinical response to infliximab in 1 study, but serum albumin is a key component, likely reflecting active disease assessment rather than malnutrition.[16] Further validation of these tools in patients with IBD is required before any specific tool can be recommended for routine clinical practice. Patients identified to be at risk for malnutrition should be referred to nutrition professionals for more comprehensive nutritional assessment and intervention.[8]

Nutrition assessment tools validated with clinical outcomes include Subjective Global Assessment and measures of sarcopenia, frequently using computed tomography of the L3 and L4 vertebrae or bioelectrical impedance analysis.[13] Although Subjective Global Assessment can be applied at the bedside and is easy to integrate into clinical practice, 2 studies that assessed Subjective Global Assessment with clinical outcomes had discordant results.[17,18] Cross-sectional measures of sarcopenia have been consistently associated with clinical outcomes. However, given the cost, resource limitations, and radiation risks from the use of cross-sectional imaging for definition, research into practical alternatives such as bedside measures of muscle health is needed.

OVERNUTRITION AND OBESITY IN INFLAMMATORY BOWEL DISEASE

Overnutrition is prevalent in patients with CD and with UC; rates of adult obesity are 15% to 40% and an additional 20% to 40% are overweight.[19] This prevalence rate is 6- to 35-fold higher than the proportion of patients with IBD with a low BMI.[20] Obesity is also observed in 20% to 30% of children with IBD, with lower rates in CD and similar rates in UC compared with the general population.[21]

Body composition is altered in many patients with IBD, with reduced lean mass and variable changes in fat compartments inaccurately predicted by BMI alone.[22] Sarcopenia can coexist with obesity,[23] otherwise known as sarcopenic obesity, compounding the impact of either entity alone. Nutrition risk screening and assessment are further complicated in obese patients, because these measures are not determined accurately by traditional assessment methods.[24]

Disease control can also be more challenging in obese patients with IBD. First, some but not other studies suggest that obesity was associated with an increased risk of persistent activity and relapse, and decreased quality of life.[25] Second, obesity may impact medical management. The hepatotoxicity associated with methotrexate may be increased in obesity-related fatty liver disease.[26] Immunomodulators can be underdosed in morbid obesity and altered drug metabolism could decrease their effectiveness.[27] For biologics, there is potential for underdosing of infliximab with increasing weight despite weight-based dosing, and underdosing of fixed dose agents.[19,28] In addition, pharmacokinetics may be altered, with rapid clearance of biologic agents and chronic inflammation in obese individuals,[29] compounding difficulties in achieving and maintaining therapeutic drug levels.[30] Third, surgical intervention is both technically difficult in obese patients (particularly stoma and pouch surgeries),[19] and has worse outcomes than in IBD surgery in nonobese patients.[31] Disease monitoring can also be more challenging, with an increase in background levels of C-reactive protein and fecal calprotectin,[32] and limitations of cross-sectional imaging particularly in morbidly obese individuals.[19] Despite the impacts of obesity on IBD including greater costs,[33] there are few studies of weight loss strategies in patients with IBD to define optimal treatments. There is interest in phentermine–topiramate and naltrexone–bupropion, which seem to be safe and effective and may have independent anti-inflammatory effects.[18] Bariatric surgery in carefully selected individuals seems to be safe and effective.[34]

MICRONUTRIENT DEFICIENCIES, ASSESSMENT, AND TREATMENT

Micronutrient deficiencies in IBD occur frequently, and may be influenced by disease location (small bowel involvement), gastrointestinal losses, and intestinal resection, and lead to symptoms and complications. Close monitoring with repletion and supplementation is essential, alongside optimizing dietary intake. **Table 2** gives an overview of micronutrients and supplementation/monitoring recommendations. Serum levels of certain micronutrients and trace elements may vary as part of an inflammatory response and not reflect total body stores. In an acute inflammatory state, both ferritin and copper levels increase as acute phase reactants, whereas serum levels of folate, zinc, selenium, albumin, and possibly vitamin D have been shown to decrease with inflammation.[28] Therefore, it is generally better to measure levels in remission. Certain medications could also impact the degree of absorption. For example, glucocorticoid therapy interferes with the absorption of calcium, phosphorus, zinc, and vitamins C and D.[2]

Iron

Anemia is highly prevalent, occurring in 27% in patients with CD and 21% of UC patients.[35] Iron deficiency is the leading cause of anemia, in 57% of cases.[36] Iron deficiency anemia in IBD is multifactorial, owing to decreased intake of foods rich in iron sources and ongoing intestinal blood loss owing to inflammation.[37] Additionally, low serum iron in patients with chronic diseases may be due to impaired absorption secondary to the effect of proinflammatory cytokines in upregulating production of liver hepcidin (a mediator of iron homeostasis), which blocks ferroportin-1 and leads intracellular iron sequestration and decreased absorption. For confirmation of iron deficiency anemia diagnosis in the setting of inflammation, a serum ferritin (<100 ng/mL) and transferrin saturation (<20%) has been suggested.[38]

Dietary iron can be found in liver, beef, fortified cereals, and baked beans. Recommendations for iron supplementation,[8] through oral or intravenous routes, are summarized in **Table 3**. Meta-analyses demonstrate that intravenous supplementation is better tolerated with a faster response[39] and should be considered first line for individuals with hemoglobin levels of less than 10 g/dL or those with active inflammation, before moving to oral therapy as needed. Treatment should be continued until hemoglobin and iron stores normalize. Individuals treated previously for iron deficiency anemia should undergo serum testing every 3 months for the first year and every 6 to 12 months thereafter.[40] Because iron is an essential nutrient for microbial growth, in vivo and in vitro studies suggest that increased colonic iron decreases beneficial commensal gut bacteria such as *Bifidobacteria* and *Lactobacilli* while increasing pathogenic enterobacteria, thereby potentially worsening inflammation in IBD.[41] In addition, iron supplementation may generate oxidative free radicals that might worsen inflammation. However, potential deleterious effects have been seen only in animal models and a negative clinical impact has not been established in humans with IBD.

Vitamin D

Vitamin D deficiency is common in the IBD population, with a reported prevalence of 55% in UC and 58% in CD.[42,43] A serum 25-hydroxyvitamin D (25-OH-D) level of less than 25 nmol/L is the threshold at which associated metabolic bone complications are

Table 2
Overview of micronutrients and recommendations

Vitamin/Trace Mineral	Normal Serum Levels	Common Deficiency States	Dietary Food Sources	Risk Factors	Supplementation Regimen	Monitoring
Iron	60–170 µg/dL	Fatigue Anemia	Red meats, fish, poultry, eggs, legumes	Small bowel disease Inadequate intake Intestinal blood loss	Hb <10 g/dL: Intravenous: iron 500–1000 mg × 3 doses PO: 1500 mg (<70 kg) and 2000 mg (>70 kg)[8] Hb: 10–13 g/dL: PO: 1000 mg (<70 kg) and 1500 mg (>70 kg)	Annually or sooner if evidence of anemia
Vitamin D	>50 nmol/L	Osteomalacia Rickets	Milk, yogurt, eggs, liver, cod liver oil, salmon	Small bowel disease Inadequate intake Prednisone usage	PO: ergocalciferol 50,000 IU/weekly for 3 mo followed by cholecalciferol 1800–3000 IU/day[51,52] IM: 300,000 IU ergocalciferol once monthly for 3 mo followed by a dose every 6–12 mo[53]	Annually or sooner/ empirically if on chronic prednisone
Calcium	8.5–10.5 mg/dL	Bone loss Tooth decay	Dairy, fish, legumes, greens, fortified foods	Active disease Inadequate intake Prednisone usage	PO: 1000–1500 mg/d[46,49]	If dietary intake likely inadequate
Vitamin B12	>220 pmol/L	Fatigue Anemia Neuropathy	Fish, meat, liver, poultry, eggs, dairy products	Decreased ileal absorption Inadequate intake	PO: 1000–2000 µg/d for 1–2 wk followed by up to 1000 µg/d[61] IM: 100–1000 µg each day or alternate day for 1–2 wk followed by 1000 µg every 1–3 mo[8]	Annually or sooner if evidence of anemia/macrocytosis or neurologic features

Zinc	0.66–1.10 μg/mL	Failure to thrive Dermatitis Poor healing Loss of taste (dysgeusia)	Some grains and vegetables, protein-containing foods	Small bowel disease Inadequate intake	PO – 40–110 mg TID for 8 wk[68,70]	If clinical concern
Folate	Serum: 2–20 ng/mL RBC: 140–628 ng/mL	Fatigue Anemia Birth defects	Dark, leafy green vegetables, beans, lentils, fortified cereals	Decreased jejunal absorption Inadequate intake Methotrexate/sulfa usage	PO: 1 mg/d[8] Those on methotrexate or sulfasalazine should receive 5 mg folic acid weekly 24–72 h following dose, or 1 mg daily for 5–6 d/wk.	Annually or sooner if evidence of anemia/macrocytosis

Abbreviations: Hb, hemoglobin; IM, intramuscularly; PO, by mouth.

Table 3
Indications and administration routes of parenteral nutrition in IBD

	Perioperative	Intestinal Failure		
		Type 1 (Short Term, Usually Self-Limiting)	Type 2 (Persistent but Recoverable)	Type 3 (Chronic)
Indications	Severely malnourished patients with IBD, typically supplemental PN together with enteral nutrition before and after surgery	Postoperative ileus Intestinal obstruction Extensive small bowel disease impairing nutrient absorption or upper GI involvement impairing intake High output ostomy	Intra-abdominal sepsis after surgery or complicated penetrating disease Enterocutaneous fistulae, including fistulizing disease and wound dehiscence Obstruction with delayed medical, endoscopic or surgical treatment, or in the context of adhesions or frozen abdomen Extensive small bowel or panenteric disease resistant to medical treatment	Sequential uncomplicated intestinal resections leading to short bowel syndrome, particularly in medically refractory or extensive disease Multiple or extensive unplanned intestinal resections, mesenteric infarction or surgical misadventure
Interventions	Central PN via peripherally inserted central catheter, tunneled catheter or dedicated port Consider peripheral PN if appropriate policy and sterility precautions		Central PN via various options, moving to longer term devices as sepsis controlled	Home PN via tunneled central catheter

likely to develop.[44] Deficiency of vitamin D may be due to decreased dietary intake, impaired absorption, decreased physical activity, UV light exposure, and an effect of chronic steroid therapy. Patients who undergo extensive small bowel resection (>200–300 cm) are more at risk. Although initial studies on the impact of vitamin D deficiency in IBD focused on calcium homeostasis and bone health, it is recognized that it may also affect intestinal inflammation through its effect on regulation of macrophage and T-cell function, as well as innate immune responses.[45,46] A randomized controlled trial by Jorgensen and colleagues[47] assessed the effect of supplemental oral vitamin D_3 (cholecalciferol) therapy compared with placebo in maintaining remission in CD, demonstrating a trend toward reduced relapse with daily supplementation with 1200 IU. A meta-analysis by Li and colleagues[48] assessed vitamin D interventions in 908 patients and demonstrated that vitamin D decreased the relapse rate by 64% in comparison with placebo. Further interventional trials are required to draw more definitive conclusions of this relationship.

Food sources of vitamin D include dairy products such as milk and yogurt, along with eggs, liver, and cod liver oil. Elimination diets including specific carbohydrate diet or lactose-restricted diet may contribute to vitamin D deficiency and patients should be counseled appropriately. Dietary intake of calcium should also be assessed and cosupplementation considered (see **Table 2**). Commercially available preparations of both vitamin D_2 (ergocalciferol) and D_3 are available for use; randomized trials have suggested that vitamin D_3 is more effective than D_2 in improving serum vitamin D level.[49] As the "sunshine" vitamin, a common recommendation for adequate vitamin D is 5 to 15 minutes of sun exposure twice weekly.[50] For patients who are deficient, a dosage of 50,000 IU weekly for 3 months is frequently used for repletion, with monitoring after 3 months to ensure improvement. For maintenance, there is wide variability in supplementation recommendations for the general population ranging from 400 to 2000 IU.[51] For those with IBD, dosages of between 1800 and 3000 IU/day may be preferred, to maintain normal serum 25-OH-D levels, and levels should be checked annually.[52,53] Those adults with severe malabsorption or in those likely to be less compliant with oral therapy, 300,000 IU ergocalciferol intramuscularly (IM) monthly for 3 months followed by a dose every 6 to 12 months is an alternative approach.[54]

Vitamin B$_{12}$

The prevalence of vitamin B_{12} deficiency in CD ranges from 5% to 38%.[55] Unlike other water-soluble vitamins, the absorption of vitamin B_{12} occurs exclusively in the terminal ileum.[56] Ileal involvement in CD increases the risk of deficiency, through impaired absorption as observed in fibrostenosing disease, active inflammation, or surgical resection, with resection lengths as short as 20 cm still a risk factor.[57] Decreased dietary intake is a risk factor for deficiency, and is especially observed among those following restrictive vegetarian and vegan diets.[58] Biomarker evidence of deficiency is a serum cobalamin level of less than 148 pmol/L.[59] Levels between 148 and 221 pmol/L are considered borderline. Confirmatory elevation in homocysteine or methylmalonic acid support intracellular B_{12} depletion and deficiency, because they are substrates of B_{12}-catalyzed reactions.[60] Cobalamin deficiency is associated with a spectrum of clinical manifestations, commonly megaloblastic anemia or neurologic symptoms.[61]

Food sources containing B_{12} are animal products such as beef, shellfish, and tuna. Serum vitamin B_{12} should be measured annually in at-risk individuals.[8] More frequent monitoring is suggested in those with extensive small bowel resection and/or extensive ileal disease or surgery. Vitamin B_{12} supplementation can be achieved through oral intake, nasal spray, or IM injection. Patients with clinical deficiency, particularly neurologic features, should receive 1000 µg IM every other day for 7 to 14 days followed by monthly injections. Traditionally prophylactic monthly injections were recommended indefinitely for those with ileal resections. However, a recent study in CD suggests that oral dosing may be sufficient even in patients with ileal involvement or resection (1 mg/d for deficiency and 2 mg twice weekly for maintenance were most often used).[62]

Zinc

Zinc is an essential trace element involved in immune function and wound repair.[63] Zinc absorption occurs along the length of the small intestine and its deficiency is most pronounced in patients with chronic diarrhea or malabsorption. Zinc deficiency is prevalent in the IBD population ranging from 15% to 65%.[64] Interpretation of serum zinc levels has been challenging.[65] Its concentration varies with factors such as inflammation, low albumin levels, fasted or non-fasted sampling, and diurnal rhythm.[66] Although more research is needed to determine a consensus regarding optimal zinc measurements, most studies use serum zinc levels, rather than plasma or urinary levels, with deficiency defined as less than 0.66 µg/mL. Zinc deficiency has been linked to poor wound healing, altered immune function, mucosal inflammation, and disease-related morbidity.[67] Decreased zinc levels may alter epithelial barrier integrity and increase permeability.[57] One prospective study identified that higher intake of zinc was associated with a lower risk of CD.[68] After 12 months of zinc supplementation in patients with inactive CD, intestinal permeability levels were decreased and 10 patients (83%) achieved normal permeability and had lower rates of disease relapse.[69] Patients with CD and patients with UC with zinc deficiency had an increased risk of adverse outcomes, including complications, hospitalizations, and surgeries, and supplementation seemed to improve disease outcomes.[70]

Zinc-rich foods include eggs, seafood, and meat such as liver. The recommended daily intake of elemental zinc for the general population is 11 mg/d for men and 8 mg/d for women. Higher doses are recommended in the IBD population (see **Table 2**).[68,71] Zinc can interfere with both copper and iron absorption and excessive intake can lead to deficiencies in these elements.

Folate

Folate is an important cofactor in DNA synthesis and erythrocyte division. In a retrospective case control study, folate deficiency was identified in 29% of CD patients and 9% of UC patients, compared with 3% of controls.[72] Factors contributing to deficiency include decreased oral intake, malabsorption, disease location (jejunal involvement), and medication effect, such as seen with sulfasalazine and methotrexate, which inhibit folate absorption.[73] Biochemical folate deficiency in adults is defined as a serum concentration of less than 3 ng/mL and erythrocyte folate of less than 140 ng/mL. Although erythrocyte folate is more expensive, its level is more stable in comparison to serum folate (which may reflect recent dietary intake), and thus the former may be preferable as an indicator of long-term folate status.[74] Deficiencies in folic acid can lead to a macrocytic megaloblastic anemia, fatigue, and neural tube defects (in pregnancy). Studies have also suggested folate deficiency may be associated with an increased risk of colorectal neoplasia[75] and supplementation may be protective.[76]

Foods rich in folate include dark, leafy greens, citrus fruits, lentils, beans, and fortified foods. We recommend annual monitoring of folate levels. In deficient states, a 1 mg/d folate supplementation dose will replenish stores within 3 weeks. Individuals on methotrexate or sulfasalazine should be prescribed 5 mg folic acid once weekly given after 24 to 72 hours, or alternatively, 1 mg/d for 5 to 6 d/wk[8]

DIET AS A RISK FACTOR FOR INCIDENT INFLAMMATORY BOWEL DISEASE OR RELAPSE IN ESTABLISHED DISEASE

An extensive review of the role of dietary factors on the pathogenesis of IBD is beyond the scope of this review, but has been recently performed.[77] Increased IBD risk has been associated with increasing intake of meat and animal protein, refined sugar including soft drinks, and certain dietary fats (unsaturated and higher omega-6/omega-3 ratio) in large prospective studies.[78,79] Diets high in fruit, vegetables, and dietary fiber, and adherence to a Mediterranean diet, may protect against incident CD.[80,81] Association of diet with IBD activity or relapse has not been as well-studied, although specific fatty acids might increase the risk of flare.[82] In addition, food additives and emulsifiers may also play a role, supported by experimental models of its effect on intestinal mucous layer, microbiome, and immune response.

DIET AND NUTRITION THERAPY

We have recently extensively reviewed dietary modification as a treatment for IBD.[3] In brief, dietary interventions may be delivered through either complete elimination of table foods (exclusive enteral nutrition [EEN]), partial dietary restriction with or without enteral supplementation (eg, CD exclusion diet, partial enteral nutrition [PEN]), or single nutrient supplementation (eg, vitamin D, zinc). Elemental (monomeric), semielemental (oligomeric), and polymeric EEN formulas are effective in achieving remission, similar or only slightly inferior to corticosteroids, and EEN is recommended as first-line treatment in children with CD. The CD-TREAT diet, an anti-inflammatory diet, was developed to mimic the effect of the EEN on the microbiome while not requiring complete elimination of table foods. In healthy volunteers, Svolos and colleagues[83] were able to replicate 48% of the changes on the microbiome induced by EEN using whole food alone and the diet demonstrated efficacy in a small open-label cohort of 5 patients with CD.

The CD exclusion diet is a novel elimination diet incorporating exclusion diet principles, together with PEN, developed by Sigall-Boneh and colleagues.[84] It is a whole food diet that allows fruits, vegetables, and meats, as well as both simple and complex carbohydrates, aiming to eliminate specific dietary components that disrupt the intestinal mucous layer or induce dysbiosis. A randomized controlled trial of the CD exclusion diet with PEN against EEN sustained remission in a greater proportion of individuals (75% vs 59%, respectively) after a 12-week trial with better tolerability (97.5%) compared with patient receiving EEN alone (73.6%).[85] Of note, the EEN arm was transitioned to receiving 75% of their calories through a free diet and 25% through PEN after week 6.

PARENTERAL NUTRITION IN INFLAMMATORY BOWEL DISEASE

Patients with IBD commonly require surgery, despite advancements in biologic therapies. In these patients, the cumulative risk of intestinal failure is increased.[86] The definition spectrum for intestinal failure, the indications for PN in IBD, and suggested administration routes are summarized in **Table 3**. Management principles in the setting of short bowel syndrome and high ostomy or fistula output are outlined in **Table 4**. A full review of these topics is beyond the scope of this article.

Preoperative nutrition assessment and management are critical to good outcomes. Although studies assessing EN in the preoperative studies have consistently shown encouraging outcomes, PN is less well-studied with a general trend toward

Table 4
Management principles in short bowel syndrome and high output ostomy/fistula

Resuscitation	Correct and monitor dehydration, electrolyte depletion, and acid–base balance
	Consider precipitating etiologies, particularly sepsis
	Multiprofessional approach including meticulous wound and stoma care
Restitution	Nutritional security typically with parenteral nutrition
	Restrict oral hypotonic and hypertonic fluids
	Oral glucose–electrolyte solutions (sodium >100 mEq/L, osmolality c.300 mOsm/kg)
	Tailored oral diet, magnesium and micronutrient supplementation
	Antimotility medications: loperamide, codeine phosphate, diphenoxylate with atropine (Lomotil)
	Consider gastric hypersecretion, bile salt diarrhea, fat malabsorption, bacterial overgrowth
Rehabilitation	Address psychological morbidity
	Support/training for home enteral and/or parenteral nutrition, consider fistuloclysis
	Imaging studies to define anatomy/fistulae
	Intestinal trophic factors, particularly glucagon-like peptide 2 analogs (teduglutide)
	Consider role/timing of surgical intervention(s), including restoration of continuity, bowel lengthening, intestinal or multivisceral transplantation

improvement in postoperative outcomes with perioperative PN use.[87] PN has been well-established as lifesaving therapy in patients with type 3, chronic intestinal failure. In contrast, less is known about supplemental PN, defined as combined use of EN together with PN in patients for whom greater than 60% of energy needs cannot be met via the enteral route. Supplemental PN for 21 days was promising in a prospective clinically controlled intervention study in 65 inpatients with IBD with improvement in serum inflammatory markers.[88]

SUMMARY

Diet and nutrition are important aspects to consider in IBD management, and their optimal integration into routine clinical care may improve clinical outcomes. Large-scale, rigorous studies expanding on the role of diet as primary and adjuvant therapy in IBD, and an optimal approach to its supportive role in admitted inpatients, are essential to help draw more firm data around its generalizability, efficacy and implementation. Clinicians are practically challenged with numerous assessments involved in IBD care and, with limited clinic time, innovative strategies are required to incorporate a thoughtful approach to diet and nutrition care. Integrating a systematic checklist, standardized protocols or inpatient order sets within each clinic or hospital visit could be one avenue for consideration, to ensure thorough consideration of malnutrition, hydration, micronutrient and dietary assessment. Shared responsibility with the patient through malnutrition self-screening[14] may prompt the clinician to further explore nutrition-focused care. Patient education tools and mobile technologies could be leveraged to disseminate education to patients and health care providers, and increase awareness of diet and nutrition in IBD management.

CLINICS CARE POINTS

- Nutritional status should be systematically and periodically assessed in all patients with inflammatory bowel diseases.
- Patients may have dietary triggers for their symptoms. Avoiding such triggers may ameliorate symptoms even without an effect on underlying inflammation.

DISCLOSURE

The authors have nothing to disclose.

REFERENCES

1. Wędrychowicz A, Zając A, Tomasik P. Advances in nutritional therapy in inflammatory bowel diseases: review. World J Gastroenterol 2016;22(3):1045–66.
2. Hwang C, Ross V, Mahadevan U. Micronutrient deficiencies in inflammatory bowel disease: from A to zinc. Inflamm Bowel Dis 2012;18(10):1961–81.
3. Sasson AN, Ananthakrishnan AN, Raman M. Diet in treatment of inflammatory bowel diseases. Clin Gastroenterol Hepatol 2019. https://doi.org/10.1016/j.cgh.2019.11.054.
4. Scaldaferri F, Pizzoferrato M, Lopetuso LR, et al. Nutrition and IBD: malnutrition and/or sarcopenia? A practical guide. Gastroenterol Res Pract 2017;2017:8646495.
5. White JV, Guenter P, Jensen G, et al. Consensus statement: Academy of Nutrition and Dietetics and American Society for Parenteral and Enteral Nutrition: characteristics recommended for the identification and documentation of adult malnutrition (undernutrition). JPEN J Parenter Enteral Nutr 2012;36(3):275–83.
6. Cruz-Jentoft AJ, Baeyens JP, Bauer JM, et al. Sarcopenia: European consensus on definition and diagnosis: report of the European Working Group on Sarcopenia in Older People. Age Ageing 2010;39(4):412–23.
7. Nguyen GC, Munsell M, Harris ML. Nationwide prevalence and prognostic significance of clinically diagnosable protein-calorie malnutrition in hospitalized inflammatory bowel disease patients. Inflamm Bowel Dis 2008;14(8):1105–11.
8. Forbes A, Escher J, Hébuterne X, et al. ESPEN guideline: clinical nutrition in inflammatory bowel disease. Clin Nutr 2017;36(2):321–47.
9. Carroll MW, Kuenzig ME, Mack DR, et al. The impact of inflammatory bowel disease in Canada 2018: children and adolescents with IBD. J Can Assoc Gastroenterol 2019;2(S1):S49–67.
10. Jo E, Lee SR, Park BS, et al. Potential mechanisms underlying the role of chronic inflammation in age-related muscle wasting. Aging Clin Exp Res 2012;24(5):412–22.
11. Zhang T, Cao L, Cao T, et al. Prevalence of sarcopenia and its impact on postoperative outcome in patients with Crohn's disease undergoing bowel resection. JPEN J Parenter Enteral Nutr 2017;41(4):592–600.
12. Sandhu A, Mosli M, Yan B, et al. Self-screening for malnutrition risk in outpatient inflammatory bowel disease patients using the Malnutrition Universal Screening Tool (MUST). JPEN J Parenter Enteral Nutr 2016;40(4):507–10.
13. Li S, Ney M, Eslamparast T, et al. Systematic review of nutrition screening and assessment in inflammatory bowel disease. World J Gastroenterol 2019;25(28):3823–37.

14. Rahman A, Williams P, Sandhu A, et al. Malnutrition Universal Screening Tool (MUST) predicts disease activity in patients with Crohn's disease. Can J Nutr 2016;2016(1):1–5.

15. Kondrup J, Rasmussen HH, Hamberg O, et al. Nutritional risk screening (NRS 2002): a new method based on an analysis of controlled clinical trials. Clin Nutr 2003;22(3):321–36.

16. Sumi R, Nakajima K, Iijima H, et al. Influence of nutritional status on the therapeutic effect of infliximab in patients with Crohn's disease. Surg Today 2016;46(8): 922–9.

17. Takaoka A, Sasaki M, Nakanishi N, et al. Nutritional screening and clinical outcome in hospitalized patients with Crohn's disease. Ann Nutr Metab 2017; 71(3–4):266–72.

18. Jansen I, Prager M, Valentini L, et al. Inflammation-driven malnutrition: a new screening tool predicts outcome in Crohn's disease. Br J Nutr 2016;116(6): 1061–7.

19. Singh S, Dulai PS, Zarrinpar A, et al. Obesity in IBD: epidemiology, pathogenesis, disease course and treatment outcomes. Nat Rev Gastroenterol Hepatol 2017; 14(2):110–21.

20. Steed H, Walsh S, Reynolds N. A brief report of the epidemiology of obesity in the inflammatory bowel disease population of Tayside, Scotland. Obes Facts 2009; 2(6):370–2.

21. Long MD, Crandall WV, Leibowitz IH, et al. Prevalence and epidemiology of overweight and obesity in children with inflammatory bowel disease. Inflamm Bowel Dis 2011;17(10):2162–8.

22. Bryant RV, Trott MJ, Bartholomeusz FD, et al. Systematic review: body composition in adults with inflammatory bowel disease. Aliment Pharmacol Ther 2013; 38(3):213–25.

23. Adams DW, Gurwara S, Silver HJ, et al. Sarcopenia is common in overweight patients with inflammatory bowel disease and may predict need for surgery. Inflamm Bowel Dis 2017;23(7):1182–6.

24. Bryant RV, Schultz CG, Ooi S, et al. Obesity in inflammatory bowel disease: gains in adiposity despite high prevalence of myopenia and osteopenia. Nutrients 2018;10(9):e1192.

25. Jain A, Nguyen NH, Proudfoot JA, et al. Impact of obesity on disease activity and Patient-Reported Outcomes Measurement Information System (PROMIS) in inflammatory bowel diseases. Am J Gastroenterol 2019;114(4):630–9.

26. Allard J, Le Guillou D, Begriche K, et al. Drug-induced liver injury in obesity and nonalcoholic fatty liver disease. Adv Pharmacol 2019;85:75–107.

27. Poon SS, Asher R, Jackson R, et al. Body Mass Index and smoking affect thioguanine nucleotide levels in inflammatory bowel disease. J Crohns Colitis 2015;9(8):640–6.

28. Gerasimidis K, Edwards C, Stefanowicz F, et al. Micronutrient status in children with IBD: true deficiencies or epiphenomenon of the systemic inflammatory response. J Pediatr Gastroenterol Nutr 2013;56:e50e1.

29. Singh S, Picardo S, Seow CH. Management of inflammatory bowel diseases in special populations: obese, old, or obstetric. Clin Gastroenterol Hepatol. 2020 May;18(6):1367–80. https://doi.org/10.1016/j.cgh.2019.11.009.

30. Harper JW, Sinanan MN, Zisman TL. Increased body mass index is associated with earlier time to loss of response to infliximab in patients with inflammatory bowel disease. Inflamm Bowel Dis 2013;19(10):2118–24.

31. Hicks G, Abdulaal A, Slesser AAP, et al. Outcomes of inflammatory bowel disease surgery in obese versus non-obese patients: a meta-analysis. Tech Coloproctol 2019;23(10):947–55.
32. Swanson SM, Harper J, Zisman TL. Obesity and inflammatory bowel disease: diagnostic and therapeutic implications. Curr Opin Gastroenterol 2018;34(2): 112–9.
33. Nguyen NH, Ohno-Machado L, Sandborn WJ, et al. Obesity is independently associated with higher annual burden and costs of hospitalization in patients with inflammatory bowel diseases. Clin Gastroenterol Hepatol 2019;17(4): 709–18.e7.
34. Hudson JL, Barnes EL, Herfarth HH, et al. Bariatric surgery is a safe and effective option for patients with inflammatory bowel diseases: a case series and systematic review of the literature. Inflamm Intest Dis 2019;3(4):173–9.
35. Rogler G, Vavricka S. Anemia in inflammatory bowel disease: an under-estimated problem? Front Med (Lausanne) 2014;1:58.
36. Filmann N, Rey J, Schneeweiss S, et al. Prevalence of anemia in inflammatory bowel diseases in European countries: a systematic review and individual patient data meta-analysis. Inflamm Bowel Dis 2014;20(5):936–45.
37. Jimenez KM, Gasche C. Management of iron deficiency anaemia in inflammatory bowel disease. Acta Haematol 2019;142:30–6.
38. Hou JK, Gasche C, Drazin NZ, et al. Assessment of gaps in care and the development of a care pathway for anemia in patients with inflammatory bowel diseases. Inflamm Bowel Dis 2017;23(1):35–43.
39. Bonovas S, Fiorino G, Allocca M, et al. Intravenous versus oral iron for the treatment of anemia in inflammatory bowel disease. Medicine (Baltimore) 2016;95: e2308.
40. Dignass AU, Gasche C, Bettenworth D, et al. European consensus on the diagnosis and management of iron deficiency and anaemia in inflammatory bowel diseases. J Crohns Colitis 2015;9:211–22.
41. Fukuda S, Toh H, Hase K, et al. Bifidobacteria can protect from enteropathogenic infection through production of acetate. Nature 2011;469(7331):543–7.
42. Sadeghian M, Saneei P, Siassi F, et al. Vitamin D status in relation to Crohn's disease: meta-analysis of observational studies. Nutrition 2016;32:505–14.
43. Blanck S, Aberra F. Vitamin D deficiency is associated with ulcerative colitis disease activity. Dig Dis Sci 2013;58:1698e702.
44. Vitamin D and health report. London: Scientific Advisory Committee on Nutrition; 2016.
45. Shang M, Sun J. Vitamin D/VDR, probiotics, and gastrointestinal diseases. Curr Med Chem 2017;24(9):876–87.
46. Chiodini I, Bolland MJ. Calcium supplementation in osteoporosis: useful or harmful? Eur J Endocrinol 2018;178(4):D13–25.
47. Jorgensen SP, Agnholt J, Glerup H, et al. Clinical trial: vitamin D3 treatment in Crohn's disease- a randomized double-blind placebo-controlled study. Aliment Pharmacol Ther 2010;32:377–83.
48. Li J, Chen N, Wang D, et al. Efficacy of vitamin D in treatment of inflammatory bowel disease: a meta-analysis. Medicine (Baltimore) 2018;97(46):12662.
49. Martineau AR, Thummel KE, Wang Z, et al. Differential effects of oral boluses of vitamin D2 vs vitamin D3 on vitamin D metabolism: a randomized controlled trial. J Clin Endocrinol Metab 2019;104(12):5831–9.
50. Sunyecz JA. The use of calcium and vitamin D in the management of osteoporosis. Ther Clin Risk Manag 2008;4(4):827–36.

51. Bordelon P, Ghetu MV, Langan R. Vitamin D Deficiency. Am Fam Physician 2009; 80(8):841–6.
52. Hlavaty T, Krajcovicova A, Payer J. Vitamin D therapy in inflammatory bowel diseases: who, in what form, and how much? J Crohns Colitis 2015;9(2):198–209.
53. Holick MF, Binkley NC, Bischoff-Ferrari HA, et al. Evaluation, treatment, and prevention of vitamin D deficiency: an endocrine society clinical practice guideline. J Clin Endocrinol Metab 2011;96:1911–30.
54. Pearce SH, Cheetham TD. Diagnosis and management of Vitamin D deficiency. BMJ 2010;340:b5664.
55. Duerksen DR, Fallows G, Bernstein CN. Vitamin B12 malabsorption in patients with limited ileal resection. Nutrition 2006;22:1210e3.
56. Kilby K, Mathias H, Boisvenue L, et al. Micronutrient absorption and related outcomes in people with inflammatory bowel disease: a review. Nutrients 2019;11(6): 1388.
57. Suwendi E, Iwaya H, Lee JS, et al. Zinc deficiency induces dysregulation of cytokine productions in an experimental colitis of rats. Biomed Res 2012;33:329–36.
58. Rizzo G, Lagana AS, Rapisarda AMC, et al. Vitamin B12 among vegetarians: status, assessment and supplementation. Nutrients 2016;8(12):e767.
59. Allen LH. How common is vitamin B12 deficiency? Am J Clin Nutr 2009;89(2): 693S–6S.
60. Battat R, Koplov U, Byer J, et al. Vitamin B12 deficiency in IBD: a prospective observational pilot study. Eur J Gastroenterol Hepatol 2017;29:1361–7.
61. Oh RC, Brown DL. Vitamin B12 deficiency. Am Fam Physician 2003;67(5):979–86.
62. Gomollón F, Gargallo CJ, Muñoz JF, et al. Oral cyanocobalamin is effective in the treatment of vitamin B12 deficiency in Crohn's disease. Nutrients 2017;9(3):e308.
63. Gîlcă-Blanariu GE, Diaconescu S, Ciocoiu M, et al. New Insights into the Role of Trace Elements in IBD. Biomed Res Int 2018;2018:1813047.
64. Filippi J, Al-Jaouni R, Wiroth JB, et al. Nutritional deficiencies in patients with Crohn's disease in remission. Inflamm Bowel Dis 2006;12:185–91.
65. Wieringa FT, Dijkhuizen MA, Fiorentino M, et al. Determination of zinc status in humans: which indicator should we use? Nutrients 2015;7(5):3252–63.
66. Lowe NM, Fekete K, Decsi T. Methods of assessment of zinc status in humans: a systematic review. Am J Clin Nutr 2009;89:2040S–51S.
67. Gammoh NZ, Rink L. Zinc in infection and inflammation. Nutrients 2017;9(6):624.
68. Ananthakrishnan AN, Khalili H, Song M, et al. Zinc intake and risk of Crohn's disease and ulcerative colitis: a prospective cohort study. Int J Epidemiol 2015;44: 1995–2005.
69. Sturniolo GC, Di Leo V, Ferronato A, et al. Zinc supplementation tightens "leaky gut" in Crohn's disease. Inflamm Bowel Dis 2001;7(2):94–8.
70. Siva S, Rubin DT, Gulotta G, et al. Zinc deficiency is associated with poor clinical outcomes in patients with inflammatory bowel disease. Inflamm Bowel Dis 2017; 23:152–7.
71. Ghishan FK, Kiela PR. Vitamins and minerals in inflammatory bowel disease. Gastroenterol Clin North Am 2017;46(4):797–808.
72. Yakut M, Ustun Y, Kabacam G, et al. Serum vitamin B12 and folate status in patients with IBD. Eur J Intern Med 2010;21:320–3.
73. Pan Y, Liu Y, Guo H, et al. Associations between folate and vitamin B12 levels and inflammatory bowel disease: a meta-analysis. Nutrients 2017;9(4):e382.
74. Galloway M, Rushworth L. Red cell or serum folate? Results from the National Pathology Alliance benchmarking review. J Clin Pathol 2003;56:924–6.

75. Subramanian V, Logan RF. Chemoprevention of colorectal cancer in inflammatory bowel disease. Best Pract Res Clin Gastroenterol 2011;25:593–606.
76. Burr NE, Hull MA, Subramanian V. Folic acid supplementation may reduce colorectal cancer risk in patients with inflammatory bowel disease: a systematic review and meta-analysis. J Clin Gastroenterol 2017;51(3):247–53.
77. Khalili H, Chan SSM, Lochhead P, et al. The role of diet in the aetiopathogenesis of inflammatory bowel disease. Nat Rev Gastroenterol Hepatol 2018;15(9):525–35.
78. Racine A, Carbonnel F, Chan SS, et al. Dietary patterns and risk of inflammatory bowel disease in Europe: results from the EPIC Study. Inflamm Bowel Dis 2016;22(2):345–54.
79. Ananthakrishnan AN, Khalili H, Konijeti GG, et al. Long-term intake of dietary fat and risk of ulcerative colitis and Crohn's disease. Gut 2014;63(5):776–84.
80. Ananthakrishnan AN, Khalili H, Konijeti GG, et al. A prospective study of long-term intake of dietary fiber and risk of Crohn's disease and ulcerative colitis. Gastroenterology 2013;145(5):970–7.
81. Khalili H, Håkansson N, Chan SS, et al. Adherence to a Mediterranean diet is associated with a lower risk of later-onset Crohn's disease: results from two large prospective cohort studies. Gut 2020. https://doi.org/10.1136/gutjnl-2019-319505.
82. Barnes EL, Nestor M, Onyewadume L, et al. High dietary intake of specific fatty acids increases risk of flares in patients with ulcerative colitis in remission during treatment with aminosalicylates. Clin Gastroenterol Hepatol 2017;15(9):1390–6.
83. Svolos V, Hansen R, Nichols B, et al. Treatment of active Crohn's disease with an ordinary food-based diet that replicates exclusive enteral nutrition. Gastroenterology 2019;156(5):1354–67.
84. Sigall Boneh R, Shabat CS, Yanai H, et al. Dietary therapy with the Crohn's Disease Exclusion Diet is a successful strategy for induction of remission in children and adults failing biological therapy. J Crohns Colitis 2017;11(10):1205–12.
85. Levine A, Wine E, Assa A. Crohn's Disease Exclusion Diet plus Partial Enteral Nutrition induces sustained remission in a randomized controlled trial. Gastroenterology 2019;157:440–50.
86. Watanabe K, Sasaki I, Fukushima K, et al. Long-term incidence and characteristics of intestinal failure in Crohn's disease: a multicenter study. J Gastroenterol 2014;49(2):231–8.
87. Stoner PL, Kamel A, Ayoub F, et al. Perioperative care of patients with inflammatory bowel disease: focus on nutrition support. Gastroenterol Res Pract 2018;2018:7890161.
88. Mańkowska-Wierzbicka D, Karczewski J, Swora-Cwynar E, et al. The clinical importance of 21-day combined parenteral and enteral nutrition in active inflammatory bowel disease patients. Nutrients 2019;11(9):e2246.

Fish Oil for Inflammatory Bowel Disease
Panacea or Placebo?

Gerard E. Mullin, MD[a],*, Berkeley N. Limketkai, MD, PhD[b],
Alyssa M. Parian, MD[a]

KEYWORDS

- Dietary supplements • Fish oil • Omega-3 fatty acids
- Inflammatory bowel disease, eicosapentaenoic acid (EPA)
- Docosahexaenoic acid (DHA) • α-Linolenic acid (ALA)

KEY POINTS

- Most Americans use dietary supplements to fortify foods and improve health outcomes.
- Fish oils may benefit patients with active ulcerative colitis and maintain remission in Crohn's disease, but the data are heterogeneous.
- Larger, randomized controlled studies are needed to further investigate the role of fish oil supplementation on inflammatory bowel disease activity.

INTRODUCTION

Due to increasing out-of-pocket health care expenses ($350 billion in 2017) and its popularization by mass media, people are using dietary supplements to promote health and mitigate disease while filling nutrient gaps in their diet.[1] The Council for Responsible Nutrition (CRN) reported that in 2019, 77% of Americans consumed dietary supplements, whereas Bailey and colleagues[2] in 2013 described the prevalence being 50%. Adults between the ages of 35 and 54 have the highest usage of dietary supplements at 81%. The most popular category is vitamins and minerals (76%), whereas the second most popular category is specialty supplements (40%), followed by herbals and botanicals (39%), sports nutrition supplements (28%), and weight management supplements (17%). According to *Nutrition Business Journal* in 2018, US retail sales of herbal supplements increased by 9.4% to a total of $8.8 billion, which represents a doubling since the year 2000. The current analysis of Reports and Data in December 2019 indicated that the global dietary supplement market was valued at

[a] Division of Gastroenterology and Hepatology, Johns Hopkins University School of Medicine, 600 North Wolfe Street, Baltimore, MD 21205, USA; [b] Division of Digestive Diseases, UCLA School of Medicine, 100 UCLA Medical Center Plaza, Suite 345, Los Angeles, CA 90095, USA
* Corresponding author.
E-mail address: Gmullin1@jhmi.edu

Gastroenterol Clin N Am 50 (2021) 169–182
https://doi.org/10.1016/j.gtc.2020.10.010
0889-8553/21/© 2020 Elsevier Inc. All rights reserved.

$140.1 billion in 2018. The global market is expected to reach $216.3 billion by 2026. There are growing concerns by health care providers about the futility[3] and potential toxicity[4] of nutraceuticals, whereas there is an accompanying increased demand for their use by the public.[5] In particular, there are growing accounts of hepatotoxicity of herbals and increased reporting of dietary supplement toxicity to poison control centers.[6,7] The regulation of dietary supplements falls under the Dietary Safety Health and Education Act of 1994 (Public Law 103–417), which permits the public seamless access and only requires the manufacturer to adhere to Good Manufacturing Practices (**Table 1**).[8] Safety data are not required unless a new ingredient (after October 15, 1994) is used in a dietary supplement.[9]

In the field of gastroenterology there are many patients who use dietary supplements along with other forms of complementary and alternative medicine (CAM). Dossett and colleagues[10] conducted a survey of individuals with a diagnosed gastrointestinal (GI) condition in the past year. Of 13,505 respondents, 42% (n = 5629) used CAM in the past year, with herbals and dietary supplements being the most common modality. Of those using CAM to address a GI condition, more than 80% felt that it was helpful. Respondents told their health care providers about use of these therapies 70% of the time. This is a shift from the past, whereby patients were reluctant to discuss alternative treatments with providers who were not familiar with integrative medicine options.[11] In the pediatric population, the use of CAM modalities appears to be high as well. In a recent study, the use of CAM for pediatric inflammatory bowel disease (IBD) was as high as 84%.[12]

Because of space limitations, this review narrows its focus on the outcomes of trials using fish oils to treat IBD.

INFLAMMATORY BOWEL DISEASE

IBD, including Crohn's disease (CD) and ulcerative colitis (UC), are autoimmune-based chronic inflammatory diseases that follow a relapsing and remitting course. The pathogenesis of IBD has yet to be fully elucidated; however, studies suggest a multifactorial process involving genetics, environmental exposures (eg, diet, smoking, and physiologic stress),[13] the gut microbiome, and immune dysregulation in innate and adaptive immunity.[14] One accepted theory is that IBD develops due to an exaggerated, uncontrolled immune response to an environmental trigger in the gut microbiota, which breaks down the gut barrier and permits the circulation of antigens into the immune system. There has been a rising incidence of IBD worldwide and experts believe a "westernized diet" is at least partially to blame.[15] A diet high in refined sugars, animal fat, and complex carbohydrates is associated with higher rates of IBD, whereas diets rich in omega-3 fatty acids, vegetables, fruits, and fiber appear to protect against development of IBD.[16] A number of alterations in the gut microbiome, such as decreased bacterial diversity and richness, are commonly found in patients with IBD when compared with the general population.[15,17] Aside from diet, gastrointestinal infections and antibiotics are known to disrupt the microbiome and have both been recognized as predisposing factors to disease and triggers of flares.[18] Aberrations in the mucosal immune system have been implicated in the pathogenesis of IBD. Patients with IBD commonly have increased intestinal permeability, which increases exposure of the intestinal immune system to luminal antigens, triggering further inflammation.[19]

FISH OIL

Humans can synthesize all polyunsaturated fatty acids (PUFAs) but 2: linoleic acid (LA) and α-linolenic acid (ALA), which are considered essential fatty acids (EFAs) and can

Table 1
Results from randomized controlled trials of fish oils for the treatment of ulcerative colitis: induction of remission

Author	Subjects, Duration	Country/Centers	Design	EFA Dose (g/d)	Clinical Remission	Endoscopic Histologic Improvement
Almallah et al,[31] 1998	18 UC proctocolitis, 6 mo	UK, Single center	Fish oil vs P DBRCT, ITT	5.6 g	3, 6 mo improved $P<.05$	Improved endoscopy $P = .013$, and histology $P = .016$
Aslan et al,[27] 1992	11 UC, 8 mo on usual meds including corticosteroid	USA, Single center	Fish oil vs P, CO, no ITT	4.2 g	Reduced disease activity index. $P<.05$, steroid sparing	No difference
Barbosa et al,[29] 2003	9 UC, 2 mo, on usual meds	Brazil Single center	Fish oil vs P, CO, no ITT	4.5 g	Not done	No difference
Lorenz et al,[33] 1989	10 UC 2 mo	Germany Single center	Fish oil vs 2 g sulfasalazine	5.4 g	Not done. Laboratory indices only.	Improved endoscopic scores with fish oil ($P<.01$)
Seidner et al,[32] 2005	121 UC corticosteroid dependent	USA MCT 5 centers	Nutritional drink including fish oil vs P, ITT	Fish oil (1.09 g EPA and 0.46 g DHA per 8 oz), 310 kcal/ 8 oz, UCNS = 33% of caloric intake*	35%–65% decrease in the mean prednisone dose UCNS vs P ($P = .03$)	No difference

(continued on next page)

Table 1
(continued)

Author	Subjects, Duration	Country/Centers	Design	EFA Dose (g/d)	Clinical Remission	Endoscopic Histologic Improvement
Stenson et al,[28] 1992	24 UC on usual meds	USA MCT	Fish oil vs P, CO, no ITT	5.4 g	Weight gain, otherwise not reported	Improved histology
Scaioli et al,[30] 2018	60 UC	Italy Single center	Fish oil vs P	1 g	100-point reduction in fecal calprotectin at 3 mo (53% vs 13%, $P = .002$) and 6 mo (63% vs 13%, $P<.001$)	Follow-up colonoscopy only performed among patients who experienced relapse

Abbreviations: CO, crossover; DBRCT, double-blind randomized controlled trial; DHA, docosahexaenoic acid; EPA, eicosapentaenoic acid; ITT, intention to treat; MCT, multicenter; Meds, medications; P, placebo; UC, ulcerative colitis.

be acquired only through dietary intake. LA is the precursor to the omega-6 (ω6) fatty acid family, and ALA is the precursor to the omega-3 (ω3) family compounds.

Fish oil is abundant in ω3 PUFAs. Long-chain ω3 PUFAs include EPA (eicosapentaenoic acid) and DHA (docosahexaenoic acid), which are found mainly in fatty fish, whereas short-chain ω3 PUFAs, such as ALA, are abundant in walnuts, chia, and flaxseeds, but are a poor source of DHA and EPA, as its conversion from ALA is inefficient in humans and may be age-dependent.[20]

ω3 PUFAs have anti-inflammatory and immunoregulatory properties both in the gut and systemically.[21] ω3 EFA downregulates the cyclooxygenase (COX) pathway (primarily COX-2), which produces prostaglandin E_2, a promoter of pain and inflammation. Arachidonic acid (AA) is the usual substrate for this pathway. EPA is a chemical homologue that differs from AA by only the presence of the n3 double bond and serves as an alternate substrate for COX and lessens AA production. Likewise, EPA inhibits the 5-lipoxygenase pathway resulting in diminished proinflammatory leukotriene B_4.[22] EPA and DHA are substrates for the formation of novel protective mediators, termed resolvins, that are produced for termination of neutrophil infiltration, stimulation of the clearance of apoptotic cells by macrophages, and promotion of tissue remodeling and homeostasis.[23] A number of autoimmune diseases have been linked to the incomplete resolution of inflammatory byproducts, thus a deficiency of EPA/DHA could promote chronic inflammation on this basis.[24]

In contrast, ω6 EFAs such as LA are more prone to proinflammatory activities and high consumption of these fatty acids is thought to be a risk factor for developing IBD.[16] ω3 fatty acids have been shown to regulate gut immunity by attenuating proinflammatory cytokines interleukin (IL)-1β and tumor necrosis factor (TNF)-α along with the peroxisome proliferator-activated receptor/nuclear transcription factor kappabeta (PPAR-γ/NF-kB) while bolstering epithelial barrier function and mucosal healing.

Numerous studies have evaluated the effects of fish oil on UC and CD (separately and together) for induction of remission and maintenance of remission. Fish oil can be administered as either raw fish oil or as an enteric-coated capsule. A dose of up to 3 g per day of EPA plus DHA has been determined to be safe for general consumption.[21,25] There are several studies demonstrating that both enteral and enema administration of fish oil induced healing and prevented colitis in animal models.[26] Although a variety of studies have been performed exploring the roles of ω3 EFA in the treatment of IBD, the methodology, endpoints, and results have been varied (see **Table 1**). For the purposes of this review, we include only randomized controlled clinical trials (RCTs). We systematically searched the world's literature using PubMed, EMBASE, SCOPUS, and Cochrane database for RCTs of fish oil for UC or CD.

Induction of Remission for Ulcerative Colitis

Seven RCTs with a small overall number of study subjects showed that fish oil induced remission in subjects with UC with active disease (see **Table 1**).[27–33]

In 1989, Lorenz and colleagues[33] reported the results of a small double-blind randomized controlled crossover trial of 10 patients with mild to moderate active UC comparing 5.4 g per day of fish oil with sulfasalazine 2 g per day. Despite lower sigmoidoscopy scores with the fish oil arm, there was no difference in histologic scores.

Aslan and Triadafilopoulos[27] in 1992 reported the results of a clinical study involving 11 patients with active mild to moderate UC. These patients were studied in an 8-month double-blind randomized controlled crossover trial of supplementation with 4.2 g of ω3 fatty acids per day versus placebo. Mean disease activity index (based on patient symptoms and sigmoidoscopic appearance) declined 56% for patients receiving fish oil and 4% for patients on placebo ($P<.05$). There were no statistically significant differences in histopathologic scores or colonic mucosal leukotriene B4 levels. All patients tolerated fish oil ingestion and showed no alteration in routine blood studies. No patient worsened; anti-inflammatory drugs could be reduced or eliminated in 8 patients (72%) while receiving fish oil.

Stenson and colleagues[28] in 1992 reported the results of a multicenter, double-blind randomized controlled crossover trail with 4-month treatment periods (fish oil and placebo) separated by a 1-month washout. Twenty-four patients with active UC entered the study and 18 patients completed it. Treatment with prednisone and sulfasalazine was continued. Fish oil supplementation consisted of 18 MaxEPA capsules daily (EPA, 3.24 g; DHA, 2.16 g). Fish oil supplementation resulted in a significant decrease in rectal dialysate levels of leukotriene B4 and total histology index. No significant changes occurred in any variable during the placebo period.

Almallah and colleagues[31] in 1998 reported the results of a double-blind RCT (DBRCT) of enteric fish oil per day versus placebo (sunflower oil) for 18 subjects with active distal proctocolitis for 6 months. Each patient received either oral fish oil extract (EPA, 3.2 g, and DHA, 2.4 g) (n = 9) or sunflower oil (placebo) (n = 9) daily. Monthly assessments of disease activity (clinical and sigmoidoscopic scores) and histologic evaluation of mucosal biopsies were carried out. After 6 months of supplementation with EFA, there was improvement in the clinical activity compared with pretreatment evaluation. There was significant reduction in the sigmoidoscopic and histologic scores in the EFA group compared with the placebo group.

Barbosa and colleagues[29] studied 4.5 g of fish oil versus placebo on 9 patients with active UC for 4 months in a crossover DBRCT. There was no improvement in sigmoidoscopy and histology scores; however, plasma oxidative stress improved and erythrocyte sedimentation rate declined when the patients used sulfasalazine plus ω3 fatty acids.

Seidner and colleagues[32] reported the results of a DBRCT with 121 patients with corticosteroid-dependent UC who either received an anti-inflammatory nutritional drink cocktail (fortified with fish oil, prebiotics fructooligosaccharides and gum arabic, and the antioxidants vitamin E, vitamin C, and selenium) or a carbohydrate-based placebo formula for 6 months. Overall, 35 subjects did not complete the trial (23 fish oil, 12 placebo) and there were a significantly greater number of patients in the nutrition supplement group who withdrew from the study compared with the placebo group ($P = .03$ Fisher exact test). It does not appear that consumption of the nutrition supplement caused the greater number of dropouts because intolerance to both formulae was similar (3 nutrition supplement, 1 placebo). No difference in clinical, endoscopic, and histologic scores were seen in those who received the nutrition supplement, but there was a more rapid reduction in corticosteroids.[32] Future studies should assess the effects of pharmaceutical-grade enteric-coated ω3 fatty acids on clinical outcomes in IBD, including requirements for corticosteroids.[34]

The most recent study to compare fish oil with placebo was performed by Scaioli and colleagues[30] in 2018. Their DBRCT included 60 adult patients with UC (29 men and 31 women) with a baseline partial Mayo score <2 and fecal calprotectin (FC) ≥150 g/g on stable therapy for at least 3 months. Patients were divided into 2 groups: 1 g daily of EPA/DHA fish oil versus placebo for 3 months. Despite the low dose of fish oil in the treatment group, significantly more subjects experienced a 100-point reduction in FC in the treatment group at 6 months from the baseline (63.3% vs 13.3%). More subjects in the treatment group also remained in clinical remission at 6 months (76.7% vs 50%). No serious adverse events were observed.

Comparing fish oil with pharmacologic therapy, a small double-blind randomized controlled crossover trial of 10 patients with mild-to-moderate active UC compared with 5.4 g per day of fish oil with 2 g per day of sulfasalazine. The study found significantly increased inflammatory markers (ie, C-reactive protein) in the fish oil arm.[35] Despite lower sigmoidoscopy scores with the fish oil arm, there was no difference in histologic scores. The study investigators, therefore, concluded that sulfasalazine, even at a low dose (2 g daily), was superior to fish oil in the treatment of mild-to-moderate active UC.

There have been several systematic reviews and meta-analyses of RCTs of ω3 fatty acids for IBD. In 2007, DeLey and colleagues[36] reported the results of a Cochrane review on 6 included RCTs of fish oils for the induction of remission for active UC (3 crossover and 3 parallel design).[27,28,31,35,37] They included one meeting abstract that was not subsequently published in article form[37] and another that was non–placebo controlled (EFA vs sulfasalazine).[35] No data were pooled for analysis due to differences in outcomes and methodology among the included studies. One small study shows a positive benefit for induction of remission (relative risk [RR] 19.00; 95% confidence interval [CI] 1.27–284.24).[31]

Maintenance of Remission for Ulcerative Colitis

In 1996, Loeschke and colleagues[38] reported the results of a trial of dietary ω3 fatty acids (5.1 g/d) for the maintenance of remission in a DBRCT of 64 patients with UC in remission and off steroids; 5-aminosalicylate (ASA) compounds were stopped 3 months after randomization and clinical disease activity was monitored for 2 years. Macroscopic and histologic activity and extension were assessed by colonoscopy at entry and at exit. Both treatment groups were well matched at start. Seventeen subjects (9 placebo, 8 ω3 EFA) stopped taking their medication prematurely and dropped out. Relapse-free survival was improved by ω3 fatty acids during months 2 and 3 ($P<.05–.01$), but cumulative relapse rate at 2 years was similar for those taking placebo (18/33 = 55%) and ω3 fatty acids (18/31 = 58%). There was also no consistent difference in clinical, macroscopic, and histologic disease activity between treatment groups. The effect of ω3 fatty acids on relapse of UC appeared to be temporary. Two other trials of ω3 fatty acids showed mixed results for the maintenance of remission for UC.[39,40]

Greenfield and colleagues[41] in 1993 reported the results of an RCT of 2 formulations of ω6 rich evening primrose oil MaxEPA (fish oil dose not reported) (n = 16), super evening primrose oil (n = 19), versus placebo (olive oil, n = 9) for 43 subjects with quiescent UC over 6 months in addition to their normal treatment. Compared with MaxEPA and placebo, super evening primrose oil significantly improved stool consistency and the difference was maintained even after treatment was discontinued. Otherwise, there was no difference in stool frequency, rectal bleeding, disease relapse, sigmoidoscopic appearance, or histology in the 3 treatment groups. Blinding was poor. Lorenz and colleagues[33] in 1989 published the results of a double-blind randomized controlled crossover trial of subjects with both UC and CD in remission. Thirty-nine patients with IBD (10 UC, 29 CD) with both active and quiescent disease were studied in a 7-month double-blind controlled crossover trial of dietary supplementation with fish oil, which provided approximately 3.2 g ω3 fatty acids per day. In patients with CD, the CD clinical activity index (CDAI) was unchanged by fish oil supplementation, and in UC, subjects' clinical disease activity decreased but "just short of being significant" without providing specific details.

Middleton and colleagues[42] in 2002 reported the results of a DBRCT study performed with a treatment duration of 12 months. Patients with quiescent UC received either trial medication (gamma-linolenic acid, 1.6 g, EPA, 270 mg, and DHA, 45 mg, per day) or placebo (sunflower oil, 500 mg/d). The primary endpoint was UC disease clinical and sigmoidoscopic disease activity. Sixty-three patients were randomized, 31 to receive essential fatty acid treatment and 32 to receive placebo. Clinical disease relapse rates at 12 months were placebo, 38%; EFAs, 55%, and were not different, as were changes in sigmoidoscopic grade from baseline.

Turner and colleagues[43] in 2007 reported a Cochrane review on the efficacy and safety of ω3 EFAs for 3 RCTs comprising 138 study subjects for maintaining remission in UC. Studies enrolled patients of any age group who were in remission at the time of recruitment, and were followed for at least 6 months. The primary outcome was relapse rate. There was heterogeneity in the use of formulation and dosing of ω3 fatty acids. The pooled analysis demonstrated that the relapse rate in the ω3 fatty acid treatment arm was similar to controls (RR 1.02; 95% CI 0.51–2.03; $P = .96$). Maintenance of remission had no statistical heterogeneity between studies ($P = .93$, $I^2 = 0\%$). No significant adverse events were recorded in any of the studies. The investigators concluded that there was no evidence supporting the use of non-enteric-coated ω3 fatty acids for maintenance of remission in UC.

Crohn's Disease

Induction
Wiese and colleagues[44] performed an open-label pilot study with 28 patients with active CD and stable medication. Eligible patients were 18 years or older (4 men and 16 women). All participants received a nutrition formula enriched with fish oil, prebiotics, and antioxidants, resulting in increased fat-free and fat mass deposition, improved vitamin D status, greater quality of life scores, and lower CD disease activity.

Maintenance of remission
The Epanova Program in Crohn's Study 1 (EPIC-1) and 2 (EPIC-2) were RCTs that recruited patients with quiescent CD from 98 centers in the United States, Canada, Europe, and Israel (**Table 2**).[45] The participants were randomized to commercial ω3 fatty acid capsules (50%–60% EPA, 15%–25% DHA) or placebo. Relapse rates were similar in both treatment arms. There have been 3 meta-analyses by the Cochrane Collaboration that evaluated the efficacy of ω3 PUFA for the maintenance of remission in CD.[46–48] The most recent Cochrane Collaboration review on this topic in 2014 was updated to include the 2 Epanova trials whose outcomes were different from the 4 prior RCTs. The primary outcome for the 2014 Cochrane pooled meta-analysis was relapse at 12 months and included 6 studies with 1039 participants. Thirty-nine percent of patients in the ω3 PUFA group relapsed at 12 months, compared with 47% of placebo patients (RR 0.77; 95% CI 0.61–0.98). The GRADE analysis rated the quality of the evidence as very low due to unexplained high heterogeneity ($I^2 = 58\%$), publication bias, and a high or unknown risk of bias for randomization and concealed allocation in the 4 RCTs that preceded the Epanova trials.[49–52] The EPIC-1 and EPIC-2 trials had no significant heterogeneity and low risk of bias when analyzed separately from the 4 prior RCTs. Overall, the protective effect of ω3 PUFA was no longer statistical significant (RR 0.88; 95% CI 0.74–1.05) with these 2 combined studies.

The efficacy of fish oil seems to be improved when combined with mesalamine therapy[50] and when used for Crohn's colitis rather than small bowel enteritis.[49] A systematic review is difficult to perform on this topic due to variation in fish oil formulations, differences in disease location, and severity. Fish oil may have its greatest effects in patients with IBD with proven essential fatty acid deficiency, and once levels are replete there may be no further benefit.[53] For the maintenance of remission in UC,

Table 2
Results from randomized controlled trials of fish oils for the treatment of Crohn's disease: maintenance of remission

Author	Intervention Duration	Country/ Centers	Design	EFA Dose (g/d)	Maintenance of Remission	Outcomes
Belluzzi et al,[51] 1996	26 Treatment 24 Placebo One year	Italy Single center, outpatient clinics	Enteric-coated fish oil capsules vs placebo, DBRCT, ITT	2.7 g	Relapse rate at 1 year: CDAI>150 or 100 points increase from baseline	41% vs 74% (P = .003)
Feagan et al,[45] 2008a	188 Treatment 186 Controls 58 wk	Multinational Multicenter	Fish oil vs placebo, DBRCT	4 g	Relapse rate at 1 year: CDAI >150 or 70 points increase from baseline	32% vs 36% (P = .30)
Feagan et al,[45] 2008b	189 Treatment 190 Controls 2 mo 58 wk	Multinational Multicenter	Fish oil vs placebo, DBRCT	4 g	Relapse rate at 1 year: CDAI>150 or 70 points increase from baseline	48% vs 49% (P = .48)
Lorenz-Meyer et al,[49] 1996	70 Treatment 65 Controls One year	Germany Multicenter	Fish oil caps vs placebo supplements, DBRCT	5 g	Relapse rate at 1 year: CDAI >200 or 60 points increase from baseline and increase in C-reactive protein by 2 standard deviations above normal	Relapse rate no different between treatment and controls (intention-to-treat analysis: placebo, 30%; active treatment, 30%; protocol-adhering patients, 29% vs 28%)
Romano et al,[50] 2005	18 Treatment 20 Controls One year	Italy Multicenter	5-ASA with fish oil vs 5-ASA with olive oil placebo	1.8 g	Relapse rate at 1 year: PCDAI >20	61% vs 95% (P = .0016)

Abbreviations: 5-ASA, 5-aminosalicylate; CDAI, Crohn's Disease Activity Index; DBRCT, double-blind randomized controlled trial; EFA, essential fatty acid; ITT, intention to treat; PCDAI, Pediatric Crohn's Disease Activity Index.

the 3 randomized trials that compared fish oil with placebo in 138 patients did not detect a difference in 1- to 2-year relapse rate.[38–40]

FISH

Fish and seafood can be rich natural sources of ω3 fatty acids, although there has so far been no RCT evaluating the effects of dietary fish consumption on clinical outcomes in IBD. A primary reason for this absence may relate to the significantly greater ease of studying standardized concentrations of ω3 fatty acids as encapsulated dietary supplements than as highly heterogeneous seafood diets. There are nonetheless observational studies that relied on self-reported dietary recall to investigate the impact of dietary patterns on risk of IBD. In a recent systematic review and meta-analysis of 6 studies (563 CD, 260 UC),[54–59] there was no association between fish consumption and overall risk of IBD[60]; however, when stratified by IBD type and using a random-effects model, there was a significant inverse association between fish consumption and risk of CD (0.54; 95% CI 0.31–0.96; $P = .03$). This association was not significant when evaluating CD with a fixed-effects model or when evaluating UC with any model. Given the inconsistency of the findings based on method of meta-analysis, substantial heterogeneity across studies, and inherent challenges at quantifying fish consumption based on diet recall, the current quality of evidence is very low and no conclusions can yet be made about fish consumption and risk of IBD.

SUMMARY

There are clear biochemical mechanisms that underlie the anti-inflammatory properties of ω3 PUFAs and to suggest that fish oil may help treat inflammation in IBD. Although RCTs have identified possible benefit of fish oil supplements for induction of remission in UC, there was no benefit found for maintenance of remission in UC. One small pilot study showed possible benefit for a fish oil–enriched nutrition formula for the induction of remission in CD. However, some major limitations include the small sample size, lack of control, and use of a nutrition formula that had other ingredients with possible anti-inflammatory properties (eg, prebiotics, antioxidants). RCTs of fish oil for maintenance of remission in CD have been inconsistent, but the large and more robust ones (GRADE assessment with moderate certainty of evidence) did not show a benefit of fish oil. The heterogeneity of effects of fish oil across indications might reflect varying modes of benefit (is fish oil more useful for induction of remission), more optimal role as adjunct therapy rather than as primary monotherapy, unclear dosing regimen, or lack of true clinical benefit. For these reasons, more investigation is needed to determine whether fish oil supplementation has or does not have a role in the treatment algorithm of IBD.

DISCLOSURE

Dr. Mullin: Grant Support: Biofilm Epidemiology and Mechanisms in Colon Cancer, National Cancer Institute, R01CA196845.

REFERENCES

1. Mullin GE. CAM safety. Nutr Clin Pract 2012;27(6):832–3.
2. Bailey RL, Gahche JJ, Miller PE, et al. Why US adults use dietary supplements. JAMA Intern Med 2013;173(5):355–61.

3. Blumberg JB, Bailey RL, Sesso HD, et al. The evolving role of multivitamin/multi-mineral supplement use among adults in the age of personalized nutrition. Nutrients 2018;10(2):248.

4. Charen E, Harbord N. Toxicity of herbs, vitamins, and supplements. Adv Chronic Kidney Dis 2020;27(1):67–71.

5. Knapik JJ, Austin KG, Farina EK, et al. Dietary supplement use in a large, representative sample of the US armed forces. J Acad Nutr Diet 2018;118(8):1370–88.

6. Roytman MM, Poerzgen P, Navarro V. Botanicals and hepatotoxicity. Clin Pharmacol Ther 2018;104(3):458–69.

7. Rao N, Spiller HA, Hodges NL, et al. An increase in dietary supplement exposures reported to US poison control centers. J Med Toxicol 2017;13(3):227–37.

8. Burnett BP, Mullin G. Therapeutic food claims: a global perspective. Curr Opin Clin Nutr Metab Care 2017;20(6):522–8.

9. Brown AC. An overview of herb and dietary supplement efficacy, safety and government regulations in the United States with suggested improvements. Part 1 of 5 series. Food Chem Toxicol 2017;107(Pt A):449–71.

10. Dossett ML, Davis RB, Lembo AJ, et al. Complementary and alternative medicine use by US adults with gastrointestinal conditions: results from the 2012 national health interview survey. Am J Gastroenterol 2014;109(11):1705–11.

11. Gallinger ZR, Nguyen GC. Practices and attitudes toward complementary and alternative medicine in inflammatory bowel disease: a survey of gastroenterologists. J Complement Integr Med 2014;11(4):297–303.

12. Phatak UP, Alper A, Pashankar DS. Complementary and alternative medicine use in children with inflammatory bowel disease. J Pediatr Gastroenterol Nutr 2019; 68(2):157–60.

13. Chen Y, Wang Y, Shen J. Role of environmental factors in the pathogenesis of Crohn's disease: a critical review. Int J Colorectal Dis 2019;34(12):2023–34.

14. Guan Q. A comprehensive review and update on the pathogenesis of inflammatory bowel disease. J Immunol Res 2019;2019:7247238.

15. Limketkai BN, Iheozor-Ejiofor Z, Gjuladin-Hellon T, et al. Dietary interventions for induction and maintenance of remission in inflammatory bowel disease. Cochrane Database Syst Rev 2019;2:CD012839.

16. Ananthakrishnan AN, Khalili H, Konijeti GG, et al. A prospective study of long-term intake of dietary fiber and risk of Crohn's disease and ulcerative colitis. Gastroenterology 2013;145(5):970–7.

17. Jacob V, Crawford C, Cohen-Mekelburg S, et al. Single delivery of high-diversity fecal microbiota preparation by colonoscopy is safe and effective in increasing microbial diversity in active ulcerative colitis. Inflamm Bowel Dis 2017;23(6): 903–11.

18. Aniwan S, Tremaine WJ, Raffals LE, et al. Antibiotic use and new-onset inflammatory bowel disease in Olmsted County, Minnesota: a population-based case-control study. J Crohns Colitis 2018;12(2):137–44.

19. Hollander D. Crohn's disease–a permeability disorder of the tight junction? Gut 1988;29(12):1621–4.

20. Patenaude A, Rodriguez-Leyva D, Edel AL, et al. Bioavailability of alpha-linolenic acid from flaxseed diets as a function of the age of the subject. Eur J Clin Nutr 2009;63(9):1123–9.

21. Parian AM, Limketkai BN, Shah ND, et al. Nutraceutical supplements for inflammatory bowel disease. Nutr Clin Pract 2015;30(4):551–8.

22. Wild GE, Drozdowski L, Tartaglia C, et al. Nutritional modulation of the inflammatory response in inflammatory bowel disease–from the molecular to the integrative to the clinical. World J Gastroenterol 2007;13(1):1–7.
23. Serhan CN, Arita M, Hong S, et al. Resolvins, docosatrienes, and neuroprotectins, novel omega-3-derived mediators, and their endogenous aspirin-triggered epimers. Lipids 2004;39(11):1125–32.
24. Abdolmaleki F, Kovanen PT, Mardani R, et al. Resolvins: emerging players in autoimmune and inflammatory diseases. Clin Rev Allergy Immunol 2020;58(1):82–91.
25. Cleland LG, James MJ, Proudman SM. Fish oil: what the prescriber needs to know. Arthritis Res Ther 2006;8(1):202.
26. Charpentier C, Chan R, Salameh E, et al. Dietary n-3 PUFA may attenuate experimental colitis. Mediators Inflamm 2018;2018:8430614.
27. Aslan A, Triadafilopoulos G. Fish oil fatty acid supplementation in active ulcerative colitis: a double-blind, placebo-controlled, crossover study. Am J Gastroenterol 1992;87(4):432–7.
28. Stenson WF, Cort D, Rodgers J, et al. Dietary supplementation with fish oil in ulcerative colitis. Ann Intern Med 1992;116(8):609–14.
29. Barbosa DS, Cecchini R, El Kadri MZ, et al. Decreased oxidative stress in patients with ulcerative colitis supplemented with fish oil omega-3 fatty acids. Nutrition 2003;19(10):837–42.
30. Scaioli E, Sartini A, Bellanova M, et al. Eicosapentaenoic acid reduces fecal levels of calprotectin and prevents relapse in patients with ulcerative colitis. Clin Gastroenterol Hepatol 2018;16(8):1268–1275 e1262.
31. Almallah YZ, Richardson S, O'Hanrahan T, et al. Distal procto-colitis, natural cytotoxicity, and essential fatty acids. Am J Gastroenterol 1998;93(5):804–9.
32. Seidner DL, Lashner BA, Brzezinski A, et al. An oral supplement enriched with fish oil, soluble fiber, and antioxidants for corticosteroid sparing in ulcerative colitis: a randomized, controlled trial. Clin Gastroenterol Hepatol 2005;3(4):358–69.
33. Lorenz R, Weber PC, Szimnau P, et al. Supplementation with n-3 fatty acids from fish oil in chronic inflammatory bowel disease–a randomized, placebo-controlled, double-blind cross-over trial. J Intern Med Suppl 1989;731:225–32.
34. Razack R, Seidner DL. Nutrition in inflammatory bowel disease. Curr Opin Gastroenterol 2007;23(4):400–5.
35. Dichi I, Frenhane P, Dichi JB, et al. Comparison of omega-3 fatty acids and sulfasalazine in ulcerative colitis. Nutrition 2000;16(2):87–90.
36. De Ley M, de Vos R, Hommes DW, et al. Fish oil for induction of remission in ulcerative colitis. Cochrane Database Syst Rev. 2007 Oct 17;(4):CD005986. DOI: https://doi.org/10.1002/14651858.CD005986.pub2
37. Stack WA, Cole AT, Makhdoom Z, et al. A randomised controlled trial of essential fatty acids (EFA) in acute ulcerative colitis (UC). Gut 1997;40:W89.
38. Loeschke K, Ueberschaer B, Pietsch A, et al. n-3 fatty acids only delay early relapse of ulcerative colitis in remission. Dig Dis Sci 1996;41(10):2087–94.
39. Hawthorne AB, Daneshmend TK, Hawkey CJ, et al. Treatment of ulcerative colitis with fish oil supplementation: a prospective 12 month randomised controlled trial. Gut 1992;33(7):922–8.
40. Mantzaris G, Archavlis E, Zografos C, et al. A prospective, randomized, placebo-controlled study of fish oil in ulcerative colitis. Hellenic Journal of Gastroenterology 1996;9(2):138–41.

41. Greenfield SM, Green AT, Teare JP, et al. A randomized controlled study of evening primrose oil and fish oil in ulcerative colitis. Aliment Pharmacol Ther 1993; 7(2):159–66.

42. Middleton SJ, Naylor S, Woolner J, et al. A double-blind, randomized, placebo-controlled trial of essential fatty acid supplementation in the maintenance of remission of ulcerative colitis. Aliment Pharmacol Ther 2002;16(6):1131–5.

43. Turner D, Steinhart AH, Griffiths AM. Omega 3 fatty acids (fish oil) for maintenance of remission in ulcerative colitis. Cochrane Database Syst Rev 2007;(3): CD006443.

44. Wiese DM, Lashner BA, Lerner E, et al. The effects of an oral supplement enriched with fish oil, prebiotics, and antioxidants on nutrition status in Crohn's disease patients. Nutr Clin Pract 2011;26(4):463–73.

45. Feagan BG, Sandborn WJ, Mittmann U, et al. Omega-3 free fatty acids for the maintenance of remission in Crohn disease: the EPIC randomized controlled trials. JAMA 2008;299(14):1690–7.

46. Lev-Tzion R, Griffiths AM, Leder O, et al. Omega 3 fatty acids (fish oil) for maintenance of remission in Crohn's disease. Cochrane Database Syst Rev 2014;2: CD006320.

47. Turner D, Zlotkin SH, Shah PS, et al. Omega 3 fatty acids (fish oil) for maintenance of remission in Crohn's disease. Cochrane Database Syst Rev 2007;(2): CD006320.

48. Turner D, Zlotkin SH, Shah PS, et al. Omega 3 fatty acids (fish oil) for maintenance of remission in Crohn's disease. Cochrane Database Syst Rev 2009;(1): CD006320.

49. Lorenz-Meyer H, Bauer P, Nicolay C, et al. Omega-3 fatty acids and low carbohydrate diet for maintenance of remission in Crohn's disease. A randomized controlled multicenter trial. study group members (German Crohn's Disease Study Group). Scand J Gastroenterol 1996;31(8):778–85.

50. Romano C, Cucchiara S, Barabino A, et al. Usefulness of omega-3 fatty acid supplementation in addition to mesalazine in maintaining remission in pediatric Crohn's disease: a double-blind, randomized, placebo-controlled study. World J Gastroenterol 2005;11(45):7118–21.

51. Belluzzi A, Brignola C, Campieri M, et al. Effect of an enteric-coated fish-oil preparation on relapses in Crohn's disease. N Engl J Med 1996;334(24):1557–60.

52. Belluzzi A, Campieri M, Belloli C, et al. A new enteric coated preparation of omega-3 fatty acids for preventing post-surgical recurrence in Crohn's disease. Gastroenterology 1997;112(4):A494.

53. Siguel EN, Lerman RH. Prevalence of essential fatty acid deficiency in patients with chronic gastrointestinal disorders. Metabolism 1996;45(1):12–23.

54. Reif S, Klein I, Lubin F, et al. Pre-illness dietary factors in inflammatory bowel disease. Gut 1997;40(6):754–60.

55. Abubakar I, Myhill DJ, Hart AR, et al. A case-control study of drinking water and dairy products in Crohn's Disease–further investigation of the possible role of Mycobacterium avium paratuberculosis. Am J Epidemiol 2007;165(7): 776–83.

56. Ananthakrishnan AN, Khalili H, Song M, et al. High school diet and risk of Crohn's disease and ulcerative colitis. Inflamm Bowel Dis 2015;21(10):2311–9.

57. Maconi G, Ardizzone S, Cucino C, et al. Pre-illness changes in dietary habits and diet as a risk factor for inflammatory bowel disease: a case-control study. World J Gastroenterol 2010;16(34):4297–304.

58. Pugazhendhi S, Sahu MK, Subramanian V, et al. Environmental factors associated with Crohn's disease in India. Indian J Gastroenterol 2011;30(6):264–9.
59. Rashvand S, Somi MH, Rashidkhani B, et al. Dietary protein intakes and risk of ulcerative colitis. Med J Islam Repub Iran 2015;29:253.
60. Mozaffari H, Daneshzad E, Larijani B, et al. Dietary intake of fish, n-3 polyunsaturated fatty acids, and risk of inflammatory bowel disease: a systematic review and meta-analysis of observational studies. Eur J Nutr 2020;59(1):1–17.

Irritable Bowel Syndrome
Food as a Friend or Foe?

Kimberly N. Harer, MD, ScM, Shanti L. Eswaran, MD*

KEYWORDS

- Diet • Carbohydrate • Fodmap • Gluten • Fructose • Lactose • Eating disorder
- Microbiome

KEY POINTS

- Irritable bowel syndrome (IBS) affects 10% to 15% of the population and is defined by symptom-based criteria, including abdominal pain associated with defecation and a change in the frequency or form of stool.
- Most patients report worsening of their symptoms with eating, and up to 90% of IBS patients exclude certain foods in the hopes of avoiding or improving their gastrointestinal symptoms.
- Among the available dietary interventions for IBS, the low FODMAP diet has the greatest evidence for efficacy.
- With the increasing use of restrictive diets to treat IBS symptoms, gastroenterologists need to be aware of the negative effects of prescribing restrictive diets and red flag symptoms of maladaptive eating patterns.
- Serum IgE and IgG testing have little to no role in diagnosing food intolerances.

INTRODUCTION

Dietary approaches for irritable bowel syndrome (IBS) have undergone countless iterations, starting from the 1970s, when Manning and colleagues[1] first explored the use of fiber for IBS. Over the years, the field moved on to elimination diets, avoiding families of foods or individual components, such as dairy, caffeine, spices, and fatty foods. Finally, in the 2010s and onward, the avoidance of gluten and FODMAPs (fermentable oligosaccharides, disaccharides, monosaccharides, and polyols) has come into vogue. In the 1990s, when these concepts were emerging, it became clear that approximately two-thirds of patients with IBS felt that their symptoms were triggered by dietary factors.[2–4] Even if patients not necessarily are looking for an all-natural approach to treating their IBS, it is a rare patient who is not interested in dietary advice for managing their symptoms.[5] A recent study utilizing Google Trends tracked patterns of interest for various IBS treatments and discovered a 117% increase in Google

Division of Gastroenterology, Department of Internal Medicine, University of Michigan, 1500 East Medical Center Drive, 3912 TC SPC 5362, Ann Arbor, MI 48109, USA
* Corresponding author.
E-mail address: seswaran@med.umich.edu

Gastroenterol Clin N Am 50 (2021) 183–199
https://doi.org/10.1016/j.gtc.2020.10.002
0889-8553/21/© 2020 Elsevier Inc. All rights reserved.

searches for the low FODMAP diet between 2014 and 2018, the largest increase in all searches for IBS treatment, quantifying the rapid rise of public interest for diet-based therapies.[6] Despite patients' clear perceptions and interest regarding diet and gastrointestinal (GI) symptoms, providers and researchers alike traditionally have turned away from the use of exclusion diets for IBS.

IRRITABLE BOWEL SYNDROME OVERVIEW AND DIAGNOSTIC CRITERIA

IBS is estimated to affect 10% to 15% of adults in North America and is the most common functional GI disorder.[7,8] Since 1989, when the first symptom-based diagnostic criteria for IBS were published, new evidence has inspired several diagnostic criteria evolutions. Currently, the Rome IV criteria are used to diagnose IBS, with 4 subtypes identified based on the predominant stool pattern abnormality. The subtypes include IBS with diarrhea (IBS-D), IBS with constipation (IBS-C), IBS with mixed symptomology (IBS-M), and unclassified IBS. The Rome IV diagnostic criteria and subtypes are outlined in **Fig. 1.**

Identifying underlying pathophysiologic mechanisms and effective treatment options for IBS has proved challenging due to the symptom-based diagnosis in concert with significant clinical heterogeneity. Despite the challenges identifying causative mechanisms, many proposed pathophysiologic mechanisms of IBS have been inspired by the growing understanding of diet and intestinal health and function. These mechanisms include visceral hypersensitivity, dysmotility, intestinal dysbiosis, and altered barrier function.[9] The connection between food and health has been known for centuries. Still, it is only recently that the underlying biological mechanisms of their interaction within the human body have begun to be recognized.

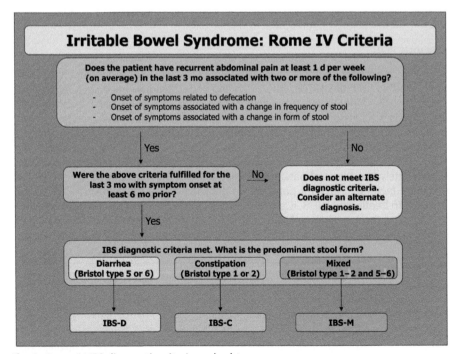

Fig. 1. Rome IV IBS diagnostic criteria and subtypes.

GENERAL MANAGEMENT

A respectful patient-physician relationship is the cornerstone of successful IBS treatment, and establishing a secure and confident diagnosis of IBS is crucial to patient acceptance of the condition. An allied relationship between patient and provider, including the use of an explanatory model regarding IBS pathophysiology, improves response to therapy, including dietary therapy.[9] The mismatch between a patient's and provider's perceptions regarding the impact of IBS can have a negative impact on the outcome of IBS treatment. Thus, goals of treatment should include improving quality of life and stress reduction, in addition to IBS symptom control. The treatment of IBS can be just as varied as the condition itself, and strategies can be symptom based or globally focused. First-line therapies, typically consisting of lifestyle modification and over-the-counter medications, generally target bowel symptoms (diarrhea or constipation) but offer only a marginal benefit for abdominal symptoms, such as pain and bloating. When these strategies fail, prescription medications often are used, including nonabsorbable antibiotics, antidepressants, and antispasmodics, but no validated treatment algorithm exists.[10,11] Unfortunately, a heterogeneous response to treatments seems to be the norm for patients with IBS, and approximately half of patients with IBS utilize complementary and alternative approaches either in addition to or instead of conventional medical therapy.[12,13]

LET FOOD BE THY MEDICINE...

Adverse reactions to both meals in general or specific foods are acknowledged by up to 45% of the general population, and GI complaints are predominant in approximately one-third to one-half of those affected.[14–16] In patients with IBS, however, this prevalence is even higher; up to two-thirds of patients report worsening of symptoms after meals.[4] Patients long have associated their IBS symptoms with the ingestion of certain foods or a meal itself, and postprandial symptoms are associated with increased disease severity and decreased quality of life.[17] Traditionally, the lack of provider training in this area coupled with inadequate data correlating IBS symptoms with specific foods has resulted in the medical community to view dietary interventions for IBS with skepticism. Additionally, the inadequate payor commitment to dietary counseling has led to a patient-directed attempts at elimination diets, ineffective at best, and nutritionally inadequate at worst.

True food allergy is uncommon in IBS patients,[18,19] although perceived food intolerances or sensitivities are more prevalent. Food allergy can be demonstrated in only a relatively small proportion of the population when double-blind food elimination and challenge studies are used, likely due to the nonspecific nature of their symptoms that are more consistent with IBS symptoms rather than a true food allergy. Up to 90% of IBS patients exclude certain foods in the hopes of avoiding or improving their GI symptoms,[20] often leading to the accumulation of trigger or culprit foods.

MECHANISMS BY WHICH FOOD CAUSES IRRITABLE BOWEL SYNDROME SYMPTOMS

Given that digestion, absorption, and elimination are the primary functions of the GI tract, it is not surprising that food ingestion leads to major changes in secretion and motility, even in healthy patients. Postprandial symptoms in IBS likely are the consequence of an abnormal physiologic response to normal stimuli, the hallmark of IBS, and also should be viewed in the context of disordered brain-gut interaction (**Fig. 2**).[21,22] Altered responses to nutrients in IBS patients include an exaggerated

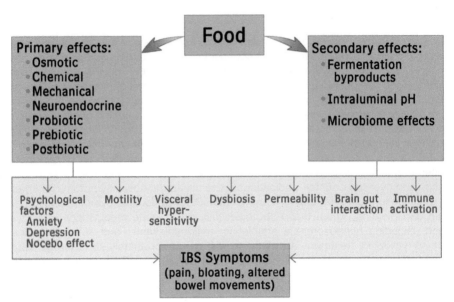

Fig. 2. Mechanisms by which food leads GI symptoms. (*Adapted from* Hookway C, Buckner S, Crosland P, Longson D. Irritable bowel syndrome in adults in primary care: summary of updated NICE guidance. BMJ. 2015;350:h701.)

gastrocolic reflex and enhanced sensitization to rectal distention after lipid ingestion. Postprandial symptoms also may be attributed to food-microbiota interactions or fermentation patterns, which may be disordered in some IBS patients.

ELIMINATION DIETS

Traditional dietary advice for IBS patients includes encouragement of regular exercise and avoidance of caffeine, alcohol, fatty foods, and spicy foods.[23] This common-sense approach is low risk, accessible, and inexpensive, providing a platform from which advanced dietary interventions can be launched if needed. A frank discussion between providers and patients about how substances found in the gut (food and bacteria) sometimes can cause GI dysfunction and lead to symptoms improves the understanding of the patient's disease process and frames the provider's recommendations for specific dietary interventions.

Fiber supplementation is a time-honored recommendation for IBS,[1] but the data supporting its use are inconsistent, likely due to variations among fiber variety and effects on specific IBS subtypes. In a meta-analysis of 15 randomized controlled trials (RCTs), bran had no significant effect on treatment of IBS (relative risk of IBS not improving 0.90; 95% CI, 0.79–1.03), but psyllium was effective in treating IBS (relative risk 0.83; 95% CI, 0.73–0.94).[11] The number needed to treat with psyllium was 7 (95% CI, 4–25). Thus, the use of soluble fiber, rather than insoluble fiber, is recommended for first-line treatment of IBS given its low cost, wide availability, and lack of serious adverse effects.[24]

Jones and colleagues[25] were among the first to demonstrate symptom improvement after an elimination diet in IBS patients in the 1980s. Based on this and other studies, some researchers began to believe that food intolerance may be a major factor in IBS symptom generation. Unfortunately, subsequent studies failed to reliably demonstrate significant response rates, contributing to the lack enthusiasm for this mode of treating IBS in the following decades. The variable response rates likely were multifactorial but likely stemmed from difficulty with blinding, poorly defined endpoints, lack of standardized protocols including the use of blinded food challenges, and under-powering. A food placebo understandably is difficult to design, and the placebo response and nocebo response are notoriously high in functional populations.[26]

Low FODMAP Diet

Although various studies have implicated the role of individual FODMAPs in IBS symptom generation (eg, fructose and lactose),[27–29] it was not until 2014 that researchers at Monash University published their seminal study grouping these carbohydrate subtypes together under the FODMAP umbrella.[30] The FODMAP food components have been identified as some of the most important dietary triggers (**Fig. 3, Table 1**). In IBS patients and in healthy controls, FODMAPs arrive undigested to the colon, where fermentation occurs, leading to the generation of short-chain fatty acids and gas production.[31] In addition, some FODMAPs (fructose) are osmotically active, drawing water into the small bowel lumen. Other potential mechanisms of symptom generation include immune activation[32,33] and effects on the GI microbiome and metabolome.[32,34]

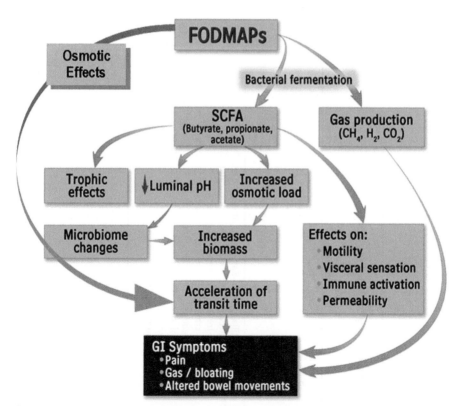

Fig. 3. Mechanisms by which FODMAPs cause GI symptoms. SCFA, short-chain fatty acid. (*Adapted from* McIntosh K, Reed DE, Schneider T, et al. FODMAPs alter symptoms and the metabolome of patients with IBS: a randomised controlled trial. Gut. 2016.)

Table 1
Examples of low and high FODMAP foods

	Grains	Fruits	Vegetables	Dairy/Plant-based Alternatives	Proteins	Beverages
High FODMAP	Wheat, rye, barley	Apples/apple juice, apricot, blackberries, cherries, dates, grapefruit, mango, pear, watermelon	Artichoke, asparagus Cauliflower, garlic, leeks, mushrooms button, portabella), onion/ shallots, sugar snap peas	Coconut milk (in the carton) Frozen yogurt, ice cream, milk, soft cheese, soy milk, yogurt	Most beans/legumes, processed meats[a]	High-fructose–containing sodas and juices Rum Tea: chamomile, oolong, fennel, and chai
Low FODMAP	Corn tortillas/ chips grits, gluten-free pastas, crackers, and breads,[a] oatmeal, potato, popcorn, rice, sourdough bread, quinoa	Banana (unripe), grapes, kiwifruit, lemon, lime, mandarin orange, orange, papaya, pineapple	Bok choy, broccoli, carrots, Chives, cucumber, Eggplant, kale, Lettuce, mushroom (oyster), olives, Radish, spinach, Tomato	Almond milk[a], Cheese (most), coconut yogurt, hemp milk,[a] lactose-free ice cream, milk yogurt,[a] cottage cheese	Beans: edamame lentils, canned/ rinsed: chickpeas, beef, chicken, egg, fish/seafood, pork, turkey, tempeh,[a] tofu–firm	Alcohol: wine (most), beer, spirits, coffee, sucrose- sweetened or diet soft drinks, tea (except those listed above), water

Not a complete list of foods. Portion size matters when it comes to FODMAPs because several foods have a specific serving size in which they would be high versus low in FODMAP.

[a] Read labels of packaged foods to ensure they do not have added high FODMAP ingredients (eg, high-fructose corn syrup, wheat, onion, and garlic).

Since its inception in the early 2000s, numerous observational studies and RCTs have reported that a majority of IBS patients (ranging from 52% to 86% of patients) experience significant improvement in their GI symptoms with the low FODMAP diet, depending on study design and clinical endpoints used. Two of the largest trials have found that both the low FODMAP diet and standard dietary advice can improve IBS symptoms. Bohn and colleagues[35] compared a dietitian-led low FODMAP diet versus standard dietary advice over 4 weeks in 75 IBS patients. Investigators found no difference in the number of patients reporting symptom reduction between the 2 diets for the primary endpoint of a reduction in IBS–Symptom Severity Score (SSS) of greater than or equal to 50 (P = .62). An American single-center RCT in 84 IBS-D patients also found no statistically significant difference in primary outcome of adequate relief of GI symptoms between 4 weeks of a dietitian-led low FODMAP diet or a diet based on modified UK National Institute for Health and Care Excellence (NICE) guidelines (52% for low FODMAP diet and 41% for modified NICE; P = .31). The low FODMAP diet did lead, however, to significant improvements in abdominal pain, bloating, and stool frequency scores compared with the modified NICE diet. In a secondary analysis from this study, the low FODMAP diet was more than twice as likely as the modified NICE diet to achieve a clinically meaningful improvement in disease-specific quality of life (52% vs 21%, respectively; P<.001).[36] Given the marginal improvement over standard dietary advice in the research setting, the NICE guidelines for adults with IBS suggest that the low FODMAP diet can be used as a second-line therapy following general lifestyle and dietary advice, such as consumption of regular meals and avoidance of suspected trigger foods.[23]

The logistical difficulties of blinding in dietary-based interventions poses a particularly unique challenge in functional GI disease, including IBS.[37] The placebo effect demonstrated in IBS medication trials is notoriously high,[26] but the opposite (nocebo effect) likely is just as powerful in dietary trials, given how closely patients link their symptoms to eating. Developing a true dietary placebo is difficult for obvious reasons but Staudacher and colleagues[38] devised a clever sham diet of equal complexity and fiber content to the low FODMAP diet. The proportion of participants reporting adequate symptom relief in the intention-to-treat analysis did not reach statistical significance (57% in the low FODMAP group vs 38% in the sham diet group; P = .051) although the difference was significant in the per-protocol analysis (61% vs 39%; P = .042). In addition, key secondary endpoints for the low FODMAP group were improved significantly compared with the sham group, including IBS-SSS (173 vs 224, respectively; P = .001), bloating (P = .001), and abdominal pain (P = .01).

Delivery of the low FODMAP diet is administered best by an experienced dietitian given the complexities and nuances involved.[24,39,40] The low FODMAP diet is composed of 3 distinct phases: (1) elimination; (2) reintroduction of foods containing individual FODMAPs to determine a person's sensitivities; and (3) personalization.[41–43] The elimination phase typically lasts approximately 2 weeks to 6 weeks and should be viewed as a diagnostic test to determine if a patient is sensitive to FODMAPs. If there is no response, the diet should be discontinued. If a therapeutic response is achieved, patients should undergo the reintroduction phase to determine sensitivities and tolerance thresholds. This information then can be used to create a personalized or maintenance version of the low FODMAP diet for long-term use. There are few data surrounding the reintroduction period, currently an ad hoc process.[44]

Given the complexities of the low FODMAP diet, there has been increasing attention on the potential role of biomarker testing as a predictor of low FODMAP diet efficacy. Baseline microbiome composition enriched in bacteria with an increased ability to metabolize carbohydrates may confer higher probability of response to the low

FODMAP diet.[45,46] Microbiome metabolites, such as volatile organic compounds, may differentiate responders versus nonresponders as well.[47]

The low FODMAP diet has several limitations that deserve discussion. Almost all the studies supporting the low FODMAP diet were performed in a research setting with education from expert registered dietitians, raising questions about generalizability to clinical practice. From a patient standpoint, the diet can be confusing, arduous, expensive, and unpalatable.[48] Access to a skilled dietitian also may be limited. The widespread availability of apps, Internet resources, and published materials can help bridge this gap and improve adherence and response.[49–51] In addition, the diet has not been well studied in Asian and African populations, and the majority of subjects enrolled in North American and European studies have been white women, bringing into the question the external validity and generalizability of this treatment strategy. Finally, most studies have only addressed the short-term effectiveness of the diet despite that IBS is a chronic condition. The entire low FODMAP process can take up to 12 weeks to complete the different phases, and it is unknown how well patients fare after the personalization phase.

Dietary interventions are considered low risk, but safety concerns about the low FODMAP diet have been raised. The elimination phase of low FODMAP diet can lead to a measurable decrease in so-called beneficial gut bacteria,[34] although these changes are not necessarily universally seen across studies. The use of a probiotic may be helpful to potentiate the negative microbiome effects of the diet.[38] Questions of nutritional adequacy also have been raised, with some studies reporting a decrease in calcium and fiber intake during the elimination phase. After correcting for calorie-adjusted nutrient intake, however, this decrease was not found to be significant.[52] It should be emphasized that the elimination phase is not meant to extend longer than 4 weeks to 6 weeks, thus any detrimental change to the microbiome or nutritional intake should be transient. A modified low FODMAP diet (after reintroduction to determine sensitivities) likely is nutritionally adequate as assessed by a longer-term study of dietary intake utilizing postal questionnaires.[53]

Gluten-Free Diet

Although gluten has been unmistakably demonstrated to be the protein triggering celiac disease, its role in symptom generation in IBS is less clear. The presence of intestinal and extraintestinal symptoms related to gluten-containing food without the diagnostic findings of celiac disease or wheat allergy has been termed, nonceliac gluten sensitivity (NCGS) or nonceliac wheat sensitivity (NCWS). The symptom complex of IBS may overlap and resemble that associated with NCGS/NCWS.[54] At present, there is no biomarker for this diagnosis; thus, the prevalence is unknown. The identification of such patients, however, is of clear clinical importance because this represents a subset of patient imminently treatable through gluten/wheat avoidance. Whether or not the culprits are gluten, amylase-trypsin inhibitors (ATIs), or the fructan component of wheat is the subject of much debate.[55]

In an online survey of IBS patients in the United States, a gluten-free diet (GFD) was the second most common diet followed by patients, with a lactose-free diet being the most common diet. Approximately one-fifth of the IBS patients in the study had followed a GFD.[56] Despite commonly used by patients with IBS, the efficacy of a GFD in IBS has not been firmly established. A 2011 double-blind RCT demonstrated that individuals with self-described NCGS experienced significant worsening of their IBS symptoms when exposed to gluten compared with a gluten-free diet.[57] Building on this study, investigators demonstrated increased stool frequency and increased intestinal permeability in IBS-D patients receiving gluten compared with a gluten-free diet, an effect that was more pronounced in HLA-DQ2/DQ8–positive patients.[58,59] Biesiekierski and colleagues[60] demonstrated, however, that once patients were on a low FODMAP diet, symptoms worsened during the study period to a similar degree regardless of how much gluten (0 g, 2 g, or 16 g) was added to their diets ($P = .001$), supporting the notion of NCWS rather than NCGS. The most recent RCT utilizing a low FODMAP diet followed by gluten versus placebo (double-blind challenge with washout and crossover), controlling for FODMAPs and ATIs.[61] Among the 30 patients who completed the study, 19% to 46% had worsening of their symptoms with gluten ingestion, depending on the criteria used. This crossover study was small with weaker clinical endpoints, but it is the first trial to demonstrate the presence of NCGS in IBS patients via this clinical trial design.

At this time, however, given the considerable heterogeneity and flaws in methodology in published studies even among double-blind placebo-controlled trials,[62] several meta-analyses and clinical guidelines have not supported the routine use of GFD in IBS patients.[11,63,64] There are no head-to-head low FODMAP diet versus GFD trials in undifferentiated IBS patients.

Low-Histamine Diet

Histamine is a biogenic amine that affects many organ systems, including the GI tract. Histamine intolerance is defined as an imbalance between excessive histamine ingestion/production and deficient histamine breakdown. Histamines are present naturally in the body but may be present in high amounts in preserved and fermented foods, such as canned foods, cheese, and alcohol.[65] The effects of histamine intolerance may be nonspecific, intestinal, or extraintestinal, including headache, rash, fatigue, dizziness, diarrhea, and abdominal pain.[66] A diagnosis of this condition requires 2 or more symptoms of histamine intolerance, with improvement after histamine avoidance and/or antihistamine medications after the exclusion of mastocytosis and IgE-mediated food allergy.[66] The prevalence is low (1% of the population) but difficult to truly estimate given the lack of biomarkers for diagnosis and nonspecific symptoms.[66,67] In particular, the role of histamine in the generation of GI symptoms and its relation to IBS is not well defined in the literature[68] and mainly anecdotal, although IBS patients commonly associate their symptoms with foods containing histamine.[17] Treatment of histamine intolerance generally involves histamine avoidance, followed by gradual reintroduction of specific histamine containing foods as tolerated.[65]

DISORDERED EATING AND EATING DISORDERS AMONG IRRITABLE BOWEL SYNDROME PATIENTS

There is growing awareness of the bidirectional relationship between chronic GI disorders and disordered eating/eating disorders. Disordered eating is defined by eating patterns that do not follow the cultural norm, including skipping meals, limiting foods, or following a restrictive diet. Disordered eating often is used by IBS patients in an attempt to avoid or prevent symptoms, and these disordered eating habits not always are harmful or pathologic. Gastroenterology patients are at increased risk, however, of maladaptive disordered eating patterns due to the frequent implementation of therapeutic diets and the potential for expansion of the dietary restrictions into pathologic exclusionary practices. In contrast to patients with disordered eating habits, patients with eating disorders demonstrate more severe eating behavior changes, may suffer with body dysmorphia as the motivating factor behind the restriction and often experience negative medical or psychosocial effects secondary to the maladaptive dietary behaviors. Eating disorders, such as anorexia nervosa, bulimia nervosa, and binge eating disorders, include maladaptive and harmful eating patterns.

A systematic review, including 9 studies, demonstrated the prevalence of disordered eating is higher among gastroenterology patients than healthy controls, with a prevalence up to 44%,[69] but there is limited evidence regarding the prevalence of eating disorders among IBS patients. Rather, much of the literature has focused on the prevalence of IBS among patients with eating disorders, with 1 study demonstrating concomitant IBS among outpatients with bulimia nervosa to be 69%.[70] Another study demonstrated that among IBS patients who were prescribed and adherent with a low FODMAP diet, 23% were classified to be at risk for eating disorder behavior.[71]

Avoidant/restrictive food intake disorder (ARFID) is an eating disorder characterized by avoidance or restriction of foods associated with clinically significant weight loss, nutritional deficiency, dependence on tube feeds/oral supplements, or significant psychosocial interference. Unlike many other eating disorders, body dysmorphia is not present. There is increasing awareness of ARFID among adult GI patients, with a prevalence of approximately 20%.[72,73] Patients with ARFID tend to identify a short list of safe foods, refuse to reintegrate other foods into their diet, and are at risk of malnutrition. Unlike orthorexia, the dietary restriction among gastroenterology patients with ARFID is driven primarily by a fear of negative consequences and desire to avoid GI symptoms rather than a compulsion with eating healthy foods. IBS patients are at particular risk for ARFID due to the high prevalence of diet-responsive symptoms, which reinforces dietary exclusion and can promote pathologic restriction.

With the increasing use of restrictive diets to treat IBS symptoms, it is imperative for gastroenterologists to be aware of the negative effects of prescribing restrictive diets and red flag symptoms of maladaptive eating patterns. Diet-controlled chronic illness is a risk factor for developing disordered eating or an eating disorder,[74] and restrictive diets are relatively contraindicated in patients with an active or prior eating disorder, underweight body mass index, or ongoing weight loss. Clinicians also should ensure the patient is not already following a restricted diet prior to prescribing a restrictive diet (eg, ensure the patient is not following a ketogenic diet prior to prescribing a low FODMAP diet).

THE ROLE OF SEROLOGIC TESTING TO PREDICT FOOD INTOLERANCE

Although the prevalence of food allergies among US adults is approximately 3.7%, 20% to 45% of adults and up to 65% of IBS patients report food sensitivities.[75] Given this, there is ongoing interest in understanding the potential role food-directed IgE and IgG antibodies play in IBS symptomatology and food hypersensitivities outside of IgE-mediated food allergies.

Several studies have provided preliminary evidence regarding the role of IgE-mediated food hypersensitivity among IBS patients.[76–80] One study evaluated 24 IBS patients, including 12 atopic and 12 nonatopic patients, who completed a 3-week low allergenic diet followed by blind dietary provocation. Fourteen of the 24 IBS patients were found to have at least 1 identified food trigger, and 9 of the 14 had elevated total serum IgE level with a positive skin prick test, and were in the atopic group. Thus, food-specific IgE may mediate a hypersensitivity reaction in a subgroup of IBS patients.

In regard to IgG-mediated food hypersensitivity, most available data suggest that IgG elevation is a result of normal immunologic response to dietary antigens.[81,82] A few studies, however, have reported improvement in GI symptoms in IBS patients by following an elimination diet based on food-specific IgG antibody testing.[83–85] The most widely cited RCT evaluated the therapeutic potential of a 12-week IgG antibody–directed exclusion diet versus sham diet in 150 IBS patients.[83] Compared with the sham diet, the IgG antibody–directed elimination diet resulted in a 10% greater reduction in IBS-SSS (*P* = .024). Among fully compliant IBS patients in the exclusion group, the reduction in severity score was 26%. After food reintroduction, the elimination diet group demonstrated worsening of IBS symptoms compared with the sham group (*P* = .047). Another study of patients who had both IBS and migraines demonstrated subjective improvement in both IBS and migraine symptoms after an IgG-based elimination diet.[86]

At this time, serum IgE testing remains an alternative to the gold standard oral food challenge for the identification of IgE-mediated food allergies.[87] Serum IgE and IgG testing, however, are considered by most experts to have little to no role in diagnosing food hypersensitivities and intolerances due to their low specificity.[87] There also is concern that increasingly popular immunoglobulin panel testing results in an increased out-of-pocket cost to the patient, overdiagnosis of food allergy, and unnecessary elimination diets.[88] Although IgE-mediated and IgG-mediated food hypersensitivities may contribute to the development of GI symptoms in a subset of IBS patients, in particular atopic patients, routine testing is not recommended at this time.

Leukocyte activation testing (LAT) garnered interest in the past couple years after a study that tested individualized LAT-directed diets in patients with IBS.[89] The parallel-group double-blind study of 58 adult IBS patients randomized patients to a 4-week diet of either elimination of positive-assay foods (with consumption of negative-assay foods) or elimination of negative-assay foods (with consumption of positive-assay foods). The group who eliminated positive-assay foods had a significantly greatly increase in mean IBS Global Improvement Scale scores at 4 weeks and 8 weeks (*P* = .02) as well as lower IBS-SSS scores at 4 weeks and 8 weeks (*P* = .03). No difference in IBS–Adequate Relief or IBS–Quality of Life scores were noted between groups at 4 weeks or 8 weeks. Interestingly, 3 of the top 5 most frequently restricted foods were also high FODMAP foods. Although larger trials are needed, this study provides preliminary evidence regarding the use of LAT-directed diets in patients with IBS and supports the increasing interest in the use of precision diet therapy in this patient population.

SUMMARY

The authors suggest that a dietary approach is best offered to patients who recognize a dietary component to their symptoms. Among the available dietary interventions for IBS, the low FODMAP diet has the greatest evidence for efficacy. The rapid and widespread adoption of the low FODMAP diet speaks not only to the research to date but also to the desperation for effective nonpharmacologic treatments for IBS. Critics of the diet, however, have pointed to high risk of bias, lack of blinding, and relatively low numbers in studies, noting "very low evidence" to support recommending a low FODMAP diet in IBS.[63] This sort of reality check is welcome and should motivate researchers to conduct larger studies with robust clinical endpoints, standard comparators, and diverse populations/cuisines.

Few clinicians and researchers would dispute that conditions like IBS, celiac disease, and lactose intolerance can be improved with diet. There likely are additional organic diseases that can be improved with specific dietary intervention, and next research steps include honing in on these to improve the therapeutic offerings to patients. Medicine has lagged behind what patients have touting for decades: that food and symptoms are linked. The use of a personalized dietary approach[90] based on fecal metabolome,[47] serum biomarkers,[89] baseline microbiome,[91] baseline symptoms, baseline diet, or genetic variants[92] may allow clinicians to predict response to allow for individually tailored dietary advice, reduce the level of dietary restriction required, and potentially be more widely applicable/appealing to patients.

DISCLOSURE

Authors state they do not have any relevant disclosures.

REFERENCES

1. Manning AP, Heaton KW, Harvey RF. Wheat fibre and irritable bowel syndrome. A controlled trial. Lancet 1977;2(8035):417–8.
2. Dalton CB, Drossman DA, Hathaway JM, et al. Perceptions of physicians and patients with organic and functional gastrointestinal diagnoses. Clin Gastroenterol Hepatol 2004;2(2):121–6.
3. Halpert A, Godena E. Irritable bowel syndrome patients' perspectives on their relationships with healthcare providers. Scand J Gastroenterol 2011;46(7–8):823–30.
4. Simrén M, Månsson A, Langkilde AM, et al. Food-related gastrointestinal symptoms in the irritable bowel syndrome. Digestion 2001;63(2):108–15.
5. Halpert A, Dalton CB, Palsson O, et al. What patients know about irritable bowel syndrome (IBS) and what they would like to know. National Survey on Patient Educational Needs in IBS and development and validation of the Patient Educational Needs Questionnaire (PEQ). Am J Gastroenterol 2007;102(9):1972–82.
6. Flanagan R, Kuo B, Staller K. Utilizing Google Trends to Assess Worldwide Interest in Irritable Bowel Syndrome and Commonly Associated Treatments. Dig Dis Sci. 2020 May 2. [Online ahead of print]
7. Hungin AP, Chang L, Locke GR, et al. Irritable bowel syndrome in the United States: prevalence, symptom patterns and impact. Aliment Pharmacol Ther 2005;21(11):1365–75.
8. Lovell RM, Ford AC. Global prevalence of and risk factors for irritable bowel syndrome: a meta-analysis. Clin Gastroenterol Hepatol 2012;10(7):712–721 e714.
9. Hungin AP, Becher A, Cayley B, et al. Irritable bowel syndrome: an integrated explanatory model for clinical practice. Neurogastroenterol Motil 2015;27(6):750–63.
10. Chey WD, Kurlander J, Eswaran S. Irritable bowel syndrome: a clinical review. JAMA 2015;313(9):949–58.
11. Ford AC, Moayyedi P, Chey WD, et al. American College of Gastroenterology Monograph on Management of Irritable Bowel Syndrome. Am J Gastroenterol 2018;113(Suppl 2):1–18.
12. El-Serag HB, Pilgrim P, Schoenfeld P. Systemic review: Natural history of irritable bowel syndrome. Aliment Pharmacol Ther 2004;19(8):861–70.
13. Lahner E, Bellentani S, Bastiani RD, et al. A survey of pharmacological and non-pharmacological treatment of functional gastrointestinal disorders. United Eur Gastroenterol J 2013;1(5):385–93.
14. Young E, Stoneham MD, Petruckevitch A, et al. A population study of food intolerance. Lancet 1994;343(8906):1127–30.
15. Monsbakken KW, Vandvik PO, Farup PG. Perceived food intolerance in subjects with irritable bowel syndrome - etiology, prevalence and consequences. Eur J Clin Nutr 2005;60(5):667–72.

16. Locke GR, Zinsmeister AR, Talley NJ, et al. Risk factors for irritable bowel syndrome: role of analgesics and food sensitivities. Am J Gastroenterol 2000; 95(1):157–65.
17. Bohn L, Storsrud S, Tornblom H, et al. Self-reported food-related gastrointestinal symptoms in IBS are common and associated with more severe symptoms and reduced quality of life. Am J Gastroenterol 2013;108(5):634–41.
18. Bischoff SC, Herrmann A, Manns MP. Prevalence of adverse reactions to food in patients with gastrointestinal disease. Allergy 1996;51(11):811–8.
19. Dainese R, Galliani EA, De Lazzari F, et al. Discrepancies between reported food intolerance and sensitization test findings in irritable bowel syndrome patients. Am J Gastroenterol 1999;94(7):1892–7.
20. Hayes P, Corish C, O'Mahony E, et al. A dietary survey of patients with irritable bowel syndrome. J Hum Nutr Diet 2014;27(Suppl 2):36–47.
21. Salvioli B, Serra J, Azpiroz F, et al. Impaired small bowel gas propulsion in patients with bloating during intestinal lipid infusion. Am J Gastroenterol 2006; 101(8):1853–7.
22. Eswaran S, Tack J, Chey WD. Food: the forgotten factor in the irritable bowel syndrome. Gastroenterol Clin North Am 2011;40(1):141–62.
23. Hookway C, Buckner S, Crosland P, et al. Irritable bowel syndrome in adults in primary care: summary of updated NICE guidance. BMJ 2015;350:h701.
24. Rajilic-Stojanovic M, Jonkers DM, Salonen A, et al. Intestinal microbiota and diet in IBS: causes, consequences, or epiphenomena? Am J Gastroenterol 2015; 110(2):278–87.
25. Jones VA, Shorthouse M, Hunter JO. Food intolerance: A major factor in the pathogenesis of irritable bowel syndrome. Lancet 1982;2(8308):1115–7.
26. Ford AC, Moayyedi P. Meta-analysis: factors affecting placebo response rate in the irritable bowel syndrome. Aliment Pharmacol Ther 2010;32(2):144–58.
27. Shepherd SJ, Parker FC, Muir JG, et al. Dietary Triggers of Abdominal Symptoms in Patients With Irritable Bowel Syndrome: Randomized Placebo-Controlled Evidence. Clin Gastroenterol Hepatol 2008;6(7):765–71.
28. Fernandez-Banares F, Rosinach M, Esteve M, et al. Sugar malabsorption in functional abdominal bloating: a pilot study on the long-term effect of dietary treatment. Clin Nutr 2006;25(5):824–31.
29. Cuatrecasas P, Lockwood DH, Caldwell JR. Lactase Deficiency in the Adult. A Common Occurrence. Lancet 1965;1(7375):14–8.
30. Halmos EP, Power VA, Shepherd SJ, et al. A diet low in FODMAPs reduces symptoms of irritable bowel syndrome. Gastroenterology 2014;146(1):67–75.e5.
31. Major G, Pritchard S, Murray K, et al. Colon Hypersensitivity to Distension, Rather Than Excessive Gas Production, Produces Carbohydrate-Related Symptoms in Individuals With Irritable Bowel Syndrome. Gastroenterology 2017;152(1): 124–33.e2.
32. McIntosh K, Reed DE, Schneider T, et al. FODMAPs alter symptoms and the metabolome of patients with IBS: a randomised controlled trial. Gut 2017;66(7): 1241–51.
33. Hustoft TN, Hausken T, Ystad SO, et al. Effects of varying dietary content of fermentable short-chain carbohydrates on symptoms, fecal microenvironment, and cytokine profiles in patients with irritable bowel syndrome. Neurogastroenterol Motil 2017;29(4).
34. Staudacher HM, Lomer MC, Anderson JL, et al. Fermentable carbohydrate restriction reduces luminal bifidobacteria and gastrointestinal symptoms in patients with irritable bowel syndrome. J Nutr 2012;142(8):1510–8.

35. Bohn L, Storsrud S, Liljebo T, et al. Diet low in FODMAPs Reduces Symptoms of Irritable Bowel Syndrome as Well as Traditional Dietary Advice: A Randomized Controlled Trial. Gastroenterology 2015;149:1399–407.e2.

36. Eswaran S, Chey WD, Jackson K, et al. A Diet Low in Fermentable Oligo-, Di-, and Mono-saccharides and Polyols Improves Quality of Life and Reduces Activity Impairment in Patients with Irritable Bowel Syndrome and Diarrhea. Clin Gastroenterol Hepatol 2017;15(12):1890–9.e3.

37. Staudacher HM, Irving PM, Lomer MCE, et al. The challenges of control groups, placebos and blinding in clinical trials of dietary interventions. Proc Nutr Soc 2017;76(3):203–12.

38. Staudacher HM, Lomer MCE, Farquharson FM, et al. Diet Low in FODMAPs Reduces Symptoms in Patients with Irritable Bowel Syndrome and Probiotic Restores Bifidobacterium Species: a Randomized Controlled Trial. Gastroenterology 2017;153(4):936–47.

39. Tuck CJ, Reed DE, Muir JG, et al. Implementation of the low FODMAP diet in functional gastrointestinal symptoms: A real-world experience. Neurogastroenterol Motil 2020;32(1):e13730.

40. O'Keeffe M, Lomer MC. Who should deliver the low FODMAP diet and what educational methods are optimal: a review. J Gastroenterol Hepatol 2017; 32(Suppl 1):23–6.

41. Whelan K, Martin LD, Staudacher HM, et al. The low FODMAP diet in the management of irritable bowel syndrome: an evidence-based review of FODMAP restriction, reintroduction and personalisation in clinical practice. J Hum Nutr Diet 2018; 31(2):239–55.

42. Liu J, Chey WD, Haller E, et al. Low-FODMAP Diet for Irritable Bowel Syndrome: What We Know and What We Have Yet to Learn. Annu Rev Med 2020;71:303–14.

43. Chey WD. Food: The Main Course to Wellness and Illness in Patients With Irritable Bowel Syndrome. Am J Gastroenterol 2016;111(3):366–71.

44. Harvie RM, Chisholm AW, Bisanz JE, et al. Long-term irritable bowel syndrome symptom control with reintroduction of selected FODMAPs. World J Gastroenterol 2017;23(25):4632–43.

45. Valeur J, Smastuen MC, Knudsen T, et al. Exploring Gut Microbiota Composition as an Indicator of Clinical Response to Dietary FODMAP Restriction in Patients with Irritable Bowel Syndrome. Dig Dis Sci 2018;63(2):429–36.

46. Chumpitazi BP, Cope JL, Hollister EB, et al. Randomised clinical trial: gut microbiome biomarkers are associated with clinical response to a low FODMAP diet in children with the irritable bowel syndrome. Aliment Pharmacol Ther 2015;42(4):418–27.

47. Rossi M, Aggio R, Staudacher H, et al. Volatile Organic Compounds Predict Response to Both Low Fodmap Diet and Probiotics in Irritable Bowel Syndrome: A Randomised Controlled Trial. Gastroenterology 2017;152(5):S713–4.

48. Trott N, Aziz I, Rej A, et al. How Patients with IBS Use Low FODMAP Dietary Information Provided by General Practitioners and Gastroenterologists: A Qualitative Study. Nutrients 2019;11(6):1313.

49. Scarlata K, Wilson D. The low-FODMAP diet: step by step. New York: Da Capo; 2017.

50. Catsos P. IBS–Free at last!: a revolutionary, new step-by-step method for those who have tried everything. Control IBS symptoms by limiting FODMAPS carbohydrates in your diet. Portland, Maine: Pond Cove Press; 2009.

51. Catsos P. The IBS elimination diet and cookbook: the proven low-FODMAP plan for EatingWell and feeling great. New York: Harmoney Books; 2017.

52. Eswaran S, Dolan R, Ball S, et al. The Impact of a 4-week Low FODMAP and mNICE Diet on Nutrient Intake in a Sample of US Adults with IBS-D. J Acad Nutr Diet 2019;120(4):641–9.
53. O'Keeffe M, Jansen C, Martin L, et al. Long-term impact of the low-FODMAP diet on gastrointestinal symptoms, dietary intake, patient acceptability, and health-care utilization in irritable bowel syndrome. Neurogastroenterol Motil 2018;30(1).
54. Potter MDE, Walker MM, Jones MP, et al. Wheat Intolerance and Chronic Gastro-intestinal Symptoms in an Australian Population-based Study: Association Between Wheat Sensitivity, Celiac Disease and Functional Gastrointestinal Disorders. Am J Gastroenterol 2018;113(7):1036–44.
55. Catassi C, Alaedini A, Bojarski C, et al. The Overlapping Area of Non-Celiac Gluten Sensitivity (NCGS) and Wheat-Sensitive Irritable Bowel Syndrome (IBS): An Update. Nutrients 2017;9(11):1268.
56. Pauls RN, Max JB. Symptoms and dietary practices of irritable bowel syndrome patients compared to controls: results of a USA national survey. Minerva Gastro-enterol Dietol 2019;65(1):1–10.
57. Biesiekierski JR, Newnham ED, Irving PM, et al. Gluten causes gastrointestinal symptoms in subjects without celiac disease: a double-blind randomized placebo-controlled trial. Am J Gastroenterol 2011;106(3):508–14 [quiz: 515].
58. Vazquez-Roque MI, Camilleri M, Smyrk T, et al. Association of HLA-DQ gene with bowel transit, barrier function, and inflammation in irritable bowel syndrome with diarrhea. Am J Physiol Gastrointest Liver Physiol 2012;303(11):G1262–9.
59. Vazquez-Roque MI, Camilleri M, Smyrk T, et al. A controlled trial of gluten-free diet in patients with irritable bowel syndrome-diarrhea: effects on bowel frequency and intestinal function. Gastroenterology 2013;144(5):903–11.e3.
60. Biesiekierski JR, Peters SL, Newnham ED, et al. No effects of gluten in patients with self-reported non-celiac gluten sensitivity after dietary reduction of ferment-able, poorly absorbed, short-chain carbohydrates. Gastroenterology 2013;145(2):320–8.e1-3.
61. Barone M, Gemello E, Viggiani MT, et al. Evaluation of Non-Celiac Gluten Sensi-tivity in Patients with Previous Diagnosis of Irritable Bowel Syndrome: A Random-ized Double-Blind Placebo-Controlled Crossover Trial. Nutrients 2020;12(3):705.
62. Molina-Infante J, Carroccio A. Suspected Nonceliac Gluten Sensitivity Confirmed in Few Patients After Gluten Challenge in Double-Blind, Placebo-Controlled Trials. Clin Gastroenterol Hepatol 2017;15(3):339–48.
63. Dionne J, Ford AC, Yuan Y, et al. A Systematic Review and Meta-Analysis Evalu-ating the Efficacy of a Gluten-Free Diet and a Low FODMAPs Diet in Treating Symptoms of Irritable Bowel Syndrome. Am J Gastroenterol 2018;113(9):1290–300.
64. Moayyedi P, Andrews CN, MacQueen G, et al. Canadian Association of Gastro-enterology Clinical Practice Guideline for the Management of Irritable Bowel Syn-drome (IBS). J Can Assoc Gastroenterol 2019;2(1):6–29.
65. Tuck CJ, Biesiekierski JR, Schmid-Grendelmeier P, et al. Food Intolerances. Nu-trients 2019;11(7):1684.
66. Maintz L, Novak N. Histamine and histamine intolerance. Am J Clin Nutr 2007;85(5):1185–96.
67. Schwelberger HG. Histamine intolerance: overestimated or underestimated? In-flamm Res 2009;58(Suppl 1):51–2.
68. Schnedl WJ, Lackner S, Enko D, et al. Non-celiac gluten sensitivity: people without celiac disease avoiding gluten-is it due to histamine intolerance? Inflamm Res 2018;67(4):279–84.

69. Satherley R, Howard R, Higgs S. Disordered eating practices in gastrointestinal disorders. Appetite 2015;84:240–50.

70. Dejong H, Perkins S, Grover M, et al. The prevalence of irritable bowel syndrome in outpatients with bulimia nervosa. Int J Eat Disord 2011;44(7):661–4.

71. Mari A, Hosadurg D, Martin L, et al. Adherence with a low-FODMAP diet in irritable bowel syndrome: are eating disorders the missing link? Eur J Gastroenterol Hepatol 2019;31(2):178–82.

72. Murray HB, Bailey AP, Keshishian AC, et al. Prevalence and Characteristics of Avoidant/Restrictive Food Intake Disorder in Adult Neurogastroenterology Patients. Clin Gastroenterol Hepatol 2019;18(9):1995–2002.e1.

73. Harer K, Baker J, Reister N, et al. Avoidant/restrictive food intake disorder in the adult gastroenterology population: an under-recognized diagnosis? Am J Gastroenterol 2018;113:S247–8.

74. Quick VM, Byrd-Bredbenner C, Neumark-Sztainer D. Chronic illness and disordered eating: a discussion of the literature. Adv Nutr 2013;4(3):277–86.

75. Park MI, Camilleri M. Is there a role of food allergy in irritable bowel syndrome and functional dyspepsia? A systematic review. Neurogastroenterol Motil 2006;18(8):595–607.

76. Andre F, Andre C, Colin L, et al. IgE in stools as indicator of food sensitization. Allergy 1995;50(4):328–33.

77. Barau E, Dupont C. Modifications of intestinal permeability during food provocation procedures in pediatric irritable bowel syndrome. J Pediatr Gastroenterol Nutr 1990;11(1):72–7.

78. Bischoff SC, Mayer J, Meier PN, et al. Clinical significance of the colonoscopic allergen provocation test. Int Arch Allergy Immunol 1997;113(1–3):348–51.

79. Bischoff SC, Mayer J, Wedemeyer J, et al. Colonoscopic allergen provocation (COLAP): a new diagnostic approach for gastrointestinal food allergy. Gut 1997;40(6):745–53.

80. Petitpierre M, Gumowski P, Girard JP. Irritable bowel syndrome and hypersensitivity to food. Ann Allergy 1985;54(6):538–40.

81. Husby S, Oxelius VA, Teisner B, et al. Humoral immunity to dietary antigens in healthy adults. Occurrence, isotype and IgG subclass distribution of serum antibodies to protein antigens. Int Arch Allergy Appl Immunol 1985;77(4):416–22.

82. Johansson SG, Dannaeus A, Lilja G. The relevance of anti-food antibodies for the diagnosis of food allergy. Ann Allergy 1984;53(6 Pt 2):665–72.

83. Atkinson W, Sheldon TA, Shaath N, et al. Food elimination based on IgG antibodies in irritable bowel syndrome: a randomised controlled trial. Gut 2004;53(10):1459–64.

84. Drisko J, Bischoff B, Hall M, et al. Treating irritable bowel syndrome with a food elimination diet followed by food challenge and probiotics. J Am Coll Nutr 2006;25(6):514–22.

85. Zar S, Mincher L, Benson MJ, et al. Food-specific IgG4 antibody-guided exclusion diet improves symptoms and rectal compliance in irritable bowel syndrome. Scand J Gastroenterol 2005;40(7):800–7.

86. Aydinlar EI, Dikmen PY, Tiftikci A, et al. IgG-based elimination diet in migraine plus irritable bowel syndrome. Headache 2013;53(3):514–25.

87. Hammond C, Lieberman JA. Unproven Diagnostic Tests for Food Allergy. Immunol Allergy Clin North Am 2018;38(1):153–63.

88. Bird JA, Crain M, Varshney P. Food allergen panel testing often results in misdiagnosis of food allergy. J Pediatr 2015;166(1):97–100.

89. Ali A, Weiss TR, McKee D, et al. Efficacy of individualised diets in patients with irritable bowel syndrome: a randomised controlled trial. BMJ Open Gastroenterol 2017;4(1):e000164.

90. Wang XJ, Camilleri M, Vanner S, et al. Review article: biological mechanisms for symptom causation by individual FODMAP subgroups - the case for a more personalised approach to dietary restriction. Aliment Pharmacol Ther 2019;50(5): 517–29.

91. Chumpitazi BP. The gut microbiome as a predictor of low fermentable oligosaccharides disaccharides monosaccharides and polyols diet efficacy in functional bowel disorders. Curr Opin Gastroenterol 2020;36(2):147–54.

92. Henstrom M, Diekmann L, Bonfiglio F, et al. Functional variants in the sucrase-isomaltase gene associate with increased risk of irritable bowel syndrome. Gut 2018;67(2):263–70.

Nutritional Care for Patients with Intestinal Failure

Laura E. Matarese, PhD, RDN, LDN, CNSC, FADA, FASPEN, FAND*, Glenn Harvin, MD

KEYWORDS

- Intestinal failure • Short bowel syndrome • Nutrition • Intestinal rehabilitation

KEY POINTS

- Short bowel syndrome is the most common form of intestinal failure and may result in numerous metabolic complications, fluid and electrolyte disturbances, and malnutrition.
- Nutrition forms the cornerstone of therapy. Interventions designed to improve nutritional status include enteral and parenteral nutrition, intestinal rehabilitation techniques, and restorative surgery. These are not competitive therapies but rather are interrelated services designed to enhance and improve nutritional status through the safest most effective manner.
- Because of heterogeneity of the patient population with intestinal failure, therapeutic options should be individualized for each patient.

INTRODUCTION

The nutritional care of patients with intestinal failure is complex. There are multiple factors to be considered and multiple nutrition therapies that can be used. Although limited, there are data to support the use of many of these therapies in this patient population. The use of these therapies is outlined in this article.

DEFINITION AND CAUSE OF INTESTINAL FAILURE

Intestinal failure is a debilitating, complex disorder that not only results in reduced quality of life but may be life-threatening.[1,2] There have been various definitions proposed, thus highlighting the complexity of this disease. The European Society for Clinical Nutrition and Metabolism has defined intestinal failure as the reduction of gut function less than the minimum necessary for the absorption of macronutrients and/ or water and electrolytes, such that intravenous (IV) supplementation is required to maintain health and/or growth.[2] It is associated with either loss of portions of the intestine or loss of intestinal function.[2,3] Short bowel syndrome (SBS) is the most

Division of Gastroenterology, Hepatology and Nutrition, Department of Internal Medicine, Brody School of Medicine, East Carolina University, 600 Moye Boulevard, Vidant MA 342, Mail Stop 734, Greenville, NC 27834, USA
* Corresponding author.
E-mail address: mataresel@ecu.edu

Gastroenterol Clin N Am 50 (2021) 201–216
https://doi.org/10.1016/j.gtc.2020.10.004
0889-8553/21/© 2020 Elsevier Inc. All rights reserved.

common form of intestinal failure. SBS generally results from extensive surgical resection because of disease, trauma, or congenital defects (**Box 1**).[2–4] Regardless of the cause, the result is an inability to maintain fluid, electrolyte, and nutrient balance from a normal diet such that IV fluids or nutrition is required.[2]

METABOLIC AND NUTRITIONAL CONSEQUENCES OF INTESTINAL FAILURE

The gastrointestinal (GI) insufficiency resulting from SBS is associated with weight loss, malnutrition, cachexia, severe diarrhea, steatorrhea, dehydration, hypovolemia, acidosis, electrolyte imbalance, renal insufficiency, and bone demineralization. Extent of the metabolic and nutritional consequences largely depends on the location and length of bowel resected.[2,5] Patients with an end jejunostomy often experience dehydration immediately following surgery. Consumption of solid foods and liquids results in increased ostomy effluent. Although the greatest risk is with fluid and electrolyte imbalance, these patients are also at risk of developing malnutrition. Those with a jejunocolic anastomosis experience weight loss and severe undernutrition often leading to a severe malnourished state. The jejunoileal anastomosis in which there is more than 10 cm of terminal ileum remaining, although less common, results in weight loss and possible development of malnutrition.

The amount of remnant intestine required to remain autonomous from parenteral nutrition (PN) is largely depended on the presence or absence of the terminal ileum and the colon.[6,7] Patients with a remnant small bowel length of greater than 60 to 90 cm and the colon, or greater than 150 cm without colon, can usually be weaned from PN.[6,7] The colon is an important factor in enhancing absorption because of its ability for fluid absorption and energy absorption by the conversion of unabsorbed carbohydrates to short-chain fatty acids.[8,9] An intact ileocecal valve, along with a portion of the ileum, results in reduced transit time with the potential for increased nutrient absorption. The ileum also has a greater ability to adapt than the jejunum and is essential for the absorption of bile acids and vitamin B_{12}.

There are other factors that affect absorption and the ability of the bowel to adapt after surgical resection (**Box 2**). For example, the younger the patient, the more likely

---

Box 1
Cause of intestinal failure

Surgical resection
- Complications of bariatric surgery
- Malignancy
- Small bowel fistulas
- Strangulated hernias
- Trauma
- Vascular catastrophes (eg, embolism, thrombus)
- Volvulus

Congenital SBS
  Functional disorders
  - Pseudo-obstruction
  - Dysmotility
  Mucosal disease
  - Crohn disease
  - Radiation enteritis
  - Refractory sprue
  - Congenital villus atrophy

Box 2
Factors that influence absorption and ability to wean from PN
Length of the remnant bowel
Presence of an ileum/ileocecal valve
Presence of entire or portion of the colon
Absence of residual disease in the remnant bowel
Age of the patient
Degree to which bowel adaptation has occurred
Duration of time on PN
Nutritional status before weaning

they are to adapt. The health of the remaining mucosa (ie, absence of mucosal disease) also influences adaptation and the presence of an intact stomach, pancreas, and liver, all of which are necessary for digestion, absorption, and metabolism of nutrients.

NUTRITIONAL INTERVENTIONS

SBS encompasses a diverse, heterogeneous group of patients. They vary in remnant GI anatomy, health of mucosa, and nutritional status. As such, treatment often requires a multipronged and dynamic approach. These therapies may be used alone or in combination with each other. Success is rarely achieved in isolation.

Parenteral Nutrition

Immediately following surgical resection, most patients require PN to promote healing and optimal management of fluids and electrolytes. Many of these patients require long-term PN and/or IV fluids. All attempts should be made to optimize the PN formula to facilitate weaning to enteral nutrition (EN) by tube and/or oral diet.[10] Patients should have PN cycled over 12 to 16 hours to allow freedom from being tethered to an IV and to encourage oral intake. In severe cases of SBS, PN and/or IV fluids may have to be infused for longer periods to prevent dehydration and damage to the kidneys. The use of PN and IV fluids does not negate the importance of initiating nutrition via the GI tract. The remnant bowel begins to adapt after surgical resection whereby it compensates to maintain nutritional homeostasis through physiologic, cellular, and molecular mechanisms.[11,12] Complex luminal nutrients are the most potent stimulus to intestinal adaptation and should be introduced as soon as possible.[13,14]

Patients who are unable to maintain nutritional status via the GI tract should be considered for home PN. It is important that the patient understands what this involves and will be compliant with the therapy. Careful discharge planning helps ensure a safe transition. The patient must have appropriate vascular access, such as a tunneled catheter, port, or peripherally inserted central catheter line. The PN formula should be prescribed so that the patient receives adequate nutrition without overfeeding and should be cycled whenever possible. Home PN has the potential for numerous complications (**Box 3**). As such, there should be emphasis on the prevention of complications of PN-dependency.[15] Complications are minimized by attempting to optimize enteral feeding, eliminate and prevent sepsis, educate the patient on good line care, and use antibiotic and ethanol locks where appropriate. Any coagulation

---

Box 3
Potential PN complications

Catheter-related
- Infection
- Loss of vascular access
- Central venous thrombosis

Liver/biliary
- Liver disease
- Steatosis
- Cholestasis
- Gallbladder sludge/stones

Metabolic
- Fluid and electrolyte abnormalities
- D-lactic acidosis
- Micronutrient deficiency
- Overfeeding/underfeeding

Bone
- Metabolic bone disease
- Osteoporosis
- Osteomalacia

Gastrointestinal
- Diarrhea
- Gastric hypersecretion
- Small bowel intestinal bacterial overgrowth

Kidney
- Nephrolithiasis
- Chronic renal failure

Quality of life
- Depression, irritability, confusion
- Reduced autonomy
- Disrupted sleep
- Diminished overall health
- Body image issues and appearance of premature aging

Financial
- High cost of care
- Some patients are unable to work

Data from Nightingale JMD. Intestinal Failure. London, England: Greenwich Medical Media; 2001:177-198 And Hofstetter S, et al. Curr Med Res Opin. 2013;29(5):495-504 And Buchman AL, Scolapio J, Fryer J. AGA Technical Review on Short Bowel Syndrome and Intestinal Transplantation. Gastroenterology. 2003;124(4):1111-1134.

---

disorders should be identified and treated to avoid thrombosis. These patients require frequent follow-up to ensure the safety and adequacy of the therapy and readiness to begin weaning.

Enteral Nutrition

Following surgical resection, patients may be advanced from PN to EN. The delivery of these formulas may be accomplished by oral supplementation, nasoenteric tube feeding, or permanent gastrostomy. In addition to providing nutrition, the use of EN also stimulates intestinal adaptation after surgical resection.[16–18] Cosnes and colleagues[19] retrospectively evaluated the effects of EN using a polymeric formula in

25 patients with severe SBS in whom malabsorption of fat ranged from 31% to 93%. All but one patient was weaned from PN. Although fecal weight increased with the use of EN, there was a significant increase in body weight and improved fluid and electrolyte balance. Eighteen of the 25 patients developed hypocalcemia and/or hypomagnesemia, which was easily controlled with oral supplementation. The authors concluded that EN can be used to stabilize most patients with severe SBS to facilitate weaning.

EN may be accomplished with the use of dual and transitional feedings. Continuous tube feeding, alone or in combination with oral feeding, has been shown to increase intestinal macronutrient nutrient absorption compared with oral feeding alone in the postoperative period.[20] There was a significant increase in total calories, lipids, and protein in patients who received enteral tube feeding and oral combined with tube feeding compared with oral feedings alone. It has been hypothesized that the benefit associated with tube feeding in this study was a result of the continuous infusion of the enteral feeds resulting in constant luminal stimulation.

The type of tube feeding formula required is largely dependent on patient tolerance and their ability to digest and absorb nutrients. Levy and colleagues[21] evaluated the use of continued EN in 62 patients with SBS. They used a semielemental formula mixed with a viscous additive to create a high-viscosity solution. They also reinfused enteric contents in some of the patients. The viscous polymeric diets were associated with good tolerance and the use of the elemental formulas was required in only a small percentage of the cases. In general, for patients with SBS, the more complex the nutrient formulation (ie, complex carbohydrates, fats, and protein), the more likely the patient will tolerate the formula and the more likely there is to be stimulation of intestinal adaptation.[11,12] For those individuals who are intolerant to complex formulas, defined formula diets that have macronutrients partially digested should be considered (**Table 1**).

Intestinal Rehabilitation

The term "intestinal rehabilitation" refers to a collection of interventions that when initiated stimulate and accelerate the natural process of intestinal adaptation resulting in enhanced absorptive capacity, improved nutritional status, and reduction in the need for PN through the use of diet, fiber supplementation, oral rehydration solutions, specialized nutrients, medications, hormonal therapy, and reconstructive surgery.[22] These techniques may be used alone but in general are used collectively.

Diet that includes complex nutrients is the foundation of therapy. It is the most potent stimulus to intestinal adaptation and is useful in controlling symptoms, such as rapid transit, osmotic diarrhea, impaired absorption, and increased losses.[23–25] Most of these patients develop hyperphagia; this should be encouraged. Although the SBS patient population is heterogeneous in nature, there are several studies that have evaluated the effects of diet composition on absorption.[8,26–32] As outlined by Byrne and colleagues,[32] the diet prescription is individualized for each patient, based on the remnant GI anatomy (**Table 2**).

The use of oral rehydration solutions may be helpful in maintaining fluid and electrolyte status. These solutions take advantage of the sodium-glucose cotransport system. To maximize absorption, the sodium content usually has to be in the range of 90 mEq/L and the carbohydrate content at 20 g/L.[33] The typical sports drink contains too much carbohydrate in the form of disaccharides and not enough sodium for patients with SBS. These are adapted with the addition of table salt to enhance absorption. There are several commercially available solutions (**Table 3**) or these are made with simple ingredients (**Box 4**).[34] In addition to the composition of these solutions it is important that the patient sip the solutions throughout the day to maximize

Table 1
Enteral formulas often used in SBS

Formula Type	Characteristics	Use in SBS
Standard polymeric	Intact nutrients, generally isotonic, 1 kcal/mL	Usually well tolerated
High-fiber polymeric	Intact nutrients, generally isotonic, 1 kcal/mL with additional fiber and prebiotics	May be useful in SBS but the high fiber content may increase output in some patients
Calorically dense polymeric	Intact nutrients, generally hypertonic, may contain 1.5–2 kcal/mL	Tolerance in SBS is variable
Blenderized formulas	Intact nutrients from whole foods; available commercially or may be prepared at home by the patient using a specific recipe strictly adhering to principles of food safety and sanitation using clean technique to avoid foodborne illness	May be useful in SBS because these formulas tend to be higher in fiber
Predigested	Formulas that contain partially digested macronutrients in the form of short-chain peptides, amino acids, glucose oligosaccharides, and medium-chain triglyceride oil	Useful in patients with SBS who are unable to digest intact nutrients

Table 2
Diet prescriptions based on GI anatomy

	Colon	No Colon
Carbohydrate	50%–60% of total calories (limit simple sugars)	40%–50% of total calories (restrict simple sugars)
Protein	20%–30% of total calories	20%–30% of total calories
Fat	20%–30% of total calories (primarily essential fats)	30%–40% of total calories (primarily essential fats)
Fluid	Isotonic fluids or hypo-osmolar fluids	Isotonic, high-sodium oral rehydration solution
Soluble fiber	5–10 g/d (if stool output is >3 L/d)	5–10 g/d (if stool output is >3 L/d)
Oxalates	Limit intake	—
Meals	5–6 meals per d	4–6 meals per d

Data from Byrne TA, Veglia L, Camelio M, et al. Beyond the prescription: optimizing the diet of patients with short bowel syndrome. Nutr Clin Pract. 2000;15:306-311.

Table 3
Examples of commercially available ORS

	CHO G/L	Na + mEq/ L	K+ mEq/ L	HCO$_3$ mEq/ L	Osmo mOsm/ L
World Health Organization ORS					
Standard formula	20	90	20	30	310
Reduced-osmolality formula	13.5	75	20	30	245
Rehydration Solutions					
Ceralyte 70 (Cera Products)	40	70	20	30	220
Cerayte 90 (Cera Products)	40	90	20	30	260
DripDrop	40	30	20		235
Jianas Brothers ORS	20	90	20	10	300
Enfalyte (Meade Johnson)	30	50	25	33	160
Pedialyte (Abbott)	25	45	20	10	250
Sports Drinks					
Gatorade	60	20	3		340
Gatorade2 + one-half teaspoon salt	29	63	3		254

Abbreviation: ORS, oral rehydration solutions.

absorption.[35] Patients should not add ice cubes because this dilutes the solution and changes the ratio of sodium, glucose, and water.

The use of soluble fiber supplements is most helpful for patients with an intact colon. The undigested fiber is metabolized by bacteria in the colon to produce short-chain fatty acids that are absorbed by colonic mucosa and used as energy. They also enhance sodium and water absorption and exert tropic effects.[36,37] Soluble fiber supplements may also be used for individuals without a colon to gelatinize the ostomy effluent.

Box 4
Recipe for oral rehydration solutions

1 L water

Three-quarter teaspoon table salt

3 tablespoons sugar (sucrose)

1 teaspoon baking powder (or one-half teaspoon baking soda)

One-half teaspoon 20% potassium chloride[a] or salt substitute[b]

Sugar-free artificial flavoring or sweetener

[a]By prescription.[b]Concentration: 7–14 mEq potassium per gram. One teaspoon: 5 g (one-sixth ounce) = 35–70 mEq potassium.

Data from Camilleri M, Prather CM, Evans MA et al. Balance studies and polymeric glucose solution to optimize therapy after massive intestinal resection. Mayo Clinic Proceedings 1992; 67(8):755-60.

Although all attempts are made to enhance absorption to the point where patients can consume and absorb enough to meet all micronutrient requirements, most require additional supplementation (**Table 4**).[38] These may be provided in the form of tablets or liquids. Of note, magnesium should be provided as lactate or gluconate. Magnesium oxide should be avoided because it is a strong cathartic and results in further magnesium losses.

Most of these patients benefit from the use of medications designed to reduce output, control acid secretion, enhance absorption, and control bacterial overgrowth (**Table 5**).[22,38,39] The best method of treating bacterial overgrowth remains unclear. The gold standard is the use of antibiotics. There is some interest in the use of probiotics to restore the natural flora. However, this has not been well studied in the short bowel model. Although some probiotics have shown to enhance intestinal adaptation in animal models, there are data to suggest that the addition of certain probiotics may actually limit adaptation and that prebiotics, such as fructooligosaccharide, may be more effective in stimulating adaptation through butyrate production.[40] Currently there is a paucity of clinical studies evaluating the efficacy, appropriate strain, and dosage of probiotics in SBS. Accordingly, administration of probiotics in this patient population should be considered only when there is strong supporting scientific evidence.

There are some patients who are also candidates for pharmacologic proadaptive treatments, such as glucagon-like peptide-2 (GLP-2) analogues and glucagon-like peptide-1 (GLP-1) agonists. GLP-2 secreted from distal small intestine and proximal colonic mucosal L-cells in response to luminal nutrients increases villus height/crypt depth by stimulating crypt cell proliferation and inhibiting enterocyte apoptosis. It also increases hexose and nutrient transporter activity, inhibits gastric acid secretion and gastric motility, increases intestinal blood flow, and decreases intestinal permeability.[41–44] Jeppesen and colleagues[45] demonstrated that meal-stimulated GLP-2 response in patients with SBS less than 150 cm of small intestine was impaired compared with normal subjects. The interest in the use of GLP-2 grew from a small, open-label trial investigating the effects of GLP-2 in humans with SBS in which eight patients received 400 µg native GLP-2 subcutaneously twice daily for 35 days.[46] Of the eight patients studied, four had a portion of colon-in-continuity and were receiving PN, whereas the other four did not have a colon and did not require PN. A modest

Table 4
Oral vitamin and mineral supplements

Nutrient	Strength	Dose
Vitamins A, D, E	25,000 IU of A 1000 IU of D 400 IU of E	1 tablet PO daily
Calcium citrate	500- to 600-mg tablet	1–2 tablets PO TID
Magnesium lactate	84-mg tablet	1–2 tablets PO TID
Magnesium gluconate	1000-mg tablet (or liquid)	1–3 tablets PO TID
Potassium chloride	20-mg tablet	1–2 tablets PO daily
Phos (NeutraPhos)	250-mg package	1 package PO TID
Sodium bicarbonate	650-mg tablet	1 tablet PO TID
Chromium	100-µg tablet	1–2 tablets PO TID
Copper	3-mg tablet	1–2 tablets PO daily
Selenium	200-µg tablet	1 tablet PO daily
Zinc sulfate	220-mg tablet	1–3 tablets PO daily

Data from Matarese LE and Steiger E. Dietary and medical management in adult patients with short bowel syndrome. J Clin Gastroenterol 2006; 40 (2): S85-93.

Table 5
Adjunctive medical management for SBS

Category	Action	Medication	Dosage
Antidiarrheal	↑ intestinal transit time	Loperamide	2-6 mg PO QID; maximum daily dose, 16 mg
		Diphenoxylate	2.5–7.5 mg PO QID; maximum daily dose, 20–25 mg
		Codeine	15–60 mg PO QID
		Opium tincture* (1% morphine anhydrous)	0.3–1 mL PO QID
Antimicrobials	↓ bacterial overgrowth	Metronidazole	250 mg PO TID for 7–14 days
		Ciprofloxacin	500 mg PO BID for 7–14 days
		Rifaximin	200–550 mg PO TID for 7–14 days
		Augmentin	500 mg PO BID for 7–14 days
		Doxycycline	100 mg PO BID for 7–14 days
		Neomycin	500 mg PO BID for 7–14 days
		Tetracycline	250–500 mg PO QID for 7–14 days
Bile Acid Sequestrants	Bind bile acids in the gut	Cholestyramine	4 grams mixed in water or other fluids 1-6 times/day
		Colestipol	5-gram packet 1-6 times/day

(continued on next page)

Table 5
(continued)

Category	Action	Medication	Dosage
GLP-2 Analogues	Increases villous height and crypt depth	Gattex	0.05 mg/kg once daily by subcutaneous injection
H₂ receptor antagonists	↓ gastric acid secretion	Famotidine	20–40 mg PO/IV BID
		Ranitidine	150–300 mg PO/IV BID
		Cimetidine	200–400 mg PO/IV QID
Pancreatic enzymes	Improve digestion	Pancrelipase	500 lipase units/kg per meal; maximum dose is 2500 lipase units/kg per meal or 10,000 lipase units/kg/d
Proton pump inhibitors	↓ gastric acid secretion	Lansoprazole	15–30 PO BID
		Pantoprazole	20–40 mg PO/IV BID
		Omeprazole	20–40 mg PO BID
		Esomeprazole	20–40 mg PO/IV BID
		Rabeprazole	20 mg PO BID
		Dexlansoprazole	30–60 mg PO BID
Somatostatin analogs	↓ secretory diarrhea	Octreotide	50–250 μg SC TID or QID
Synthetic conjugated bile acid	↑ fat absorption	Conjugated bile acids (OTC)	1–2 capsules per meal
	↓ diarrhea	Cholylsarcosine (not available in the US)	2–4 g per meal

* Not to be confused with paregoric, which is much less concentrated.
Data from Refs.[22,38,39]

increase in overall energy absorption, decrease in fecal wet weight, slowing of gastric emptying, and nonsignificant trend toward increased jejunal villus height and crypt depth were demonstrated. However, native GLP-2 has a half-life of only 7 minutes, which limits its clinical utility. Substituting a single amino acid of alanine to glycine at the second position of the N-terminus resulted in a longer-acting analogue (teduglutide) with an extended half-life of 1.3 hours. This was shown in an open-label study to be safe, well-tolerated, intestinotrophic, and significantly increased intestinal wet weight absorption, but not energy absorption in 16 patients with SBS with an end-jejunostomy or a colon-in-continuity.[47] Teduglutide was then studied in two phase III multinational, randomized, double-blind, placebo-controlled trials that included a total of 169 PN- or parenteral fluid–requiring patients with SBS in an outpatient setting. In the first study, 83 patients with SBS were separated into three treatment arms (placebo, 0.05 mg/kg/d, and 0.10 mg/kg/d administered subcutaneously once daily) for 6 months. The lower teduglutide dose significantly reduced PN requirements (46% for 0.05 mg/kg/d vs 6% for placebo), and three patients were completely weaned from PN.[48] Additionally, teduglutide restored the structural integrity of the mucosa as evidenced by increased villus height, plasma citrulline concentration, and lean body mass.[49] After discontinuation of teduglutide at the end of the 24-week treatment period, some patients (15/37) required an increase in their fluids, whereas others (22/37) were able to maintain adequate fluid status.[50] A long-term study that included an additional 28 weeks of treatment in 52 patients demonstrated 68% of the 0.05 mg/kg/d and 52% of the 0.10 mg/kg/d dose group had a greater than or equal to 20% reduction in PN, with a reduction of 1 or more days of PN dependency in 68% and 37%, respectively.[51] The most frequent GI side effects included abdominal pain, nausea, stomal changes, abdominal distention, and peripheral edema. Because teduglutide is a growth factor, the only contraindication to its use is active GI neoplasia. Teduglutide is a daily injection. Glepaglutide, a new long-acting GLP-2 analogue that is given as a daily injection, is currently being studied in a randomized phase 2 trial.[52,53] To date, it has been shown to be safe and well tolerated resulting in increased transit time and mucosal growth, and a significant decrease in fecal output and an increase in intestinal absorption of wet weight, sodium, potassium, and macronutrients. A larger phase 3 trial has been initiated. To lengthen the duration of time between injections, another GLP-2 analogue, apraglutide was tested in a pig model and shown to increase intestinal adaptation and length.[54] A trial of weekly apraglutide in adults with SBS was just completed with results pending.[55]

GLP-2 is rapidly inactivated by dipeptidyl peptidase IV (DPP4). In one study, orally active DPP4 inhibitor administered to mice after 50% proximal small bowel resection stimulated epithelial cell proliferation in the jejunum and ileum at all time points and led to greater morphologic adaptive changes, some increase in villus height, with a predominant increase in crypt depth. Adaptation continued up to 90 days postresection, with a peak at 30 days, as did GLP-2 plasma levels.[56] These data led to the hypothesis that DPP4-I treatment may amplify the effects of GLP-2 and prove to be a viable option for accelerating intestinal adaptation in patients with SBS. In a placebo-controlled study of the acute effects of continuous infusions of GLP-1, GLP-2, and the combination GLP-1 and GLP-2 on intestinal absorption in patients with SBS, GLP-1 decreased diarrhea and fecal excretions in patients with SBS, but it seemed less potent than GLP-2. The combination of GLP-1 and GLP-2 provided additive effects on intestinal absorption compared with either peptide given alone. All treatments significantly reduced energy, nitrogen, and losses compared with placebo.[57]

In addition to the dietary and medical therapies, there are nontransplant surgical procedures that used to augment SBS. In some cases, isolated loops of bowel are

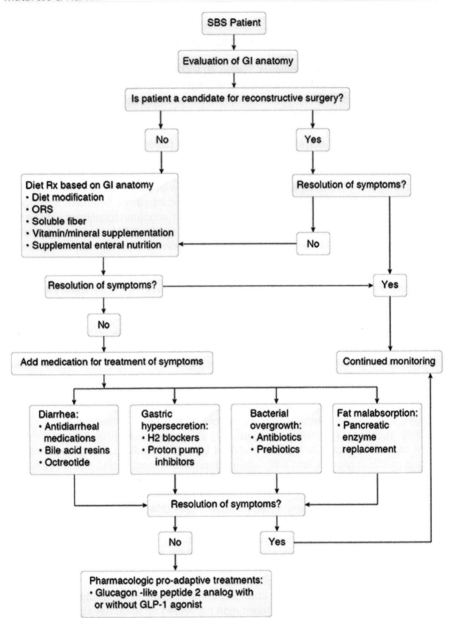

Fig. 1. Algorithm for the management of patients with SBS (*Adapted from* Matarese LE. Nutrition and Fluid Optimization for Patients with Short Bowel Syndrome. JPEN J Parenter Enteral Nutr. 2013; 37(2)161 – 170.)

placed back into circuit. Dilated bowel can undergo tapering, stricturoplasty, or lengthening procuress to provide more surface area.[58]

APPROACH TO PATIENT CARE

Because of the complexity and heterogeneity of this patient population nutrition care should be individualized. A coordinated approach that considers all therapeutic possibilities is helpful (**Fig. 1**). This algorithm provides a stepwise approach in determining the best nutrition interventions for these patients. In reality, these often occur simultaneously and multiple therapies may be used together. It is important to understand the patient's remnant anatomy. If the patient has isolated loops of bowel that can be put into circuit or is a candidate for a lengthening procedure, a referral to surgery should be made. Diet is the foundation of therapy. Diet alone may not be sufficient to ensure nutritional autonomy but it may aid in the optimization of PN therapy. In most cases standard medications are required along with diet to enhance absorption. Supplemental EN may also be used. When these attempts fail, use of pharmacologic proadaptive treatments should be considered. The importance of continued monitoring cannot be overemphasized as the patient's bowel continues to adapt and the clinical condition changes.

SUMMARY

The care of patients with SBS is complex. Complex luminal nutrients should be initiated as soon as possible following surgical resection to enhance intestinal adaptation. The nutrition interventions may include PN and EN, diet modification, standard medications, hormonal therapy, and/or reconstructive surgery. The goal is always to enhance absorption in the safest, most effective manner.

DISCLOSURE

The authors have nothing to disclose.

REFERENCES

1. Hofstetter S, Stern L, Willet J. Key issues in addressing the clinical and humanistic burden of short bowel syndrome in the US. Curr Med Res Opin 2013;29(5): 495–504.
2. Pironi L, Arends J, Baxter J, et al. ESPEN endorsed recommendations. Definition and classification of intestinal failure in adults. Clin Nutr 2015;34(2):171–80.
3. Nightingale JMD. The short bowel. In: Nightingale JMD, editor. Intestinal failure. London (United Kingdom): Greenwich Medical Media; 2001. p. 177–98.
4. Buchman AL. The clinical management of short bowel syndrome: steps to avoid parenteral nutrition. Nutrition 1997;13:907–13.
5. Nightingale J, Woodward JM. Guidelines for management of patients with a short bowel. Gut 2006;55(suppl 4):iv1–12.
6. Carbonnel F, Cosnes J, Chevret S, et al. The role of anatomic factors in nutritional autonomy after extensive small bowel resection. JPEN J Parenter Enteral Nutr 1996;20:275–80.
7. Messing B, Crenn P, Beau P, et al. Long-term survival and parenteral nutrition dependence in adult patients with the short bowel syndrome. Gastroenterology 1999;117:1043–50.
8. Nordgaard I, Hansen BS, Mortensen PB. Colon as a digestive organ in patients with short bowel. Lancet 1994;343:373–6.
9. Nightingale JM, Lennard-Jones JE, Gertner DJ, et al. Colonic preservation reduces need for parenteral therapy, increases incidence of renal stones, but does not change high prevalence of gall stones in patients with a short bowel. Gut 1992;33:1493–7.
10. Matarese LE. Nutrition and fluid optimization for patients with short bowel syndrome. JPEN J Parenter Enteral Nutr 2013;37(2):161–70.

11. Tappenden K. Intestinal adaptation following resection. JPEN J Parenter Enteral Nutr 2014;38:S23–31.
12. Weale AR, Edwards AG, Bailey M, et al. Intestinal adaptation after massive intestinal resection. Postgrad Med J 2005;81:178–84.
13. Tappenden KA. Mechanisms of enteral nutrient-enhanced intestinal adaptation. Gastroenterology 2006;130:S93–9.
14. Young EA, Cioletti LA, Winborn WB, et al. Comparative study of nutritional adaptation to defined formula diets in rats. Am J Clin Nutr 1980;33:210610.
15. Pironi L, Arends J, Bozzetti F, et al. ESPEN guidelines on chronic intestinal failure in adults. Clin Nutr 2016;35:247–307.
16. Feldman FT, Dowling RH, McNaughton J, et al. Effect of oral versus intravenous nutrition on intestinal adaptation after small bowel resection. Gastroenterology 1976;70:712–9.
17. Wilmore DW, Dudrick SJ, Daly JM, et al. The role of nutrition in the adaptation of the small intestine after massive resection. Surg Gynecol Obstet 1971;132:673–80.
18. Weser E. Nutritional aspects of malabsorption: short gut adaptation. Clin Gastroenterol 1983;12:443–60.
19. Cosnes J, Gendre JP, Evard D, et al. Compensatory enteral hyperalimentation for management of patients with severe short bowel syndrome. Am J Clin Nutr 1985;41:1002–9.
20. Joly F, Dray X, Corcos O, et al. Tube feeding improves intestinal absorption in short bowel syndrome patients. Gastroenterology 2009;136:824–31.
21. Levy E, Frileux P, Sandrucci S, et al. Continuous enteral nutrition during the early adaptive stage of the short bowel syndrome. Br J Surg 1988;75:549–53.
22. Matarese LE, O'Keefe SJ, Kandil HM, et al. Short bowel syndrome: clinical guidelines for nutrition management. Nutr Clin Pract 2005;20(6):493–502.
23. Weser E, Babbitt J, Hoban M, et al. Intestinal adaptation. Different growth responses to disaccharides compared with monosaccharides in rat small bowel. Gastroenterology 1986;91:1521–7.
24. Bines JE, Taylor RG, Justice F, et al. Influence of diet complexity on intestinal adaptation following massive small bowel resection in a preclinical model. J Gastroenterol Hepatol 2002;17:1170–9.
25. Ford WD, Boelhouwer RU, king WW, et al. Total parenteral nutrition inhibits intestinal adaptive hyperplasia in young rates: reversal by feeding. Surgery 1984;96:527–34.
26. Woolf GM, Miller C, Kurian R, et al. Nutritional absorption in short bowel syndrome: evaluation of fluid, calorie, and divalent cation requirements. Dig Dis Sci 1987;32:8–15.
27. Andersson H. Fat-reduced diet in the symptomatic treatment of patients with ileopathy. Nutr Metab 1974;17:102–11.
28. Hessov I, Andersson H, Isaksson B. Effects of a low-fat diet on mineral absorption in small-bowel disease. Scand J Gastroenterol 1983;18:551–4.
29. Woolf GM, Miller C, Kurian R, et al. Diet for patients with a short bowel: high fat or high carbohydrate? Gastroenterology 1983;84:823828.
30. Jeppesen PB, Mortensen PB. The influence of a preserved colon on the absorption of medium chain fat in patients with small bowel resection. Gut 1998;43:478–83.
31. Ovesen L, Chu R, Howard L. The influence of dietary fat on jejunostomy output in patients with severe short bowel syndrome. Am J Clin Nutr 1983;38:270–7.

32. Byrne TA, Veglia L, Camelio M, et al. Beyond the prescription: optimizing the diet of patients with short bowel syndrome. Nutr Clin Pract 2000;15:306–11.

33. Rodrigues CA, Lennard-Jones JE, Thompson DG, et al. What is the ideal sodium concentration of oral rehydration solutions for short bowel patients. Clin Sci 1988; 74(suppl18):69.

34. Camilleri M, Prather CM, Evans MA, et al. Balance studies and polymeric glucose solution to optimize therapy after massive intestinal resection. Mayo Clin Proc 1992;67(8):755–60.

35. Fortrand JS. Stimulation of active and passive sodium absorption by sugars in the human jejunum. J Clin Invest 1975;55(4):728–37.

36. Jeppesen P, Mortensen PB. Colonic digestion and absorption of energy from carbohydrates and medium-chain fat in small bowel failure. JPEN 1999;23:S101–5.

37. Royall D, Wolever T, Jeejeebhoy K. Evidence for colonic conservation of malabsorbed carbohydrate in short bowel syndrome. Am J Gastroenterol 1992;87:751.

38. Matarese LE, Steiger E. Dietary and medical management in adult patients with short bowel syndrome. J Clin Gastroenterol 2006;40(2):S85–93.

39. Kumph VJ. Pharmacologic management of diarrhea inpatients with short bowel syndrome. JPEN 2014;38(suppl 1):38S–44S.

40. Barnes JL, Hartmann B, Holst JJ, et al. Intestinal adaptation is stimulated by partial enteral nutrition supplemented with the prebiotic short-chain fructooligosaccharide in a neonatal intestinal failure piglet model. JPEN 2012;36:524–37.

41. Drucker DJ, Erlich P, Asa SL, et al. Induction of intestinal epithelial proliferation by glucagon-like peptide 2. Proc Natl Acad Sci U S A 1996;93:7911–6.

42. Ghatei MA, Goodlad RA, Taheri S, et al. Proglucagon-derived peptides in intestinal epithelial proliferation. Glucagon-like peptide-2 is a major mediator of intestinal epithelial proliferation in rats. Dig Dis Sci 2001;46:1255–63.

43. Scott RB, Kirk D, MacNaughton WK, et al. GLP-2 augments the adaptive response to massive intestinal resection in rat. Am J Phys 1998;275:G911–21.

44. Wojdemann M, Wettergren A, Hartmann B, et al. Glucagon-like peptide-2 inhibits centrally induced antral motility in pigs. Scand J Gastroenterol 1998;33:828–32.

45. Jeppesen PB, Hartmann B, Hansen BS, et al. Impaired meal stimulated glucagon-like peptide 2 response in ileal resected short bowel patients with intestinal failure. Gut 1999;45(4):559–763.

46. Jeppesen PB, Hartmann B, Thulesen J, et al. Glucagon-like peptide 2 improves nutrient absorption and nutritional status in short-bowel patients with no colon. Gastroenterology 2001;120:806–15.

47. Jeppesen PB, Sanguinetti EL, Buchman A, et al. Teduglutide (ALX-0600), a dipeptidyl peptidase IV resistant glucagon-like peptide analogue, improves intestinal function in short bowel syndrome patients. Gut 2005;54:1224–2123.

48. Jeppesen PB, Gilroy R, Pertkiewicz M, et al. Randomised placebo-controlled trial of teduglutide in reducing parenteral nutrition and/or intravenous fluid requirements in patients with short bowel syndrome. Gut 2011;60:902–14.

49. Tappenden KA, Edelman J, Joelsson B. Teduglutide enhances structural adaptation of the small intestinal mucosa in patients with short bowel syndrome. J Clin Gastroenterol 2013;47:602–7.

50. Compher C, Gilroy R, Pertkiewicz M, et al. Maintenance of parenteral nutrition volume reduction, without weight loss, after stopping teduglutide in a subset of patients with short bowel syndrome. JPEN J Parenter Enteral Nutr 2011;35:603–9.

51. O'Keefe SJ, Jeppesen PB, Gilroy R, et al. Safety and efficacy of teduglutide after 52 weeks of treatment in patients with short bowel intestinal failure. Clin Gastroenterol Hepatol 2013;11:815–23.

52. Naimi RM, Hvistendahl M, Enevoldsen LH, et al. Glepaglutide, a novel long-acting glucagon-like petide-2 analogue, for patients with short bowel syndrome: a randomized phase 2 trial. Lancet Gastroenterol Hepatol 2019. https://doi.org/10.1016/S2469-1253(19)300779.

53. Hvistendahl MK, Naimi RM, Enevoldsen LH, et al. Effect of glepaglutide, a long-acting glucagon-like peptide-2 analog, on gastrointestinal transit time and motility in patients with short bowel syndrome: findings from a randomized trial. JPEN 2020. https://doi.org/10.1002/jpen.1767.

54. Slim GM, Lansing M, Wizzard P, et al. Novel long-acting GLP-2 analogue, FE203799 (Apraglutide), enhances adaptation and linear intestinal growth in a neonatal piglet model of short bowel syndrome with total resection of the ileum. JPEN J Parenter Enteral Nutr 2019;43(7):891–8.

55. Jeppeson PB. Safety, Efficacy, PD of FE203799 in Short Bowel Syndrome on Parenteral Support. ClinicalTrials.gov Identifier: NCT03415594.

56. Sueyoshi R, Woods Ignatoski KM, Okawada M, et al. Stimulation of intestinal growth and function with DPP4 inhibition in a mouse short bowel syndrome model. Am J Physiol Gastrointest Liver Physiol 2014;307:G410–9.

57. Madsen KB, Askov-Hansen C, Naimi RM, Brandt CF, Hartmann B, Holst JJ, Mortensen PB, Jeppesen PB. Acute effects of continuous infusions of glucagon-like peptide (GLP)-1, GLP-2 and the combination (GLP-1+GLP-2) on intestinal absorption in short bowel syndrome (SBS) patients. A placebo-controlled study. Regul Pept 2013;184:30–9.

58. Iyer K. Surgical management of short bowel syndrome. JPEN 2014; 38(Supplement 1):53S–9S.

The Impact of Dietary Patterns and Nutrition in Nonalcoholic Fatty Liver Disease

Ahyoung Kim, MD, Arunkumar Krishnan, MBBS, James P. Hamilton, MD, Tinsay A. Woreta, MD, MPH*

KEYWORDS

- Nonalcoholic fatty liver disease • Diet • Macronutrients • Micronutrients • Nutrition
- Dietary recommendations

KEY POINTS

- Nonalcoholic fatty liver disease (NAFLD) is the leading cause of chronic liver disease worldwide. NAFLD is a spectrum of disease with clinical-histological phenotypes from nonalcoholic fatty liver (NAFL) to nonalcoholic steatohepatitis (NASH), which can progress to cirrhosis.
- The trends in NAFLD prevalence parallel the rising prevalence of obesity and metabolic syndrome, and the pathogenesis of NAFLD is complex, heterogeneous, and multifactorial.
- Dietary intervention is an effective treatment for NAFLD and remains the mainstay in the management. A 7% to 10% weight loss and its sustainability is the goal in patients with NAFLD.
- Current evidence suggests the importance of well-balanced specific dietary macronutrients and micronutrients that may help prevent the manifestation of processes involved in NAFLD pathogenesis and progression.
- A Mediterranean low-carbohydrate diet has been shown to be beneficial in reducing hepatic steatosis and is recommended as the first-line dietary intervention in individuals with NAFLD. In addition, caloric restriction has been found to be an essential component of dietary interventions for NAFLD.

INTRODUCTION

Nonalcoholic fatty liver disease (NAFLD) is one of the most common liver diseases in the world, affecting 25% to 30% of the global population and approximately one-third of the population in the United States.[1,2] NAFLD is defined as an excess accumulation of lipids within hepatocytes, detected either by histology or imaging, in the absence of excessive alcohol use or other causes of chronic liver disease.[3] These patients may

Division of Gastroenterology and Hepatology, Johns Hopkins University School of Medicine, Baltimore, MD, USA
* Corresponding author. 600 North Wolfe Street, Hal 407, Baltimore, MD 21287.
E-mail address: tworeta1@jhmi.edu

Gastroenterol Clin N Am 50 (2021) 217–241
https://doi.org/10.1016/j.gtc.2020.10.013
0889-8553/21/© 2020 Elsevier Inc. All rights reserved.

gastro.theclinics.com

present with hepatic steatosis observed on imaging studies and/or elevated liver enzymes with clinical features of metabolic syndrome, which includes prediabetes, type 2 diabetes mellitus (T2DM), hypertension, dyslipidemia, and central obesity.[1,4–7] NAFLD affects 15% of nonobese patients (body mass index [BMI] <30), 65% of obese patients (BMI 30–39), and 85% of extremely obese patients (BMI ≥40).[8] However, considerable numbers of lean individuals with NAFLD have also been reported in the literature.[9–11] The prevalence was initially described in Asian populations, and studies in Western countries show that NAFLD occurs in 7% to 9% of the lean population.[12,13] However, the pathophysiology of NAFLD in lean individuals remains poorly characterized.

NAFLD is histologically categorized as nonalcoholic fatty liver (NAFL) or nonalcoholic steatohepatitis (NASH).[4,7,14] This distinction can be made only with liver biopsy, the current gold standard for diagnosing NAFLD. NAFL is characterized by ≥5% hepatic steatosis without hepatocyte injury, whereas NASH is characterized by ≥5% hepatic steatosis with evidence of hepatocyte injury in the form hepatocyte ballooning, with or without the presence of fibrosis.[14] NASH is the most severe type of NAFLD and is more likely to progress to cirrhosis and its associated complications, including hepatocellular carcinoma.[4,6] NAFL progresses to cirrhosis in approximately 2% to 3% of individuals over 10 to 20 years, and NASH progresses to cirrhosis in 15% to 20% of persons over 10 to 20 years.[6,8]

The exact mechanism for the development of NAFLD is unclear, although the current evidence indicates that it is likely a complex interplay among neurohormones, intestinal dysbiosis, nutrition, and genetics.[15] Insulin resistance plays a key role in NAFLD pathophysiology. Insulin resistance causes increased adipocyte lipolysis, resulting in the circulation of more free fatty acids that are available for hepatic uptake. Gluconeogenesis is increased, and glycogen storage is reduced, often even with concomitant hyperglycemia. All these effects of insulin resistance result in increased free fatty acid accumulation in hepatocytes, exposing cells to the lipotoxic environment and downstream effects of impaired insulin signaling, oxidative damage, inflammation, and fibrosis.[15,16]

Obesity, insulin resistance, and T2DM are commonly found in patients with NAFLD.[15,17] The presence of metabolic syndrome, T2DM, persistently elevated aspartate aminotransferase (AST) and alanine aminotransferase (ALT) levels, increasing age, and BMI have also been well documented to correlate with the presence of NASH.[6] Given these risk factors in patients with NAFLD, the initial treatment often focuses on the treatment of obesity, insulin resistance, and metabolic syndrome. Lifestyle modifications such as weight loss, a healthy diet, and cardiovascular exercise are recommended as the first-line treatment.[14,18,19]

CURRENT GUIDELINES

Currently, there is no approved pharmacologic option for the treatment of NAFLD.[19,20] Current guidelines on NAFLD emphasize the importance of lifestyle modifications for all patients with NAFLD, given the strong evidence suggesting the correlation between unhealthy lifestyle and NAFLD. Weight loss is considered the most effective treatment of NAFLD.[21] Weight reduction of 7% to 10% body weight is associated with histologic improvement, resolution of liver fat, necroinflammation, and fibrosis. The American Association of the Study of Liver Diseases (AASLD) broadly outlines that increased physical activity and hypocaloric diet with weight loss are helpful in the NAFLD population.

Similarly, the European Association for the Study of the Liver (EASL) recommends the following: healthy diet and physical activity, 7% to 10% of weight loss in overweight/obese patients, energy restriction, avoidance of processed food and food/beverages high in fructose, and macronutrient components of a Mediterranean diet. Both guidelines recommend a "healthy diet" without suggesting one standardized diet, which leads to variability in the interpretation of this broad term. In addition, there is a scarcity of high-quality literature on the optimal diet for lean individuals with NAFLD. Lifestyle modification is also reportedly helpful in remission of steatosis among lean individuals in studies conducted in Asian populations.[22] This review focuses on the currently available data supporting the recommendations for macro and micronutrients in NAFLD.

MACRONUTRIENTS AND DIFFERENT DIET PATTERNS
Mediterranean Diet

The Mediterranean diet has been one of the most recommended diets for patients with NAFLD based on robust data supporting its role in the treatment of NAFLD.[20] It slightly varies between regions and cultures, but it generally consists of fresh vegetables, fruits, whole-grain cereals, legumes, olive oil, moderate intake of dairy products and wine, low intake of red and processed meats, and restricted intake of foods containing high amounts of added sugar.[2,21,23] The Mediterranean diet is known for its high content of antioxidants, fiber, and monosaturated fatty acids (MUFA)/balanced polyunsaturated fatty acids (PUFA), and low content of saturated fat/cholesterol and simple sugars.[7,21] This combination of factors results in antioxidant, anti-inflammatory, and antifibrotic effects, decreased oxidative stress and cytokine expression, and prevention of cell injury. Clinically, the Mediterranean diet modulates visceral obesity, insulin resistance, dyslipidemia, chronic inflammation, hepatic steatosis, and elevation of AST/ALT.[21,24]

Several cross-sectional studies suggest the beneficial effects of the Mediterranean diet on NAFLD and are summarized in **Table 1**. Kontogianni and colleagues[25] first described the association between the Mediterranean diet and NAFLD in a cross-sectional study. Seventy-three adults with NAFLD were instructed to follow the Mediterranean diet, and their adherence to the Mediterranean diet was measured by MedDietScore. The investigators concluded that better adherence to the Mediterranean diet improved ALT, insulin level, insulin resistance index, and the severity of hepatic steatosis. A 1-unit increase in MedDietScore was associated with a 36% lower likelihood of having NASH.[25] Similarly, Aller and colleagues[26] conducted a cross-sectional study on 82 patients with biopsy-proven NAFLD and showed that greater adherence to the Mediterranean diet as assessed by a 14-item Mediterranean Diet Assessment Tool score was significantly associated with less steatosis and steatohepatitis on histology along with a lower degree of insulin resistance. In a study involving 532 patients with NAFLD diagnosed by ultrasound and 667 patients without NAFLD, Trovato and colleagues[27] demonstrated that a poorer adherence to the Mediterranean diet profile strongly predicted the occurrence of NAFLD independent of the overweight/obesity status. Baratta and colleagues[23] assessed hepatic steatosis and dietary habits in 584 outpatients with 1 or more cardiovascular risk factors (T2DM, arterial hypertension, overweight/obesity, dyslipidemia) and found an inverse relationship between adherence to the Mediterranean diet and prevalence of NAFLD. On a larger scale, a cross-sectional analysis of data from 2 population-based adult cohorts, one from England (n = 9645) and the other from Switzerland (n = 3957), showed that greater adherence to the diet as assessed by Mediterranean diet scores was

Table 1
Mediterranean diet studies (cross-sectional studies)

Authors	Study Type	Number of Patients	Intervention	Control	Results	Limitations
Kontogianni et al,[25] 2014	Cross-sectional analysis	73 patients with NAFLD (34 with liver biopsies)	Mediterranean Diet Score (MedDietScore) was calculated from food frequency questionnaire	No	MedDietScore was negatively correlated with ALT, insulin levels, insulin resistance index, and severity of steatosis.	• No control • Observational study • Not all patients had a liver biopsy
Aller et al,[26] 2015	Cross-sectional analysis	82 biopsy-proven patients with NAFLD	14-item Mediterranean Diet Assessment Tool	No	Greater adherence to the Mediterranean diet was significantly associated with less steatosis and steatohepatitis.	• No control • Observational study
Trovato et al[27] 2016	Cross-sectional analysis	532 patients with NAFLD and 667 non-NAFLD patients	Baecke questionnaire: 1 wk recall computerized questionnaire including physical activity	Yes	Poorer adherence to the Mediterranean diet profile strongly predicted the occurrence of NAFLD.	• Observational study • Reliance on recall for questionnaire • Lack of histology for NAFLD diagnosis
Baratta et al,[23] 2017	Cross-sectional analysis	584 patients with 1 or more cardio-vascular risk factors (T2DM, arterial hypertension, overweight/obesity, dyslipidemia)	Short 9-item validated dietary questionnaire	No	There was an inverse relationship between adherence to the Mediterranean diet and prevalence of NAFLD.	• Observational study • Lack of histology for NAFLD diagnosis
Khalatbari-Soltani et al,[24] 2019	Cross-sectional analysis	9645 patients in England cohort and 3957 patients in Switzerland cohort	Cohort-specific food frequency questionnaire	No	Greater adherence to the Mediterranean diet was associated with a lower prevalence of hepatic steatosis.	• Lack of histology for NAFLD diagnosis

Abbreviations: ALT, alanine aminotransferase; NAFLD, nonalcoholic liver disease; T2DM, type 2 diabetes mellitus.

associated with a lower prevalence of hepatic steatosis. The presence of hepatic steatosis was determined by ultrasound and fatty liver index (FLI) in the England cohort and FLI and NAFLD liver fat score in the Switzerland cohort.[24] FLI is a score calculated using BMI, waist circumference, triglyceride, and gamma-glutamyl transferase (GGT). NAFLD liver fat score is an algorithm including the presence of metabolic syndrome, presence of T2DM, fasting insulin, AST, and ALT ratio.

There are multiple longitudinal studies demonstrating the effect of the Mediterranean diet in patients with NAFLD (**Table 2**). In a 6-week crossover study of patients with biopsy-proven NAFLD, a Mediterranean diet high in MUFA effectively reduced hepatic steatosis when compared with an isocaloric low-fat, high-carbohydrate diet.[3] Twelve patients who participated in this study showed a reduction in hepatic steatosis on nuclear magnetic resonance (NMR) spectroscopy, improved peripheral insulin sensitivity, and reduced circulating insulin concentrations even without weight loss.[3] In another study, 28 overweight and obese patients with ultrasonography-proven NAFLD and abnormal liver enzymes were randomly assigned to the Mediterranean diet group and control group. Their level of adherence to the Mediterranean diet was assessed by the MedDietScore. Although there was no evaluation of hepatic steatosis at the end of the 6-month study period, body weight, BMI, waist circumference, Homeostatic Model Assessment of Insulin Resistance (HOMA-IR), and ALT were all significantly reduced.[28] The same group of investigators conducted a single-blinded, randomized, controlled, clinical trial on 63 overweight/obese patients with NAFLD; these patients were assigned to a control group, Mediterranean diet group, and Mediterranean lifestyle group for 6 months.[29] Both the Mediterranean diet group and the Mediterranean lifestyle group received nutritional counseling, whereas only the Mediterranean lifestyle group received counseling on physical activity. At the end of the study period, patients in both the Mediterranean diet group and Mediterranean lifestyle group showed a significant improvement in liver stiffness as measured by elastography.[29] Trovato and colleagues[30] studied the effect of Mediterranean diet intervention in 90 patients with nonalcoholic and nondiabetic hepatic steatosis diagnosed on ultrasonography. These patients with NAFLD showed a significant decrease in Bright Liver Score (a score measuring the severity of steatosis/echogenicity on ultrasonography) after 6 months of the Mediterranean diet. The differences at 1 month and 3 months were not significant, although there was still a significant decrease in BMI and HOMA-IR.[30] Misciagna and colleagues[31] randomized 98 patients with a moderate or severe ultrasound-diagnosed NAFLD into a low-glycemic Mediterranean diet and the healthy diet recommended by the World Health Organization (WHO). At 3 months and 6 months of evaluation, patients in the low-glycemic Mediterranean diet group showed a greater reduction in NAFLD score on ultrasonography and FLI. ALT decreased in both the low-glycemic Mediterranean diet and the healthy diet recommended by WHO, but the GGT level decreased only in the low-glycemic Mediterranean diet.[31] In a separate study, 46 adults with NAFLD received a clinical and dietary intervention in the form of a Mediterranean diet for 6 months. Steatosis grade ≥ 2 reduced from 93% to 48% of patients, whereas steatosis completely regressed in 20% of patients at the end of the study term; 7% weight reduction was achieved in 25 patients. There was a significant improvement in AST, ALT, GGT, BMI, and waist circumference. FLI, Kotronen score (used as a predictor of liver fat percentage), NAFLD liver fat score, and visceral adiposity index were all reduced as well.[32] Ma and colleagues[33] performed a prospective study on second-generation and third-generation cohorts of the Framingham Heart Study and showed that liver fat decreased by 0.57 for each standard deviation increase in Mediterranean-style diet

Table 2
Mediterranean diet studies (longitudinal studies)

Authors	Study Type	Number of Patients	Intervention	Diet Composition	Study Duration	Results	Limitations
Ryan et al.[3] 2013	Crossover randomized trial	12 nondiabetic with biopsy-proven NAFLD	Mediterranean diet vs control diet (low-fat–high-carbohydrate diet)	*Mediterranean diet:* 40% fat (MUFA and omega 3 PUFA), 40% carbohydrate, 20% protein. *Low-fat and high-carbohydrate diet:* 30% fat, 50% carbohydrate, 20% protein	6-wk intervention with the first diet followed by 6-wk washout period followed by 6-wk intervention with the second diet	Mediterranean diet resulted in a relative reduction in hepatic steatosis	• Sample size
Katsagoni et al, (abstract only)[28] 2016	Cohort	28 overweight/obese patients with NAFLD	Mediterranean diet group and control group	Mediterranean diet group attended intensive group counseling sessions. The control group was provided with relevant written recommendations.	6 mo	An increase in adherence to the Mediterranean diet and weight loss improved liver function in NAFLD.	• Full article not available • Details of intervention unknown • Compounded by weight loss

Katsagoni et al,[29] 2018	Randomized controlled trial	63 overweight/obese patients with NAFLD	Mediterranean diet group vs Mediterranean lifestyle group vs control group	All groups received instructions on energy restriction with carbohydrates 45%, protein 20%, lipids 35%, 1500 kcal for women and 1800 kcal for men. *Control group:* general written dietary guidelines. *Mediterranean diet group and Mediterranean lifestyle group:* 60-min small group sessions on the diet. *M lifestyle group:* additional guidance on physical activity and sleep habits.	6 mo	Mediterranean diet group and Mediterranean lifestyle group showed significant improvement in liver stiffness.	• Lack of histology for NAFLD diagnosis • Compounded by weight loss
Trovato et al,[30] 2015	Cohort	90 nondiabetic patients with NAFLD	All patients received an intervention	Counseling intervention on diet and physical activity	6 mo	Adherence to the Mediterranean diet significantly improved Bright Liver Score.	• No control • Lack of histology for NAFLD diagnosis

(continued on next page)

Table 2
(continued)

Authors	Study Type	Number of Patients	Intervention	Diet Composition	Study Duration	Results	Limitations
Misciagna et al,[31] 2017	Randomized controlled trial	98 patients with moderate to severe NAFLD	Low–Glycemic Index Mediterranean diet (n = 50) vs control diet (n = 48)	*Control:* recommended by the World Health Organization and followed by INRAN. *Low-glycemic M diet:* 10% of total daily calories from saturated fats, high in MUFA from olive oil and containing omega-3 PUFA from plant and marine sources	6 mo	Low–Glycemic Index Mediterranean Diet decreased NAFLD score	• Lack of histology for NAFLD diagnosis
Gelli et al,[32] 2017	Observational	46 patients with NAFLD	All patients received clinical and nutritional counseling	*M diet:* low to moderate amounts of wine, 55%–60% of carbohydrates (80% complex carbohydrates), 10%–15% of proteins about 60% of animal origin, 25%–30% fat	6 mo	MedDietScore was significantly and inversely correlated with steatosis grade.	• No control • Lack of histology for NAFLD diagnosis • Compounded by weight loss

| Ma et al,[33] 2018 | Cohort | 1521 patients with NAFLD | All patients completed the questionnaire | Validated, self-administered semiquantitative 126-item Harvard food frequency questionnaire | Average follow-up of 6 y | Improved diet quality was associated with reduced liver fat accumulation. | • No control
• Lack of histology for NAFLD diagnosis
• Reliance on recall for questionnaire |

Abbreviations: INRAN, Istituto Nazionale di Ricerca per gli Alimenti e la Nutrizione (Italian:National Institute of Research on Foods and Nutrition); MUFA, mono-saturated fatty acid; NAFLD, nonalcoholic liver disease; PUFA, polyunsaturated fatty acid.

score. In summary, all studies on the Mediterranean diet and NAFLD suggest that the Mediterranean diet improves hepatic steatosis (see **Table 2**).

Monounsaturated fatty acids/Polyunsaturated fatty acids

MUFA and PUFA are essential components of the Mediterranean diet. Hazelnuts, macadamia nuts, pecans, and pistachios are high in MUFA, whereas walnuts, flax-seed, and soybeans are high in PUFA.[34] Several studies have specifically assessed the effect of these components in patients with NAFLD. In a factorial 2 × 2 randomized parallel-group design, 37 men and 8 women with T2DM were assigned to 8 weeks of isocaloric diets (high-carbohydrate/high-fiber/low–glycemic index diet vs high-MUFA diet vs high-carbohydrate/high-fiber/low–glycemic index diet plus physical activity vs high MUFA diet plus physical activity). The investigators noted a greater decrease in hepatic steatosis in MUFA diet groups compared with a high-carbohydrate diet group with or without exercise. Liver fat content measured by ^{1}H NMR spectrometry was significantly decreased in the MUFA group with and without exercise.[35] Similarly, adherence to a Mediterranean diet supplemented with extra virgin olive oil (a form of MUFA) showed reduced prevalence of hepatic steatosis among older individuals at high cardiovascular risk. The follow-up period was an average of 3 years in this study. No recommendations were made regarding physical activity or weight loss. The patients following a Mediterranean diet supplemented with extra virgin olive oil showed a trend toward lower liver fat as determined by NMR spectrometry without changes in adiposity, energy expenditure, or macronutrient intake during follow-up.[36] In a study by Capanni and colleagues,[37] 42 patients with NAFLD consumed n-3 PUFA 1-g capsules daily for 12 months. PUFA supplementation significantly decreased serum AST, ALT, GGT, transpeptidase, triglycerides, and fasting glucose. Ultrasonography showed an improvement in liver echotexture and an increase of Doppler perfusion index after PUFA supplementation. No significant changes were observed in the control group.[37] Spadaro and colleagues[38] studied 40 patients with NAFLD who were randomized into 2 groups: one group received the American Heart Association (AHA) recommended diet and PUFA 2 g/d, and the other group received only the AHA regular diet. Fatty liver was assessed by abdominal ultrasound. After 6 months of intervention, the PUFA group showed a decrease in ALT and HOMA-IR. Complete fatty liver regression was observed in 33.4%, and an overall reduction of hepatic steatosis was observed in 50% in the PUFA group. There was no regression of hepatic steatosis in the AHA diet alone group.[38] In a randomized controlled trial by Zhu and colleagues,[39] Group A received recommended diet and 2 g n-3 PUFA from seal oils 3 times daily, and Group B received recommended diet and 2 g placebo 3 times daily. The recommended diet was composed of 50% carbohydrate, 20% protein, and 30% fat. Hepatic steatosis was assessed by ultrasound. In Group A, complete fatty liver regression was observed in 19.70%, and an overall reduction was observed in 53.03%. In Group B, complete regression was observed in only 7.35%, and some improvement of fatty liver was observed in 35.29%.[39] A synthetic form of PUFA, ethyl-eicosapentaenoic acid (EPA-E), has also been studied in a phase 2 trial. Thirty-seven sites in North America included patients with NASH and NAFLD activity scores ≥4, with minimum scores of 1 for steatosis and inflammation, along with either ballooning or at least stage 1a fibrosis. A total of 243 subjects were randomly assigned to groups given a placebo, low dose EPA-E (1800 mg/d), or high dose EPA-E (2700 mg/d) for 12 months. Interestingly, EPA-E had no significant effects on steatosis, inflammation, ballooning, or fibrosis score.[40] The current data on MUFA and PUFA appear beneficial for patients with NAFLD but are inconclusive.

Mediterranean diet recommendations

- Moderate to high carbohydrate intake (45%–65% of total daily calories; high preference for whole grains and low–glycemic index foods)[2]
- Low to moderate fat intake (<30–35% of total calories with a low proportion of saturated and trans-fat and a higher proportion of MUFA and omega-3 PUFAs)
- Protein intake (15%–20% of total daily calories with minimization of red meat intake and increased consumption of poultry, fish, low-fat or nonfat dairy products)
- A blend of vegetable protein sources
- Increased consumption of fruits and vegetables
- Prebiotic fiber

Carbohydrate-Restricted Diet

Carbohydrate-restricted diet has been described to decrease hepatic steatosis.[6] In a study by Browning and colleagues,[41] 18 patients were assigned to a calorie-restricted diet (1200–1500 kcal/d) or carbohydrate-restricted diet (<20 g/d) without calorie restriction for 2 weeks. Intrahepatic triglyceride was measured by magnetic resonance spectroscopy. At the end of the study period, the patients on the carbohydrate-restricted diet showed a rapid decrease of intrahepatic triglyceride content by approximately 42% after 4.3% weight loss.[41] The degree of reduction of intrahepatic triglycerides was more significant in patients on the carbohydrate-restricted diet compared with patients on the calorie-restricted diet, despite the similar weight loss achieved in both groups.[41] Tendler and colleagues[42] conducted a pilot study to assess the effect of low-carbohydrate and ketogenic diet on obesity associated with fatty liver disease. Five patients with a mean BMI of 36.4 kg/m^2 and biopsy-proven fatty liver were instructed to follow the prescribed diet (<20 g/d carbohydrate) with nutritional supplementation for 6 months. The patients were allowed unlimited amounts of meats, unlimited eggs, cheese (up to 4 oz/d), salad vegetables (2 cups/d), and low-carbohydrate vegetables (1 cup/d). There was no limit on the caloric intake. At the end of the study period, 4 of 5 posttreatment liver biopsies showed histologic improvements in steatosis, inflammatory grade, and fibrosis.[42]

More recently, a study by Gepner and colleagues[43] showed that a Mediterranean low-carbohydrate diet reduced the hepatic fat content more effectively than the low-fat diet. A total of 278 patients were included in the study with diet intervention for 18 months. The patients in the Mediterranean low-carbohydrate diet had a significantly more decrease in hepatic fat content as determined by MRI even after controlling for visceral adipose tissue loss. As outlined previously, current studies on a carbohydrate-restricted diet are small in number but are suggestive of positive effects in patients with NAFLD (**Table 3**).

Carbohydrate diet recommendation

- Limit carbohydrate consumption to less than 20 g/d

Calorie-Restricted Diet

On the other hand, several studies have illustrated that macronutrient composition may not be as pivotal as a total caloric restriction in the management of patients with NAFLD. Twenty-two obese patients with BMI greater than 35 were randomized to low-fat and high-carbohydrate (>180 g/d) diet or low-fat and low-carbohydrate (<50 g/d) diet for 3 months.[44] All patients in this study were calorie restricted. Within 48 hours of the study, intrahepatic triglyceride content decreased by 30% in the

Table 3
Carbohydrate-restricted diet studies

Authors	Study Type	Number of Patients	Intervention	Diet Composition	Duration	Results	Limitations
Browning et al,[41] 2011	Randomized controlled trial	18 patients with NAFLD	Carbohydrate-restricted diet vs calorie-restricted diet	*Carbohydrate-restricted diet:* limit carbohydrate intake to <20 g/d. *Calorie-restricted diet:* reduced energy to ~1200 kcal/d for women and ~1500 kcal/d for men	2 wk	Reductions of hepatic triglycerides were significantly higher in carbohydrate-restricted groups than the calorie-restricted group.	• No control • Lack of histology for NAFLD diagnosis
Tendler et al,[42] 2007	Single-arm clinical pilot trial	5 patients with biopsy-proven NAFLD	All patients received a dietary intervention	*Low-carbohydrate ketogenic diet:* <20 g/d carbohydrate, unlimited amounts of meats, unlimited eggs, cheese (4 oz/d), salad vegetables (2 cups/d) and low-carbohydrate vegetables (1 cup/d). No predetermined limit on the amount of caloric intake.	6 mo	There was a significant improvement in liver histology after dietary intervention.	• No control • Small sample size
Gepner et al,[43] 2019	Randomized controlled trial	278 patients with abdominal obesity/dyslipidemia	Low-fat diet vs Mediterranean diet/low-carbohydrate diet with or without physical activity	*Low-fat diet:* total fat 30% of calories (≤10% of saturated fat), ≤300 mg/d of cholesterol, increase dietary fiber. *Mediterranean low-carbohydrate diet:* <40 g/d in the first 2 mo, and gradual increase up to 70 g/d, increase protein and fat intake + 28 g of walnuts/d starting from the third month.	18 mo	Mediterranean diet/low-carbohydrate diet showed a more significant decrease in hepatic steatosis than a low-fat diet.	• A small number of women (12%) • Lack of histology for NAFLD diagnosis

Abbreviation: NAFLD, nonalcoholic liver disease.

low-carbohydrate group compared with 10% in the high-carbohydrate group. Interestingly, the patients in both groups achieved a 7% weight loss and reduced intrahepatic fat content similarly by 40% after approximately 11 weeks of intervention. Other parameters, such as AST and ALT, did not significantly change after 48 hours or 11 weeks in both groups.[44] A separate study of 170 obese patients with BMI greater than 30 were randomized to reduced carbohydrate or reduced-fat diet for 6 months. All patients had a total energy-restricted diet, which was defined as 30% less energy intake compared with before the study.[45] Intrahepatic fat content was assessed by magnetic resonance tomography. All patients, regardless of their assigned diet group and their initial intrahepatic fat content, showed a similar decrease in intrahepatic lipid content.[45] Thirty-one patients with NAFLD received a diet that is 500 to 1000 kcal/d less compared with their baseline diet, with 15% protein, 55% carbohydrates, and 30% fat for 6 months.[46] Adherence to the prescribed diet was determined by weight loss of at least 5%. At the end of the study period, the patients who were adherent to the prescribed diet showed a decrease in ALT and an improvement of hepatic fat on follow-up computed tomography.[46] Similarly, 12 patients with NAFLD received a diet intervention that restricted energy, fat, and iron intake. All patients under the intervention arm decreased their energy intake from 150 kJ/kg per day to 104 kJ/kg per day and lost, on average, 3 kg over a 6-month period. AST and ALT significantly improved at the end of the study.[47] Although AST and ALT could be used as the surrogate markers for inflammation in the liver, neither liver biopsy nor imaging study was completed to confirm the reduction in hepatic steatosis or steatohepatitis after the intervention.

Jin and colleagues[48] evaluated the efficacy of dietary modification with caloric restriction and exercise on the degree of steatosis in a study of 1365 patients with nonobese NAFLD. After lifestyle modification, they found an 86% improvement in the degree of steatosis at the time of follow-up biopsy. On multivariate analysis, weight reduction of $\geq$5%, higher baseline steatosis, and total cholesterol reduction of $\geq$10% were significantly associated with steatosis improvement in nonobese patients with NAFLD.[48] One proposed mechanism for this finding was that reduction in weight in nonobese patients with NAFLD resulted in a reduction of body fat, especially visceral fat, although body composition was not reported in this study. Similarly, Wong and colleagues[22] conducted a single-blind randomized controlled trial comparing a community-based lifestyle intervention consisting of caloric restriction and exercise to standard care in patients with NAFLD. A total of 154 patients with NAFLD were randomized to receive lifestyle intervention (n = 77) or standard care (n = 77). The diagnosis of fatty liver was made using proton-magnetic resonance spectroscopy and transient elastography. The investigators found that the reduction in body weight and waist circumference predicted remission of NAFLD in nonobese patients. The degree of weight reduction further correlated with NAFLD remission in a dose-dependent manner. Importantly, although all nonobese patients achieved remission of NAFLD with $\geq$10% weight reduction, 70% of those with 5% to 10% weight reduction also achieved remission of NAFLD. The proportion of nonobese patients achieving remission of NAFLD with modest weight reduction was higher than that in obese patients.[22] These studies suggest that weight loss can be particularly helpful in a subset of lean patients with NAFLD, particularly in those with visceral obesity.

A study of 8 patients with T2DM studied the effect of a weight-reduction diet (50% carbohydrate, 43% protein, 3% fat, 12 g fiber) that was supplemented with fruits and vegetables to a total of approximately 1200 kcal/d.[49] These patients had an average of 8 kg weight loss or an average of 8% of their body weight loss over an average of 7-

Table 4
Calorie-restricted diet studies

Authors	Study Type	Number of Patients	Intervention	Diet Composition	Duration	Results	Limitations
Kirk et al,[44] 2009	Randomized controlled trial	22 obese patients	High-carbohydrate diet vs low-carbohydrate diet	Average total daily energy intake ~1100 kcal. *High-carbohydrate diet:* ≥180 g carbohydrates/d and ~65% of total daily energy intake as carbohydrates, 20% as fat, and 15% as protein *Low-carbohydrate diet:* ≤50 g carbohydrates/d and ~10% of daily energy intake as carbohydrates, 75% as fat, 15% as protein	11 wk	Both groups achieved similar rates of weight loss and reduction in intrahepatic fat content.	• No control • Lack of histology for NAFLD diagnosis
Haufe et al,[45] 2011	Randomized controlled trial	170 overweight and obese patients	Hypocaloric diet: reduced carbohydrate diet vs reduced-fat diet	All patients, regardless of their assigned group, had a hypocaloric diet that was 30% less in total energy (minimum 1200 kcal/d). *Reduced carbohydrate group:* ≤90g carbohydrates, 0.8 g protein/kg body weight, minimum of 30% fat *Reduced-fat group:* fat content ≤20% of total energy intake, 0.8 g protein/kg body weight, remaining energy by carbohydrates	6 mo	Intrahepatic lipid content decreased similarly in both diet groups.	• Lack of histology for NAFLD diagnosis
Elias et al,[46] 2010	Cohort	31 patients with NAFLD	All patients received a dietary intervention	Diet with a reduction of 500–1000 kcal/d containing 15% protein, 55% carbohydrates, 30% fat	6 mo	Adherence to the prescribed diet showed improvement in hepatic fat content.	• Lack of histology for NAFLD diagnosis

| Yamamoto et al,[47] 2007 | Randomized controlled trial | 27 patients with NAFLD | Diet group (n = 12) vs follow-up group (n = 10) | *Diet group:* 126 kJ/kg/d, fat energy fraction 20%, ≤6 mg/d iron, 1.1–1.2 g/kg/d protein. *Follow-up group:* no specific treatment was administered | 6 mo | AST and ALT were significantly decreased in the diet group | • AST/ALT as surrogates for hepatic steatosis at the end of the study |
| Petersen et al,[49] 2005 | Cohort - prospective | 8 obese diabetic patients | All patients received a dietary intervention | Isocaloric diet of 35 kcal/kg; 60% carbohydrate, 20% protein, 20% fat | ~3 mo | An average of 8 kg weight loss or an average of 8% body weight loss was associated with a reduction in intrahepatic lipid. | • Lack of histology for NAFLD diagnosis |

Abbreviations: ALT, alanine aminotransferase; AST, aspartate aminotransferase; NAFLD, nonalcoholic liver disease.

week period, which was associated with 81% reduction in intrahepatic lipid as assessed on NMR.[49]

All these studies suggest that calorie restriction is a key component of the dietary recommendations for patients with NAFLD[45,50] (**Table 4**).

Calorie-restricted diet recommendation

- Restrict caloric intake to 1100 to 1200 kcal/d minimum or reduce the total caloric intake by 500 to 1000 kcal/d.

Vegetarian Diet

Vegetarian diets have been shown to be protective against metabolic diseases, but the data for NAFLD are conflicting. Chiu and colleagues[51] conducted a cross-sectional study, including 2127 nonvegetarians and 1273 vegetarians. Fatty liver and fibrosis were determined using ultrasonography and NAFLD fibrosis score. Diet was assessed using a validated food frequency questionnaire. The investigators concluded that the vegetarian diet was associated with lower odds of fatty liver, although the effect was attenuated after adjusting for BMI. The vegetarians also had less severe fibrosis and NAFLD.[51]

On the other hand, Choi and colleagues[52] conducted a cross-sectional, retrospective study demonstrating that the vegetarian diet does not confer protection against NAFLD. They studied 615 Buddhist priests who strictly followed a vegetarian diet and 615 age-matched and gender-matched controls who did not follow a vegetarian diet. The diagnosis of fatty liver was made by abdominal ultrasonography. At the end of the study, the investigators found that the prevalence of NAFLD was not statistically different between the 2 groups (29.9% vs 25.05%). The Buddhist group also had higher serum AST, ALT, and triglyceride levels.[52] The verdict on the effect of a vegetarian diet on NAFLD is yet to be determined.

Dark Chocolate

Dark chocolate consumption is associated with lowering lipid peroxidation by inhibiting reactive oxygen species (ROS) and reducing downstream proinflammatory response. Loffredo and colleagues,[53] in a crossover trial, randomized 19 patients with NASH and 19 age, gender, BMI-matched controls to 20 g dark chocolate or milk chocolate twice a day for 2 weeks with a 1-week washout period in between. After dark chocolate consumption for 2 weeks, there was a significant reduction in serum levels of soluble nicotinamide adenine dinucleotide phosphate-oxidase 2 (NOX2) derivative peptide and serum isoprostanes, which are markers of oxidative and inflammatory signaling. The same effect was not observed after milk chocolate administration.[53] A follow-up study also concluded that the endothelial function improved after dark chocolate consumption, as assessed by flow-mediated dilation suggestive of a reduction in ROS production and proinflammatory response.[54] However, the markers studied by Loffredo and colleagues[54] are not liver-specific.[55] More studies assessing the effect of dark chocolate on hepatic steatosis are needed.

MICRONUTRIENTS

Micronutrients are required in minimal amounts to supplement a well-balanced macronutrient diet and have antioxidative and anti-inflammatory effects that may help in preventing the development of NAFLD.[56]

Vitamin E

Vitamin E is synthesized in vegetables and is mostly present in seeds, nuts, vegetable oils, green leafy vegetables, and fortified cereals.[57] It is a potent antioxidant and has been shown to suppress lipid peroxidation and oxidative stress while improving inflammation and fibrosis in patients with NASH.[58,59] In the landmark PIVENS (Pioglitazone vs Vitamin E vs Placebo for the Treatment of Non-diabetic patients with NASH) trial, high-dose vitamin E (800 IU/d) reduced hepatocyte ballooning and lobular inflammation and facilitated the resolution of NASH when compared with pioglitazone and placebo supplementation (43% vs 34% vs 19%, respectively). There was no improvement in the liver fibrosis score.[60] In the Treatment of NAFLD in Children (TONIC) trial, vitamin E improved hepatocellular ballooning and resolved NASH more frequently compared with placebo.[61] Despite these positive effects of vitamin E, both the PIVENS and TONIC trials excluded patients with diabetes and cirrhosis. Therefore, the AASLD and EASL guidelines suggest vitamin E supplementation as an effective short-term treatment option for nondiabetic patients with biopsy-proven NASH. Recently, Bril and colleagues[62] found that vitamin E alone appeared to not be as effective in patients with T2DM, as it failed to meet the primary outcome of a 2-point reduction in the NAFLD activity score from 2 different parameters, without worsening of fibrosis. However, when vitamin E was combined with pioglitazone, more patients on combination therapy achieved the primary outcome versus placebo (54% vs 19%, P = .003), although the efficacy did not seem to be greater than that with pioglitazone alone observed in previous trials (143, 148). Resolution of NASH occurred in both groups compared with placebo (combination group: 43% vs 12%, P = .005; vitamin E alone: 33% vs 12%, P = .04).[62]

Further confirmatory trials are necessary to assess the effectiveness and safety of vitamin E in NAFLD, especially in populations with diabetes and cirrhosis.

Vitamin C

Vitamin C is an antioxidant that has a central role in the prevention of oxidative stress. A cross-sectional study of 3471 patients revealed an inverse association between ultrasound-diagnosed NAFLD and dietary vitamin C intake.[63] Vitamin C deficiency has also been associated with reduced activity of various antioxidant enzymes leading to increased oxidative stress, which may play an essential role in NAFLD.[64] However, the effect of vitamin C supplementation on the treatment of NAFLD remains to be further elucidated.

Vitamin D

Vitamin D is a fat-soluble vitamin with anti-inflammatory and antifibrotic properties.[65,66] The active form vitamin D is 1,25-dihydroxy vitamin D, which is derived from either vitamin D2 (ergocalciferol, acquired through dietary sources such as dairy products, fish, and fish oils) or vitamin D3 (cholecalciferol; acquired through sun exposure). A meta-analysis showed patients with NAFLD were 26% more likely to present vitamin D deficit than controls.[67] In animal models, vitamin D supplementation showed improvements in insulin sensitivity and anti-inflammatory effects in the liver.[68] A large study from the NASH Clinical Research Network group reported that vitamin D deficiency was associated with histologic severity of NAFLD, definitive diagnosis of NASH, increased lobular inflammation and ballooning, and the presence of fibrosis independent of BMI or metabolic syndrome.[69] However, the supplementation of high-dose vitamin D (cholecalciferol 2000 IU/d) did not improve hepatic steatosis, liver enzymes, or insulin resistance in patients with NAFLD with T2DM.[70] Further clinical studies are needed to evaluate the association of vitamin D and NAFLD.

Probiotics

Probiotics are live bacteria or yeast with the capacity of conferring a health benefit on the host by regulating intestinal microbial flora. The changes in the intestinal microbiome can contribute to the pathogenesis of obesity and NAFLD/NASH.[71] In NAFLD, the intestinal microbiome enhances the intestinal permeability by direct activation of inflammatory cytokines via the release of lipopolysaccharide (LPS), which favors the absorption of endotoxins and production of endogenous ethanol.[72–74] Gut-derived LPS may cross intestinal tight junctions inducing liver injury through Kupffer cell activation, thus contributing to the onset of liver fibrosis.[75,76] Therefore, gut microbiota may play a significant role in the development of NAFLD and NASH.

Probiotics have multiple clinical properties that include improvement of serum ALT, lipid levels, hepatic steatosis, inflammation, liver fibrosis, oxidative stress, and insulin resistance.[75–78] In NAFLD animal models, probiotics have been shown to prevent liver fibrosis even in the absence of significant changes in inflammatory markers and in liver steatosis.[66] Paolella and colleagues[79] conducted a randomized controlled study to assess the role of probiotics in NAFLD and found that there were improvements in transaminases and hepatic steatosis. Aller and colleagues[80] investigated the impact of probiotics in patients with NAFLD in a randomized, double-blind, placebo-controlled trial and found that the administration of probiotics for 3 months showed a significant reduction in serum aminotransferases and GGT levels in patients with NAFLD. Eslamparast and colleagues[81] reported a study with a substantial improvement in ALT, AST, GGT, inflammatory markers, and liver stiffness assessed by transient elastography when lifestyle intervention was supplemented with a probiotic for 6 months. A recent meta-analysis of 1309 patients from 25 studies supported the potential use of microbial therapies, including prebiotics and probiotics, for NAFLD by demonstrating a significant reduction in BMI, liver enzymes, serum cholesterol, and triglycerides, although there was no change in inflammation.[82] Currently, there is insufficient evidence to recommend the use of probiotics in the treatment of NAFLD.

Coffee

Caffeine intake reduces inflammatory cytokines, alters adipose tissue gene expression, and reduces liver fat and collagen deposition. It has been shown to lower the risk of NAFLD.[83–85] Birerdinc and colleagues[86] conducted an observational study using the data from 4 continuous cycles of National Health and Nutrition Examination Surveys (NHANES 2001–2008), including 1782 patients with NAFLD and 16,768 control subjects. Multivariate analysis showed an inverse correlation between caffeine consumption and the prevalence of NAFLD, even after adjusting for race, gender, and metabolic syndrome. An extra cup of caffeine consumption was also shown to lower the odds of NAFLD.[86] In a cross-sectional study by Molloy and colleagues,[87] a total of 306 patients were categorized into ultrasonography-negative controls, patients with bland steatosis/not NASH, patients with NASH stage 0 to 1 fibrosis, and patients with NASH stage 2 to 4 fibrosis. Their caffeine consumption was studied via a validated caffeine questionnaire. This study concluded that there was a significant reduction in fibrosis risk among patients with NASH with coffee caffeine consumption.[87] Anty and colleagues[88] distributed a questionnaire specifically examining the various types of coffee, caffeinated drinks, and chocolate consumption among 195 severely obese patients undergoing bariatric surgery. The investigators found that regular coffee consumption, but not espresso consumption, was an independent protective factor against fibrosis, presence of NASH, presence of metabolic syndrome, and the level of HOMA-IR.[88] In a systemic review, coffee consumption was shown to be inversely related to the severity of steatohepatitis in patients with NAFLD. There was also a decreased risk of progression to cirrhosis, lowered mortality rate in cirrhotic patients, and a reduced rate of hepatocellular carcinoma development.[89] Further longitudinal studies are needed to confirm these effects and determine the quantity associated with histologic improvements in NAFLD.

Limitations

Although the studies assessing the association between NAFLD and dietary modification exist, it is challenging to draw a definitive conclusion regarding the optimal diet for patients with NAFLD given the heterogeneity of studies. Mediterranean diet, low-carbohydrate diet, and low-calorie diet are much-generalized umbrella terms. The dietary intervention used in each study was slightly different. The sample size and study population varied widely among studies. The sample size calculation was often not clearly explained or included in smaller studies. Some studies were observational studies without control groups. Body composition was not reported in many studies, which is important in understanding the mechanism by which dietary modification may benefit lean individuals with NAFLD. Hepatic steatosis, the hallmark that defines NAFLD, was also measured in different ways. Some studies used AST/ALT as the proxy of hepatic steatosis and steatohepatitis, whereas some other studies used imaging studies, such as ultrasound or MRI, to assess the NAFLD status. None of these methods has a 100% sensitivity or specificity, leaving room for overestimating or underestimating the effect of the studied dietary intervention. Liver biopsy is the gold standard for diagnosing NAFLD because some of these other methods cannot truly assess the presence of steatohepatitis and fibrosis, and it was not consistently performed in most studies. Ultimately, liver fibrosis stage is an important clinical outcome, as it is directly related to mortality in patients with NAFLD. Finally, the long-term (>5 years) effect of these dietary interventions is not known. Current studies on nutrition for patients with NAFLD included in this review were limited by nonstandardization of diets, heterogeneous study population, and the lack of histopathology before and after the study intervention.[21] More rigorous and long-term trials are needed in this field to determine the optimal diet for patients with NAFLD and provide more-specific dietary recommendations to patients with NAFLD in guidelines and clinical practice.

SUMMARY

In summary, NAFLD is a significant global health burden, which remains inadequately understood. It is a complex disease with increasing prevalence, and evidence suggests that healthy dietary modifications can improve NAFLD. However, the ability to give specific nutritional recommendations is limited at this time, given the heterogeneity of the available studies. Currently there is no effective medical treatment for the disease. Thus, nutritional intervention is key in the treatment for NAFLD, and it is a preventive measure for the associated diseases and resulting complications. The Mediterranean diet has the most evidence advocating for its role in NAFLD and perhaps should be recommended as the first-line dietary intervention. In addition, carbohydrate restriction, calorie restriction by at least 30% or by 500 to 1000 kcal/d (approximately 1200–1500 kcal/d for individuals <115 kg and approximately 1500–1800 kcal/d for individuals >115 kg), and weight loss should also be recommended.[6,14] Additional benefits of the low-carbohydrate diet include improved diabetes control, increase in insulin sensitivity, reduction in triglycerides, and increase in high-density lipoprotein cholesterol. Furthermore, a low-carbohydrate diet may be as effective as a calorie-restricted Mediterranean diet in improving NAFLD in patients with diabetes, and may be beneficial for individuals who cannot exercise. Based on the current evidence, reduced intake of carbohydrates and saturated and trans-fatty acids, and increased intake of PUFAs, MUFAs, antioxidants, and other micronutrients are beneficial. Weight loss remains the backbone of therapy in all patients with NAFLD and overweight/obesity, but regular physical activity should also be emphasized in patients with NAFLD who are lean.

Attaining macronutrient and micronutrient balance will be fundamental to improving diets that promote weight loss and can be a successful treatment option for patients with NAFLD. However, although weight loss can be an effective treatment for most patients, it is a challenging goal to achieve and maintain. Thus, additional interventions are also needed that are not entirely dependent on weight loss to obtain benefits on NAFLD pathogenesis and progression. Larger randomized controlled trials are required to investigate the precise macronutrient and micronutrient dietary compositions that will benefit individuals with NAFLD.

COMPETING INTERESTS

All authors declare no competing interests relevant to this article.

REFERENCES

1. Younossi ZM, Koenig AB, Abdelatif D, et al. Global epidemiology of nonalcoholic fatty liver disease—meta-analytic assessment of prevalence, incidence, and outcomes. Hepatology 2016;64(1):73–84.

2. Eslamparast T, Tandon P, Raman M. Dietary composition independent of weight loss in the management of non-alcoholic fatty liver disease. Nutrients 2017; 9(8):800.

3. Ryan MC, Itsiopoulos C, Thodis T, et al. The Mediterranean diet improves hepatic steatosis and insulin sensitivity in individuals with non-alcoholic fatty liver disease. J Hepatol 2013;59(1):138–43.

4. Matteoni CA, Younossi ZM, Gramlich T, et al. Nonalcoholic fatty liver disease: a spectrum of clinical and pathological severity. Gastroenterology 1999;116(6): 1413–9.

5. Ratziu V, Giral P, Charlotte F, et al. Liver fibrosis in overweight patients. Gastroenterology 2000;118(6):1117–23.

6. Rinella ME, Sanyal AJ. Management of NAFLD: a stage-based approach. Nat Rev Gastroenterol Hepatol 2016;13(4):196–205.

7. Suarez M, Boque N, Del Bas JM, et al. Mediterranean diet and multi-ingredient-based interventions for the management of non-alcoholic fatty liver disease. Nutrients 2017;9(10):1052. LID - E1052 [pii] LID - 10.3390/nu9101052 [doi]. (2072-6643 (Electronic)).

8. Schugar RC, Crawford PA. Low-carbohydrate ketogenic diets, glucose homeostasis, and nonalcoholic fatty liver disease. Curr Opin Clin Nutr Metab Care 2012;15(4):374–80.

9. Leung JCF, Loong TCW, Wei JL, et al. Histological severity and clinical outcomes of nonalcoholic fatty liver disease in nonobese patients. Hepatology 2017;65(1): 54–64.

10. Feng R-N, Du S-S, Wang C, et al. Lean-non-alcoholic fatty liver disease increases risk for metabolic disorders in a normal weight Chinese population. World J Gastroenterol 2014;20(47):17932.

11. Akyuz U, Yesil A, Yilmaz Y. Characterization of lean patients with nonalcoholic fatty liver disease: potential role of high hemoglobin levels. Scand J Gastroenterol 2015;50(3):341–6.

12. Browning JD, Szczepaniak LS, Dobbins R, et al. Prevalence of hepatic steatosis in an urban population in the United States: impact of ethnicity. Hepatology 2004; 40(6):1387–95.

13. Younossi ZM, Stepanova M, Negro F, et al. Nonalcoholic fatty liver disease in lean individuals in the United States. Medicine 2012;91(6):319–27.

14. Chalasani N, Younossi Z, Lavine JE, et al. The diagnosis and management of nonalcoholic fatty liver disease: practice guidance from the American Association for the Study of Liver Diseases. Hepatology 2018;67(1):328–57.

15. Carr RM, Oranu A, Khungar V. Nonalcoholic fatty liver disease: pathophysiology and management. Gastroenterol Clin North Am 2016;45(4):639–52.

16. Petta S, Gastaldelli A, Rebelos E, et al. Pathophysiology of non alcoholic fatty liver disease. Int J Mol Sci 2016;17(12):2082.

17. Haas JT, Francque S, Staels B. Pathophysiology and mechanisms of nonalcoholic fatty liver disease. Annu Rev Physiol 2016;78:181–205.

18. Thoma C, Day CP, Trenell MI. Lifestyle interventions for the treatment of non-alcoholic fatty liver disease in adults: a systematic review. J Hepatol 2012; 56(1):255–66.

19. Noureddin M, Anstee QM, Loomba R. Review article: emerging anti-fibrotic therapies in the treatment of non-alcoholic steatohepatitis. Aliment Pharmacol Ther 2016;43(11):1109–23.

20. European Association for the Study of the Liver (EASL); European Association for the Study of Diabetes (EASD); European Association for the Study of Obesity (EASO). EASL–EASD–EASO clinical practice guidelines for the management of non-alcoholic fatty liver disease. J Hepatol 2015;64(6):1388–402.

21. Anania C, Perla FM, Olivero F, et al. Mediterranean diet and nonalcoholic fatty liver disease. World J Gastroenterol 2018;24(19):2083–94.

22. Wong VW-S, Wong GL-H, Chan RS-M, et al. Beneficial effects of lifestyle intervention in non-obese patients with non-alcoholic fatty liver disease. J Hepatol 2018; 69(6):1349–56.

23. Baratta F, Pastori D, Polimeni L, et al. Adherence to Mediterranean diet and non-alcoholic fatty liver disease: effect on insulin resistance. Am J Gastroenterol 2017; 112(12):1832–9.

24. Khalatbari-Soltani S, Imamura F, Brage S, et al. The association between adherence to the Mediterranean diet and hepatic steatosis: cross-sectional analysis of two independent studies, the UK fenland study and the swiss colaus study. BMC Med 2019;17(1):19.

25. Kontogianni MD, Tileli N, Margariti A, et al. Adherence to the Mediterranean diet is associated with the severity of non-alcoholic fatty liver disease. Clin Nutr 2014; 33(4):678–83.

26. Aller R, Izaola O, de la Fuente B, et al. Mediterranean diet is associated with liver histology in patients with non alcoholic fatty liver disease. Nutr Hosp 2015;32(6): 2518–24.

27. Trovato FM, Martines GF, Brischetto D, et al. Neglected features of lifestyle: their relevance in non-alcoholic fatty liver disease. World J Hepatol 2016;8(33):1459.

28. Katsagoni CN, Egkomiti A, Papageorgiou M, et al. Improvement in liver function after an intervention based on the Mediterranean diet in patients with non alcoholic fatty liver disease (NAFLD). 2016;13:e57. https://doi.org/10.1016/j.clnesp.2016.03.012.

29. Katsagoni CN, Papatheodoridis GV, Ioannidou P, et al. Improvements in clinical characteristics of patients with non-alcoholic fatty liver disease, after an intervention based on the Mediterranean lifestyle: a randomised controlled clinical trial. Br J Nutr 2018;120(2):164–75.

30. Trovato FM, Catalano D, Martines GF, et al. Mediterranean diet and non-alcoholic fatty liver disease: the need of extended and comprehensive interventions. Clin Nutr 2015;34(1):86–8.

31. Misciagna G, del PD, Caramia DV, et al. Effect of a low glycemic index Mediterranean diet on non-alcoholic fatty liver disease. A randomized controlled clinici trial. J Nutr Health Aging 2017;21(4):404–12.

32. Gelli C, Tarocchi M, Abenavoli L, et al. Effect of a counseling-supported treatment with the Mediterranean diet and physical activity on the severity of the non-alcoholic fatty liver disease. World J Gastroenterol 2017;23(17):3150.

33. Ma J, Hennein R, Liu C, et al. Improved diet quality associates with reduction in liver fat, particularly in individuals with high genetic risk scores for nonalcoholic fatty liver disease. Gastroenterology 2018;155(1):107–17.

34. Kris-Etherton PM. Monounsaturated fatty acids and risk of cardiovascular disease. Circulation 1999;100(11):1253–8.

35. Bozzetto L, Prinster A, Annuzzi G, et al. Liver fat is reduced by an isoenergetic MUFA diet in a controlled randomized study in type 2 diabetic patients. Diabetes care 2012;35(7):1429–35.

36. Pintó X, Fanlo-Maresma M, Corbella E, et al. A Mediterranean Diet rich in extra-virgin olive oil is associated with a reduced prevalence of nonalcoholic fatty liver disease in older individuals at high cardiovascular risk. J Nutr 2019;149(11):1920–9.

37. Capanni M, Calella F, Biagini MR, et al. Prolonged n-3 polyunsaturated fatty acid supplementation ameliorates hepatic steatosis in patients with non-alcoholic fatty liver disease: a pilot study. Aliment Pharmacol Ther 2006;23(8):1143–51.

38. Spadaro L, Magliocco O, Spampinato D, et al. Effects of n-3 polyunsaturated fatty acids in subjects with nonalcoholic fatty liver disease. Dig Liver Dis 2008;40(3):194–9.

39. Zhu F-S, Liu S, Chen X-M, et al. Effects of n-3 polyunsaturated fatty acids from seal oils on nonalcoholic fatty liver disease associated with hyperlipidemia. World J Gastroenterol 2008;14(41):6395–400.

40. Sanyal AJ, Abdelmalek MF, Suzuki A, et al. No significant effects of ethyl-eicosapentanoic acid on histologic features of nonalcoholic steatohepatitis in a phase 2 trial. Gastroenterology 2014;147(2):377–84.e1.

41. Browning JD, Baker JA, Rogers T, et al. Short-term weight loss and hepatic triglyceride reduction: evidence of a metabolic advantage with dietary carbohydrate restriction. Am J Clin Nutr 2011;93(5):1048–52.

42. Tendler D, Lin S, Yancy WS, et al. The effect of a low-carbohydrate, ketogenic diet on nonalcoholic fatty liver disease: a pilot study. Dig Dis Sci 2007;52(2):589–93.

43. Gepner Y, Shelef I, Komy O, et al. The beneficial effects of Mediterranean diet over low-fat diet may be mediated by decreasing hepatic fat content. J Hepatol 2019;71(2):379–88.

44. Kirk E, Reeds DN, Finck BN, et al. Dietary fat and carbohydrates differentially alter insulin sensitivity during caloric restriction. Gastroenterology 2009;136(5): 1552–60.

45. Haufe S, Engeli S, Kast P, et al. Randomized comparison of reduced fat and reduced carbohydrate hypocaloric diets on intrahepatic fat in overweight and obese human subjects. Hepatology 2011;53(5):1504–14.

46. Elias MC, Parise ER, Carvalho Ld, et al. Effect of 6-month nutritional intervention on non-alcoholic fatty liver disease. Nutrition 2010;26(11–12):1094–9.

47. Yamamoto M, Iwasa M, Iwata K, et al. Restriction of dietary calories, fat and iron improves non-alcoholic fatty liver disease. J Gastroenterol Hepatol 2007;22(4): 498–503.

48. Jin YJ, Kim KM, Hwang S, et al. Exercise and diet modification in non-obese non-alcoholic fatty liver disease: analysis of biopsies of living liver donors. J Gastroenterol Hepatol 2012;27(8):1341–7.

49. Petersen KF, Dufour S, Befroy D, et al. Reversal of nonalcoholic hepatic steatosis, hepatic insulin resistance, and hyperglycemia by moderate weight reduction in patients with type 2 diabetes. Diabetes 2005;54(3):603–8.

50. Boden G. High- or low-carbohydrate diets: which is better for weight loss, insulin resistance, and fatty livers? Gastroenterology 2009;136(5):1490–2.

51. Chiu TH, Lin M-N, Pan W-H, et al. Vegetarian diet, food substitution, and nonalcoholic fatty liver. Ci Ji Yi Xue Za Zhi 2018;30(2):102.

52. Choi SH, Oh DJ, Kwon KH, et al. A vegetarian diet does not protect against nonalcoholic fatty liver disease (NAFLD): a cross-sectional study between Buddhist priests and the general population. Turk J Gastroenterol 2015;26(4):336–43.

53. Loffredo L, Del Ben M, Perri L, et al. Effects of dark chocolate on NOX-2-generated oxidative stress in patients with non-alcoholic steatohepatitis. Aliment Pharmacol Ther 2016;44(3):279–86.

54. Loffredo L, Baratta F, Ludovica P, et al. Effects of dark chocolate on endothelial function in patients with non-alcoholic steatohepatitis. Nutr Metab Cardiovasc Dis 2018;28(2):143–9.

55. Malhi H, Loomba R. Editorial: dark chocolate may improve NAFLD and metabolic syndrome by reducing oxidative stress. Aliment Pharmacol Ther 2016;44(5): 533–4.

56. de Wit NJ, Afman LA, Mensink M, et al. Phenotyping the effect of diet on non-alcoholic fatty liver disease. J Hepatol 2012;57(6):1370–3.

57. Niki E, Traber MG. A history of vitamin E. Ann Nutr Metab 2012;61(3):207–12.

58. Musso G, Gambino R, De Michieli F, et al. Dietary habits and their relations to insulin resistance and postprandial lipemia in nonalcoholic steatohepatitis. Hepatology 2003;37(4):909–16.

59. Lavine JE. Vitamin E treatment of nonalcoholic steatohepatitis in children: a pilot study. J Pediatr 2000;136(6):734–8.

60. Sanyal AJ, Chalasani N, Kowdley KV, et al. Pioglitazone, vitamin E, or placebo for nonalcoholic steatohepatitis. N Engl J Med 2010;362(18):1675–85.

61. Lavine JE, Schwimmer JB, Van Natta ML, et al. Effect of vitamin E or metformin for treatment of nonalcoholic fatty liver disease in children and adolescents: the TONIC randomized controlled trial. JAMA 2011;305(16):1659–68.

62. Bril F, Biernacki DM, Kalavalapalli S, et al. Role of vitamin E for nonalcoholic steatohepatitis in patients with type 2 diabetes: a randomized controlled trial. Diabetes Care 2019;42(8):1481–8.

63. Wei J, Lei G-h, Fu L, et al. Association between dietary vitamin C intake and non-alcoholic fatty liver disease: a cross-sectional study among middle-aged and older adults. PloS one 2016;11(1):e0147985.

64. Ipsen DH, Tveden-Nyborg P, Lykkesfeldt J. Does vitamin C deficiency promote fatty liver disease development? Nutrients 2014;6(12):5473–99.

65. Kitson MT, Roberts SK. D-livering the message: the importance of vitamin D status in chronic liver disease. J Hepatol 2012;57(4):897–909.

66. Abramovitch S, Dahan-Bachar L, Sharvit E, et al. Vitamin D inhibits proliferation and profibrotic marker expression in hepatic stellate cells and decreases thioacetamide-induced liver fibrosis in rats. Gut 2011;60(12):1728–37.

67. Eliades M, Spyrou E, Agrawal N, et al. Meta-analysis: vitamin D and non-alcoholic fatty liver disease. Aliment Pharmacol Ther 2013;38(3):246–54.

68. Mazzone G, Morisco C, Lembo V, et al. Dietary supplementation of vitamin D prevents the development of western diet-induced metabolic, hepatic and cardiovascular abnormalities in rats. United European Gastroenterol J 2018;6(7): 1056–64.

69. Nelson JE, Roth CL, Wilson L, et al. Vitamin D deficiency is associated with increased risk of nonalcoholic steatohepatitis in adults with nonalcoholic fatty liver disease: possible role for MAPK and NF-kB? Am J Gastroenterol 2016; 111(6):852.

70. Barchetta I, Del Ben M, Angelico F, et al. No effects of oral vitamin D supplementation on non-alcoholic fatty liver disease in patients with type 2 diabetes: a randomized, double-blind, placebo-controlled trial. BMC Med 2016;14(1):92.

71. Kolodziejczyk AA, Zheng D, Shibolet O, et al. The role of the microbiome in NAFLD and NASH. EMBO Mol Med 2019;11(2):e9302.

72. Duseja A, Chawla YK. Obesity and NAFLD: the role of bacteria and microbiota. Clin Liver Dis 2014;18(1):59–71.

73. Ma Y-Y, Li L, Yu C-H, et al. Effects of probiotics on nonalcoholic fatty liver disease: a meta-analysis. World J Gastroenterol 2013;19(40):6911.

74. Sáez-Lara MJ, Robles-Sanchez C, Ruiz-Ojeda FJ, et al. Effects of probiotics and synbiotics on obesity, insulin resistance syndrome, type 2 diabetes and non-alcoholic fatty liver disease: a review of human clinical trials. Int J Mol Sci 2016;17(6):928.

75. Velayudham A, Dolganiuc A, Ellis M, et al. VSL# 3 probiotic treatment attenuates fibrosis without changes in steatohepatitis in a diet-induced nonalcoholic steatohepatitis model in mice. Hepatology 2009;49(3):989–97.

76. Yadav H, Jain S, Sinha P. Antidiabetic effect of probiotic dahi containing *Lactobacillus acidophilus* and *Lactobacillus casei* in high fructose fed rats. Nutrition 2007; 23(1):62–8.

77. Ma X, Hua J, Li Z. Probiotics improve high fat diet-induced hepatic steatosis and insulin resistance by increasing hepatic NKT cells. J Hepatol 2008;49(5):821–30.

78. Li Z, Yang S, Lin H, et al. Probiotics and antibodies to TNF inhibit inflammatory activity and improve nonalcoholic fatty liver disease. Hepatology 2003;37(2): 343–50.

79. Paolella G, Mandato C, Pierri L, et al. Gut-liver axis and probiotics: their role in non-alcoholic fatty liver disease. World J Gastroenterol 2014;20(42):15518.

80. Aller R, De Luis D, Izaola O, et al. Effect of a probiotic on liver aminotransferases in nonalcoholic fatty liver disease patients: a double blind randomized clinical trial. Eur Rev Med Pharmacol Sci 2011;15(9):1090–5.

81. Eslamparast T, Poustchi H, Zamani F, et al. Synbiotic supplementation in nonalcoholic fatty liver disease: a randomized, double-blind, placebo-controlled pilot study. Am J Clin Nutr 2014;99(3):535–42.

82. Loman BR, Hernández-Saavedra D, An R, et al. Prebiotic and probiotic treatment of nonalcoholic fatty liver disease: a systematic review and meta-analysis. Nutr Rev 2018;76(11):822–39.

83. Murase T, Misawa K, Minegishi Y, et al. Coffee polyphenols suppress diet-induced body fat accumulation by downregulating SREBP-1c and related molecules in C57BL/6J mice. Am J Physiol Endocrinol Metab 2011;300(1):E122–33.

84. Vitaglione P, Morisco F, Mazzone G, et al. Coffee reduces liver damage in a rat model of steatohepatitis: the underlying mechanisms and the role of polyphenols and melanoidins. Hepatology 2010;52(5):1652–61.

85. Yesil A, Yilmaz Y. Coffee consumption, the metabolic syndrome and non-alcoholic fatty liver disease. Aliment Pharmacol Ther 2013;38(9):1038–44.

86. Birerdinc A, Stepanova M, Pawloski L, et al. Caffeine is protective in patients with non-alcoholic fatty liver disease. Aliment Pharmacol Ther 2012;35(1):76–82.

87. Molloy JW, Calcagno CJ, Williams CD, et al. Association of coffee and caffeine consumption with fatty liver disease, nonalcoholic steatohepatitis, and degree of hepatic fibrosis. Hepatology 2012;55(2):429–36.

88. Anty R, Marjoux S, Iannelli A, et al. Regular coffee but not espresso drinking is protective against fibrosis in a cohort mainly composed of morbidly obese European women with NAFLD undergoing bariatric surgery. J Hepatol 2012;57(5):1090–6.

89. Saab S, Mallam D, Cox GA, et al. Impact of coffee on liver diseases: a systematic review. Liver Int 2014;34(4):495–504.

Moving?

Make sure your subscription moves with you!

To notify us of your new address, find your **Clinics Account Number** (located on your mailing label above your name), and contact customer service at:

Email: journalscustomerservice-usa@elsevier.com

800-654-2452 (subscribers in the U.S. & Canada)
314-447-8871 (subscribers outside of the U.S. & Canada)

Fax number: 314-447-8029

Elsevier Health Sciences Division
Subscription Customer Service
3251 Riverport Lane
Maryland Heights, MO 63043

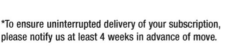
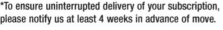

*To ensure uninterrupted delivery of your subscription, please notify us at least 4 weeks in advance of move.

ELSEVIER